Religion, Devotion and Medicine in North India

ALSO AVAILABLE FROM BLOOMSBURY

Bloomsbury Companion to Hindu Studies, Jessica Frazier
Hinduism and the 1960s, Paul Oliver
South Asian Sufis, Clinton Bennett

Religion, Devotion and Medicine in North India

The Healing Power of Śītalā

FABRIZIO M. FERRARI

BLOOMSBURY
LONDON • NEW DELHI • NEW YORK • SYDNEY

Bloomsbury Academic
An imprint of Bloomsbury Publishing Plc

50 Bedford Square
London
WC1B 3DP
UK

1385 Broadway
New York
NY 10018
USA

www.bloomsbury.com

First published 2015

British Library Cataloguing-in-Publication Data
A catalogue record for this book is available from the British Library.

ISBN: HB: 978-1-4411-4829-2
PB: 978-1-4411-6380-6
ePDF: 978-1-4725-9871-4
ePub: 978-1-4725-9872-1

Library of Congress Cataloging-in-Publication Data
A catalogue record for this book is available from the Library of Congress.

Typeset by Fakenham Prepress Solutions, Fakenham, Norfolk NR21 8NN

Contents

List of illustrations vii
Acknowledgements ix
Note on transliteration xi
Abbreviations xiii
Months in north India xvii
Introduction xix

1 Śītalā, the Cold Mother 1

The goddess Śītalā in Indian literature 5
Purāṇas and *dharmanibandhas* 8
Tantric and āgamic literature 19
The Bengali *Śītalāmaṅgalkāvyas* 23
Bhakti gīti 27
Concluding remarks 34

2 Visions of the goddess: The iconography of Śītalā 41

Aniconic *mūrtis* 41
Ethnographic vignette 1: Śrī Mātā Śītalā Devī Mandir, Gurgaon (*Haryana*) 44
The water pitcher 49
The broom and the winnower 50
Cephalomorphic *mūrtis* 51
Ethnographic vignette 2: The Agam Kuāṅ, Patna (Bihar) 52
Ethnographic vignette 3: The Choṭa Mā Yātrā, Salkia (West Bengal) 54
Zoomorphic and phytomorphic *mūrtis* 57
Equestrian *mūrtis* 59
The ass *vāhana* 67
Ethnographic vignette 4: Śrī Dakṣiṇī Ādi Śītalā (Buṛhiyā Māī) Mandir, Banaras (Uttar Pradesh) 74
Concluding remarks 80

3 Hosting Mā, feeding Mā. Controversies around *Śītalāpūjā* 87

Ethnographic vignette 5: Animal sacrifice: feeding and thanking the goddess 88
Ethnographic vignette 6: Possession: bearing the visit of the goddess 93
Ethnographic vignette 7: Mortification of the flesh: Śītalā meets Māriyammaṉ 99
Concluding remarks 103

4 The smallpox myth and the creation of the goddess of smallpox 113

Ethnographic vignette 8: The Baṛī Śītalā Mandir of Adalpura (Uttar Pradesh) 114
Disease and ambiguity: The construction of the 'other' in the Bengali *maṅgalkāvyas* 119
The consolidation of the smallpox myth: The struggle against smallpox 131
Concluding remarks 144

5 The legacy of Śītalā 151

After smallpox. The AIDS myth? 153
Śītalā's shade in Calcutta: On a contemporary *maṅgal* novel 156
The Durgāfication of the goddess. Śītalā in pop-devotional culture 160
Concluding remarks 167

Concluding reflections 171
Appendix A. *Śrīśītalāsaptamīvratakathā* 175
Appendix B. *Śrīśītalāsaptamīvrata* of *Skandapurāṇa* 179
Appendix C. *Śītalāsaptamīvratakathā* of *Bhaviṣyapurāṇa* 181
Appendix D. *Śītalāpūjāpaddhati* of *Picchilātantra* 185
Bibliography 191
Index 211

List of illustrations

The following images were reproduced with kind permission. The author has made every effort to trace the copyright holders and to obtain permission to reproduce images. This has not been possible in every case; however, any omissions brought to our attention will be remedied in future editions.

Fig. 1.1 Śītalā Mātā, postcard (author's collection). 2
Fig. 1.2 Śītalā Mātā, front page of vintage calendar (author's collection). The invocation reads: *sarva duḥkhāntakāriṇī śrī śītalādevyai namaḥ* (Skt. 'Obeisance to the goddess Śītalā, the destroyer of all sufferings'). 4
Fig. 1.3 Dakṣiṇāśītalā, Kāl Bhairo Mandir, Banaras (photo by author). 7
Fig. 1.4 Jvarāsura, Śītalā Mandir, Kolkata (photo by author). 25
Fig. 2.1 Punjabi mother with child, *muṇḍan khānā*, Śrī Mātā Śītalā Devī Mandir, Gurgaon (photo by author). 45
Fig. 2.2 Śītalā Devī, Gurgaon Mandir, Gurgaon, poster (author's collection). 47
Fig. 2.3 *Śītalākuṇḍa*, Gurgaon Mandir, Gurgaon (photo by author). 49
Fig. 2.4 Standing couple, black stone, Baṛī Śītalā Dhām, Adalpura (photo by author). 53
Fig. 2.5 Choṭa Mā, Śrī Śrī Choṭa Śītalā Mātā Mandir, Salkia (photo by author). 55
Fig. 2.6 Baṛo Mā on palanquin, Choṭa Mā Yātrā, Salkia (photo by Jayanta Roy). 56
Fig. 2.7 Mejo Mā on palanquin, Choṭa Mā Yātrā, Salkia (photo by Jayanta Roy). 56
Fig. 2.8 Sejo Mā, Śrī Śrī Śītalā Mātār Mandir, Salkia (photo by Jayanta Roy). 57
Fig. 2.9 Śītalā, figure in Kapili niche, north, Sūrya Mandir, Maḍhkeda (Madhya Pradesh), ninth century (courtesy and copyright of Michael W. Meister). 59
Fig. 2.10 Śītalā, sandstone, detail of the exterior, Saccikamātā Mandir, Osiañ (Rajasthan), c.ca twelfth century (courtesy of American Institute of Indian Studies). 60
Fig. 2.11 Śītalā, buff sandstone standing figure, 58 x 49 cm, Gandhisagar (Madhya Pradesh), c.ca fourteenth century (courtesy of American Institute of Indian Studies). 62
Fig. 2.12 Śītalā riding an ass, greyish sandstone standing figure, 54.5 x 37 cm, Allahabad Museum, c.ca fourteenth century (courtesy of American Institute of Indian Studies). 62
Fig. 2.13 Parṇaśavarī, stone, eleventh century, Vikrampur, Dacca district, E67.319, Department of History and Classical Art, National Museum of

Bangladesh, Dhaka (Photograph by John C. Huntington Courtesy of The Huntington Photographic Archive at The Ohio State University) 63
Fig. 2.14 Detail: Śītala, from Parṇaśavarī stele, black stone, h. 121.92, eleventh century, Vajrayogini, Munshiganj, Dhaka district, E.67.031, Department of History and Classical Art, National Museum of Bangladesh, Dhaka (Photograph by John C. Huntington Courtesy of The Huntington Photographic Archive at The Ohio State University) 64
Fig. 2.15 Śītalā, Kālīghāṭ painting, opaque watercolour on paper, Calcutta, c.ca 1885, Victoria and Albert Museum, IS.607-1950 (Courtesy of Victoria and Albert Museum, London). 66
Fig. 2.16 Goddess Shitala, *Icons and Illusions*, oil on canvas, by Shuvaprasanna (courtesy of Shuvaprasanna Bhattacharjee). 66
Fig. 2.17 Śītala (left), Śani (right) and Caṇḍī (aniconic), Bandhaghat, Salkia (photo by author). 70
Fig. 2.18 Śrī Avināś Paṇḍey at Śrī Dakṣiṇī Ādi Śītalā Mandir, Banaras (photo by author). 75
Fig. 2.19 Particular, Śrī Dakṣiṇī Ādi Śītalā Mandir, Banaras (photo by author). 76
Fig. 2.20 Śītalā, posterior shrine, Śrī Dakṣiṇī Ādi Śītalā Mandir, Banaras (photo by author). 76
Fig. 2.21 Śītalā, posterior shrine, Śrī Dakṣiṇī Ādi Śītalā Mandir, Banaras (photo by author). 77
Fig. 2.22 Śītalā *pratimās*, particular, posterior shrine, Śrī Dakṣiṇī Ādi Śītalā Mandir, Banaras (photo by author). 77
Fig. 2.23 Śrī Dakṣiṇī Ādi Śītalā, grotto, Śrī Dakṣiṇī Ādi Śītalā Mandir, Banaras (photo by author). 79
Fig. 3.1 *Hijṛa* devotee waiting for *chāg utsarga*, Śrī Śrī Baṛo Śītalā Māyer Mandir, Salkia (photo by Jayanta Roy). 90
Fig. 3.2 *Balidān*, Śrī Śrī Baṛo Śītalā Māyer Mandir, Salkia (photo by Jayanta Roy). 92
Fig. 3.3 Young woman during an episode of *bhar*, Choṭa Mā Yātrā, Salkia (photo by Jayanta Roy). 95
Fig. 3.4 Daṇḍīkāṭā, Choṭa Mā Yātrā, Salkia (photo by Jayanta Roy). 97
Fig. 4.1 Baṛī Śītalā surrounded by *māllah pūjārī*s (mother and son), Śītalā Dhām, Adalpura (UP) (photo by author). 115
Fig. 4.2 Baṛī Śītalā, Adalpura, poster (author's collection). 116
Fig. 4.3 Actors impersonating monsters, Salkia (photo by Jayanta Roy). 126
Fig. 5.1 Śītalā with Hanumān (top left) and Bhairava (top right), poster (author's collection). 161
Fig. 5.2 Śītalā Mātā (1981), directed by Ramgopal Gupta, VCD cover (author's collection). 164

Acknowledgements

It took many years to collect the material that informed this book. During this time, my work has been facilitated in many ways by the patience, support, love and encouragement of my extended family, particularly my wife. Grazie di cuore!

Many friends and colleagues took their time to assist me in various ways, comment on my work and give advice. I wish to remember: Alex McKay, Amy Allocco, Anjum Katyal, Anthony Cerulli, Asko Parpola, Assa Doron, Bill Harman, David Arnold, Devanshi Chanchani, Francesco Brighenti, Frank Korom, Fred Smith, Gavin Flood, Hans Bakker, István Keul, Ivette Vargas-O'Bryan, Jacqueline Suthren Hirst, James Mallinson, Jinah Kim, Joyce Flueckiger, June McDaniel, Loriliai Biernacki, Lucia Dolce, Mario Russo, Mehreen Chida-Razvi, Michael Slouber, Naveen Kishore, Nick Barnard, Nilima Chitgopekar, Paolo Scarpi, Ralph Nicholas, Ruby Sain, Sanjoy Bhattacharyya, Sarit Chaudhuri, Shaman Hatley, Simon Brodbeck, Sohini Dey, Stefano Beggiora, Thomas Dähnardt, Ülo Valk, Xenia Zeiler. My teachers deserve special mention: William Radice, for he continues to be a source of inspiration in all possible ways, and Mariola Offredi, because I owe her more than she may think. My deep gratitude to Hena Basu, Krishna Mohan Mishra and Gianni Pellegrini, who assisted me with translations from, respectively, Bengali, Hindi and Sanskrit. (It goes without saying that I am solely responsible for any mistakes.) I am grateful to Michael Meister, Vandana Sinha (American Institute of Indian Studies) and Greg Shonk (The Huntington Archive) for granting permission to reprint visual material. For the beautiful stories they narrate, and for their readiness to help me, thanks to Amitav Ghosh and Shuvaprasanna. Jayanta Roy is the photographer anyone would have on fieldwork: *dhonnobad*! While in Banaras, I received the hospitality of Vijay and Padma Dvivedi, whose friendship I treasure very much. I am also thankful to Prasant Vyas, who guided me in and around Bhaironāth Mandir, and Vijay Vajpay, for introducing me to the world of Bhojpuri *devī-gīti*. Many friends in India have supported me with their hospitality, friendship and willingness to help. Along with them, countless *mahānt*, *pūjārī*, *sevāit*, *purohit* and devotees of the goddess have helped me and shared their knowledge throughout the years. Among them, special thanks to Maharaji and the ladies of Causaṭṭī Yoginī Devī Mātā Mandir. All these persons are more than just 'informants'. The book is dedicated to them.

Note on transliteration

Throughout this book, I adopt a simplified version of the standard system for the transliteration from Sanskrit, unless specified otherwise. Each Indian modern language would require a modified transliteration system. It will be impractical, hence my choice. Below is a general guide to the pronunciation of Sanskrit phonemes.

a	b*u*t
ā	f*a*r
i	s*i*t
ī	d*ee*p
u	p*u*t
ū	b*oo*m
ṛ	*ri*sk
e	pr*ay*
ai	m*y*
o	h*o*pe
au	s*ou*nd
k	*k*ettle
kh	aspirated k
g	*g*olf
gh	aspirated g
ṅ	a*n*ger
c	*ch*ain
ch	aspirated c
j	*j*oy
jh	aspirated j
ñ	pu*n*ch
ṭ ṭh ḍ (ṛ) ḍh (ṛh) ṇ	These sounds do not exist in English. Consonants are retroflex: the tip of the tongue should touch the palate.

t	pes*t*er
th	aspirated t
d	*d*isco
dh	aspirated d
n	*n*ame
p	*p*raise
ph	aspirated p
b	*b*oy
bh	aspirated b
m	*m*other
y	*y*ou
r	no English equivalent (as in Italian: b*r*avo)
l	*l*ens
v	*w*ine
ś	*sh*ame
ṣ	retroflex sh
s	fa*s*t
h	*h*alt

When reporting from vernacular contexts (e.g. ethnographic vignettes), it should be implied I use the local language, unless otherwise specified. One should be aware that in modern north Indian languages, the final *–a* vowel is not pronounced. The word *darśana* is thus pronounced *darshan*; Rāma is Rām, etc. In Bengali only, the inherent vowel 'a' is pronounced 'o' (ɔ, ô); all sibilant consonants are pronounced 'sh', and the semi-vowel 'v' is always pronounced 'b'. Therefore the words *vaiṣṇava*, *darśana*, Śītalā are pronounced respectively: *boishnob*; *dorshon* and Sheetola.

Abbreviations

AB	*Aitareyabrāhmaṇa*
AHS	*Aṣṭāṅgahṛdayasaṃhitā*
AV	*Atharvaveda*
AVP	AV. Paippalāda recension
AVŚ	AV. Śaunaka recension
BMKI	*Bāṁlā Maṅgalkāvyer Itihās* (Bhaṭṭācārya, 1998)
BaŚ	*Baṅgīya Śabdakoṣa* (Bandyopādhyāy 2001)
BŚS	*Baudhāyana Śrautasūtra*
BhP	*Bhāgavatapurāṇa*
BhPr	*Bhāvaprakāśa*
BhaP	*Bhaviṣyapurāṇa*
CC	*Calcutta Chromosome (The)*
CaS	*Carakasaṃhitā*
Cik	*Cikitsāsthāna*
DBP	*Devībhāgavatapurāṇa*
DM	*Devīmāhātmya*
H.ŚMK	*Harideva, Śītalāmaṅgalkāvya*
HV	*Harivaṃśa*
KāP	*Kālikāpurāṇa*
Ka	*Kalpasthāna*
KKh	*Kāśīkhaṇḍa*
J.ŚMK	Kavi Jagannāth, *Śītalāmaṅgalkāvya*
KKG	*Kriyākālaguṇottaratantra*
KD.ŚMK	Kṛṣṇarām Dās, *Śītalāmaṅgalkāvya*
MN	*Mādhavanidāna*
Ma	*Madhyakhaṇḍa*
MBh	*Mahābhārata*
Manu	*Mānavadharmaśāstra* or *Manusmṛti*
MG.ŚMK	Mānikrām Gāṅgulī, *Śītalāmaṅgalkāvya*
MMK	*Mañjuśrīmūlakalpa*
MaP	*Matsyapurāṇa*
Nā	*Nālandā Viśāl Śabd Sagar* (Navaljī 1994)
NāP	*Nāradapurāṇa*
Ni	*Nidānasthāna*

NC.ŚMK	Nityānanda Cakravartī, *Śītalāmaṅgalkāvya*
NC.ŚMK-B	*Nityānander (Kavi) Śītalā Maṅgal*, in Bera 2001
PiT	*Picchilātantra*
Rām	*Rāmāyaṇa*
RV	*Ṛgveda*
ŚKD	*Śabdakalpadruma* (Deva 1967)
SPP	*Sarvadevadevīpūjāpaddhati*
ŚB	*Śatapathabrāhmaṇa*
ŚC	*Śītalācālīsā*
ŚMK	*Śītalāmaṅgalkāvya*
ŚAS	*Śītalāṣṭakastotra*
ŚVK	*Śītalāvratakathā*
SkP	*Skandapurāṇa*
SuS	*Suśrutāsaṃhitā*
Sū	*Sūtrasthāna*
TS	*Taittirīyasaṃhitā*
Utt	*Uttarasthāna* or *Uttaratantra*
VS	*Vajasaneyisaṃhitā*
VR	*Vratarāja*

Historical records

BVA	Bengal Legislative Department (India), *The Bengal Vaccination Act, 1880.*
BSR	*Bengal Sanitary Reports*
BMJ	*British Medical Journal*
BSC	*First Annual Report of the Sanitary Commission for Bengal, 1864–65*
ICM	International Congress of Medicine, 17th, 1913, London (1914). *The history of inoculation and vaccination for the prevention and treatment of disease: lecture memoranda*
RSC	*Report of the smallpox commissioners, appointed by government, with an appendix*, Calcutta, 1st July 1850

Languages

A	Arabic
B	Bengali
Bhp	Bhojpuri
F	Farsi (Persian)
Gr	Greek

G	Gujarati
H	Hindi
M	Marathi
P	Punjabi
Skt	Sanskrit
T	Tamil
Tib	Tibetan

Months in north India

There is no such thing as a single 'Hindu calendar'. Lunar and solar calendars are used along with regional and confessional variants. I use here a simplified version:

Caitra (March/April)
Vaiśākha (April/May)
Jyeṣṭha (May/June)
Āṣāḍha (June/July)
Śrāvaṇa (July/August)
Bhādra(pada) (August/September)
Āśvina (September/October)
Kārtika (October/November)
Agrahāyaṇa (November/December)
Pauṣa (December/January)
Māgha (January/February)
Phālguna (February/March)

Introduction

Health narratives and healing rituals pervade Indian literature. A variety of gods and goddesses are summoned and praised for protection against chaos, misfortune and disease. Among them, the goddess Śītalā holds a unique position. Though she is neither a pan-Hindu goddess nor she is celebrated extensively in authoritative texts, she is ardently worshipped by Hindus, Muslims, Sikhs, Buddhists, Christians and *ādivāsī*s (members of 'indigenous' communities) in villages, towns and large urban centres of Pakistan, north India, Nepal and Bangladesh. Śītalā is a women's goddess, and a protector of children. In particular, she cures them of fevers and exanthemata and, until 1979, the dreaded smallpox.

I first met Śītalā in a small temple in Kaulagarh Road, Dehradun (Uttarakhand), in 1997. Having heard and read a variety of stories on the Indian 'smallpox goddess', her temperamental nature and her power to inflict diseases, I did not know what to expect. To my surprise, I witnessed an offering (*pūjā*) of water, sweets, fruits and flowers, and listened to women singing songs of praise to the Mother (Mā). Śītalā was not worshipped out of fear. In fact, she is invoked because she is gentle, compassionate and loving. As any mother, she protects her children from all imbalances: illness, poverty, injustice, misfortune, etc. I was intrigued; everything I read about her pointed in a different direction.

Scholarly literature portrays Śītalā – whose name means 'Cold [Lady]' – as a goddess who causes and heals smallpox. She is often described as the deification of smallpox. Victims of smallpox are said to be possessed by her. Reports from the colonial epoch onwards tell stories of devotees who, fearing the rage of Śītalā, strenuously resisted vaccination and preferred the goddess's visitation (i.e. smallpox). My experience, and the words of my informants, says otherwise. Śītalā is a benevolent mother, and a goddess of hygiene. She is predominantly worshipped by women, whom she blesses with fertility, healthy sons and decent husbands.

This book questions renditions of Śītalā as an ambiguous and capricious 'goddess of smallpox' invariably associated with folk/village Hinduism. In so doing, it is primarily a critique of the construction of myth. In order to counter this dominating – and now consolidated – trend, I trace a genealogy of Śītalā built on a 'nomadology of narratives' (Mukharji 2012: 96–101). Beside data on ritual and devotional culture collected in over ten years of fieldwork in north India, Nepal and Bangladesh, I show the way in which Śītalā has been portrayed in: a) Sanskrit texts like *purāṇa*s, *dharmanibandha*s, āyurvedic compendia, *vratakathā*s, *tantra*s and ritual manuals; b) Hindi, Bhojpuri and Bengali songs,[1] hymns and oral myths; c) the Bengali *Śītalāmaṅgalkāvya*s and their theatrical renditions; d) records of the colonial and post-colonial struggle against smallpox; and e) contemporary renditions of Śītalā in scholarly literature and popular culture (films, open theatre, pop music, novels, blogs, video-clips, smart-phone apps).

Along with a study of textual sources, I have conducted an analysis of Śītalā's iconography starting from her earliest appearance in the subcontinent (circa ninth century) to contemporary online *bhakti* culture. This has permitted to counter the argument that Śītalā is a village/folk goddess. The divide between 'popular' (Skt. *laukika*) or 'village' (*grāmya*) culture as opposed to *vaidika* (i.e. derived from the Vedas) or *mārgīya* (< Skt. *mārga*, 'path,' 'doctrine') knowledge is fictional, just like the 'smallpox myth'. When discussing restricted vernacular realities, I will do so by calling them *āñcal*s.

In Hindi, the *āñcal* is the 'hem' (of the sari) and, by extension, the periphery of a wider map. The idea of *āñcal* was initially used in Hindi literature to indicate rural settlements isolated from urban centres. (In Phaṇīśvar Nāth Reṇu's 1954 Hindi novel *Mailā Āñcal*, there are no heroes. The protagonist is a Bihari village, with its different, often contrasting, characters and cultures.) But *āñcalik saṃskṛti* is not necessarily insular. The *āñcal* is a polyphonic territory informed by the coexistence of different social sectors with diverse expertise, knowledge, capital, authority, charisma, history, languages and heritage. In line with this, the book offers a description of Śītalā moving from the many voices that have informed her culture. Concepts like Sanskrit and vernacular culture are blurred labels that do not suggest a historical problematization of texts and social dynamics (cf. Pollock 2006: 19–30). Likewise, my book eschews either/orism. As per my fieldwork, I recur to ethnographic vignettes, but I will not engage with 'thick descriptions'. This may be a disadvantage. Yet my strategy has permitted me to highlight two consistent patterns: the pervasiveness of the protective goddess, and the marginality of the 'smallpox myth', a fabrication some would call an Orientalist construction.

Representations of Śītalā have suffered from uncritical (and partial) readings of Indian texts. They also have been affected by colonial and post-colonial agendas, and the personal fixations and infatuations of authoritative narrators. All these aspects converge in the rendering of Śītalā as a 'disease goddess' rather than a 'healing mother'. The difference, as I will show, is not academic. With very few exceptions (e.g. Wadley 1980), the goddess has been consistently spectacularized and pathologized, an exercise that has resulted in the misrepresentation of an important devotional culture. This does not surprise. Indian medical texts too have systematically eschewed discourses on devotion (*bhakti*).

The earliest references to healing practices in India are found in the oral tradition preserved in the *Ṛgvedasaṃhitā* (c.ca 1,700–1,000 BCE) and, more emphatically, in the *Atharvavedasaṃhitā* (c.ca 1,000–800 BCE). The *bhaiṣajya* (medical) section of the *Kauśikasūtra* (the ritual part of AV) is the main source of information on healing in Vedic culture. Along with ritualists such as the *āṅgirasas*, *bhārgavas* and later the *ātharvaṇas*, whose work was functional to the maintenance of the natural and social order (*ṛtám*, *dhárman*), a class of medicine men or healers affirmed, the *bhiṣáj*. Conversant in the art of spells and ritual dancing, and therefore known as 'shakers' (*vipra*) or 'chanters' (*kavi*), the *bhiṣáj* developed a rich corpus of rituals and mantras to dispel harmful gods and spirits, and their negative effects on humans, domestic animals (primarily cattle) and crops (AVŚ 2.32). Demons are feared, but also equated to the gods (AVŚ 6.20.2; AVP 19.12.11 and 1.45.1) for their capacity to heal (AVŚ 1.2.9: 5–6; 1.6.20). Since they cannot be destroyed, they are transferred into the bodies of animals, into water, under the ground, or into the bodies of competitors, enemies or faraway people (AVŚ 5.22: 1–14; RV 1.50: 11–13). With very few exceptions,[2] anatomical knowledge is wanting in the practice of the Vedic medicine man, just like devotional piety. Some hymns, however, show feelings such as surrender and cries for forgiveness. In this case, the *bhiṣáj* invokes the name of the afflicted person, the symptoms of illness, the names of the demon(s), and the name of the god(s) (AVŚ 4.13: 1–7). The duty of the healer is to assess symptoms, to identify their origin and to make them go away. Therapeutic exorcism requires the use of herbs (RV 10: 97), water (AVŚ 1.2.3; 1.6.24; 1.6.91), amulets (AVŚ 1.2.9; 1.2.4; 1.6.85; 1.19.34–35; 2.4.10, 3.10.3; 4.6.81), sympathetic magic (AVŚ 1.1.22; 1.7.116), dancing, recitation of mantras and the capacity to experience visions.[3]

Echoes of Vedic medicine reverberate in the later Āyurveda ('knowledge', *veda*, of 'long life', *ayus*). The foundational āyurvedic collections can be divided in two groups. The great trio (*bṛhattrayī*) consists of: *Carakasaṃhitā* (circa first–second centuries CE), *Suśrutasaṃhitā* (circa third–fourth centuries CE), *Aṣṭāṅgahṛdayasaṃhitā* (attributed to Vāgbhaṭa, circa sixth–seventh centuries CE). The little trio (*laghutrayī*) is made of: *Mādhavanidāna* (attributed to Mādhavakara, eighth century CE), *Śārṅgadharasaṃhitā* (fourteenth century) and the *Bhāvaprakāśa* of Bhāvamiśra (sixteenth century).[4] Āyurveda is a fragmented tradition where many theories converge. According to the prevalent one, health is a matter of balance, or equilibrium, between bodily humours (*doṣa*). The human body, it is posited, is crossed by three humours (Skt. *tridoṣa*): wind (*vāta*), bile (*pitta*) and phlegm (*śleṣman* or *kapha*). The balance between these humours ensures the correct functioning of the body's digestive processes, a series of activities that permit the birth and successive development of the human physical structure (bones, marrow, tissues, blood, etc.). Āyurvedic compendia indicate health as a state of satisfaction, self-content or comfort (*svāsthya*). It is the condition of being free from disease (*ārogya*). Conversely, disease (*roga*, *vyādhi*) is discussed as a situation of imbalance, often resulting from actions in breach of right conduct (*sadvṛtti*). Just like health reflects order (*dharma*), illness is a form of chaos (*adharma*). The perpetration of actions (*karma*) contrary to *dharma*, besides causing an accumulation of demerit (*pāpa*), inevitably affects the *tridoṣas*.[5] Along with the *tridoṣavidyā*, or humoral theory, there exist a variety of approaches that look at disease as resulting from (*pravṛtta*): heredity (*ādibala*); congenital fault (*janambala*); offence against wisdom (*prajñāparādha*); failure of the seven bodily supports (*saptadhātu*); divine wrath (*daivaroga*); contact (*upasarga*) and the ruler's immorality (*rājayakṣmana*). Pluralism did not just feature diagnostics, but therapeutics. Āyurvedic physicians (*vaidya*s) developed a rich pharmacopeia informed by the knowledge of farmers, herders, hunters, monks and forest-dwellers (CaS.Sū 1.120-123; SuS.Sū 36: 10).[6]

Successive to Āyurveda is tantric medicine, a ritual tradition that bears witness to a continuation with the magical culture of AV, the practice of asceticism, the cultivation of powers (*siddhi*) and the influence of philosophical systems such as Yoga and Sāṃkhya. Tantric medical literature consolidates itself around the tenth century. Disease is diagnosed by examining the passage of winds (*prāṇa*) through a series of channels (*nāḍi*) that intersect sites of energy (*cakra*). The earliest evidence of this method can be found in the *Kubjikāmātātantra* and the *Mālinīvijayottaratantra* (Wujastyk 2003b: 398). Tantric physiology is built around concepts of *sthūla śarīra* (gross body) and *sūkṣma śarīra* (subtle body), whereas therapeutics is a coercive exercise of power. Healers are *siddha*s, accomplished teachers and masters in arts such magic spells, alchemy and *yoga*.

These and other (notably Yūnānī medicine and 'Western' biomedicine) medical systems in north India rely on the knowledge of specialist practitioners. Outcomes are overtly practical, and there is little, if any, space for devotion (*bhakti*). There are few exceptions to such trend. One such case is a *stotra* (Skt. 'hymn') included in the work of Bhāvamiśra, a sixteenth-century physician from Banaras (Vāraṇāsī, Kāśī). Miśra confesses the uselessness of medical science in front of smallpox (Skt. *masūrikā*, *visphoṭa*). There is one and only remedy: firm devotion and faith in Śītalā.

Two major differences with medical culture emerge. First, *bhakti* does not depend upon a class of specialized healers or ritualists. Second, the healer is *de facto* a god or a goddess. Devotional moods such as love, piety and repentance are core elements in *bhakti* culture. They serve to attract the attention of a deity, often a goddess, and to give voice publicly to personal suffering. Health is negotiated by means of a variety of practices such as vows, scheduled fasts and associated rituals, vegetarian and non-vegetarian offerings, austerities, etc. Annual festivals and pilgrimages are the occasion for spectacular celebrations of devotion, and for the enactment of public commitment to the goddess. Devotion is ultimately associated to *śraddhā*, usually translated as 'faith',[7] and *viśvāsa*, belief. Both concepts show that *bhakti* in general, and the *sakāma* (Skt. 'with desires [attached]') nature of devotional practices associated to Śītalā in particular, continue to be a way to achieve health and wellbeing, rather than a mystical disposition or a theological notion.

But the voices of Śītalā's devotees, their texts and their material culture have been suffocated by the truth-claims of powerful, external door-keepers. Uncritical and incomplete versions have proliferated, nurtured by the fixation of much scholarship with the deconstruction of knowledge and authority, an exercise that has increasingly transformed critique into convention, and, ultimately, into fashion. (Or, as René Girard recently noted, 'a disappointing academic routine' [2011: 3].) With this in mind, one could legitimately ask whether discourses on Orientalism and cultural colonialism have been actually digested. This study rejects such conventions. Some believe that 'to pursue excellence scholars must be free to ask any question, to offer any interpretation, and to raise any issue' (Board of Directors, AAR 2014). The excellence of a scholar is not worth the misrepresentation of real people and their beliefs.

Notes

1 The choice depends exclusively on my familiarity with the above languages, and the regions where I conducted fieldwork. Narratives and songs from Gujarat, Punjab, etc. have been examined in their translated forms.

2 See for instance AVP 4: 15, where the knowledge of plants is accessory to the healing of an open fracture (Staal 2008: 137–8). Unlike the physicians of the post-Vedic tradition, *bhiṣáj*s acquired their knowledge from observation of animal sacrifices or natural phenomena (e.g. decomposition of bodies in the open). Because of their impure profession, medicine men were not allowed to perform rituals (ŚB. 4.1.5: 14; cf. Manu 3: 152). The use of anatomical terminology was borrowed from the hymns pronounced by the *hotṛ* (the specialist in RV formulae), and the observation of their rituals. The same criteria of exclusion apply to the Aśvins, the physicians of the gods (TS. 6.4.9: 2). The impurity of doctors disappears completely with Āyurveda, where medical science is paralleled to *śruti* (CaS. Sū. 30: 21), and medical treatment is equated to mantra (SuS.Cik. 1: 75–6).

3 Formulae to contrast the evil charm of sorcerers and evil eye are scattered in AV, particularly Book 3 (e.g. 1.7–8; 1.16; 4.17–19; 5.14; 5.31; 7.70).

4 Other relevant Āyurvedic compendia are the *Bhelasaṃhitā* (circa first century) and the *Kāśyapasaṃhitā* (seventh century), almost entirely dealing with paediatrics and gynaecology.

5 Cf. Das 2000: 66 on *adharma* in relation to transmissible diseases such as *masūrikā* in Gayadāsa's commentary to Suśruta.

6 Medicines are derived from plants and animals (e.g. SuS.Sū. 46: 53–135.). They may contain ingredients as exotic as crushed bones, teeth, fangs and nails, horns, hairs, bile, skin, urine, dung, etc. of domestic and semi-domestic (goat, donkey, cow, buffalo, dog, cat, parrot) and feral (leopard, elephant, alligator, tiger, monkey, owl, vulture, tortoise) animals (CaS.Cik. 9: 49–51; 10: 39–40; SuS.Utt. 60: 29–50).

7 The word *śraddhā* means 'to place the hearth', and is 'the "confidence" in the efficacy of the ritual, i.e. its ability to motivate counter-gifts and to lead to heaven' (Witzel 2003: 79).

1

Śītalā, the Cold Mother

Indian medical culture depends on the knowledge and practices of physicians, surgeons, ritualists, healers, magicians, astrologers, ascetics, yogis, fakirs, etc. These specialists derive their authority from education, consortium, lineage, or divine designation. Alongside, there exists a series of healing measures that do not require the skills of specialized personnel. Such is the case of rites informed by faith (*śraddhā*), belief (*viśvāsa*) and devotion (*bhakti*). Within this context, an unsystematic, and often undocumented, healing culture has emerged. Rather than on knowledge, authority and tradition, this relies on the capacity of devotees to move powerful and holistic healers: the gods. One such deity is the goddess Śītalā.

The name *śītalā* is a *tatsama śabda* (identical loanword) derived from the Sanskrit root *śīta*, 'cold'. It can be a noun ('cold', 'coldness') or an adjective ('cold', 'cool', 'cooling', 'refreshing', 'calm', 'gentle', 'mild', 'free from passion'). The goddess is 'Coldness', or the 'Cold [Lady]'. Śītalā, who is principally a women's goddess, is visualized as a mother (*mā*, *mātā*) who protects children from paediatric ailments, notably exanthemata. She is also a fertility goddess, who helps women in finding good husbands and conceiving healthy sons. Her auspicious presence ensures the wellbeing of the family, and protects sources of livelihood. Being cold, Śītalā is summoned to ensure regular refreshing rains, and to prevent famines, droughts and cattle diseases. The worship of Śītalā is not just functional to protection. It has served for centuries to learning and disseminating basic hygienic norms for the wellbeing of the household.

Śītalā Devī is easily distinguishable. According to a consolidated iconography, she sits side-saddle on an ass, holds a broom and carries in the crook of her left arm a big pitcher. Textual sources agree with a standard description: the three-eyed goddess is a white-complexioned naked (*digambara*, 'sky-clad') young lady with long black dishevelled hair and a winnowing basket on her head. All these objects bear witness to her skills in managing and controlling diseases. The vessel contains cold healing water. With the broom the goddess wipes 'dirt' away. The winnower, a reminder of her agricultural origin, is used to throw fresh air at those burning with fevers. In modern and contemporary renditions, Śītalā wears a red sari, is heavily bejewelled and is adorned with a gold tiara.[1]

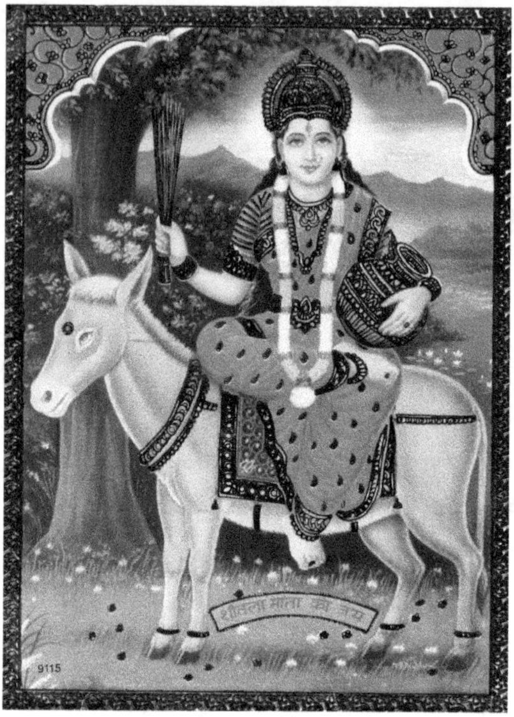

FIGURE 1.1 *Śītalā Mātā, postcard (author's collection).*

The description is that of a reassuring goddess. Yet from the eighteenth century, Śītalā begins to be represented consistently as a capricious, dangerous and disease-inflicting deity. It is the beginning of the myth of the 'goddess of smallpox'. Stories of a powerful yet lesser goddess of Indian peasantry originally emerge in a minor chapter of the Bengali premodern *maṅgalkāvyas* (B. auspicious poems). In the *Śītalāmaṅgalkāvyas*, Śītalā is an intimidating presence who distributes infected pulses in village markets, or sends hordes of disease-demons, thus causing outbreaks of smallpox and other contagious illnesses. Only when properly worshipped does she agree to heal her victims. This mythology has been enthusiastically received. Unfamiliar to the rest of India, it has been celebrated by Bengali intellectuals as genuine folk poetry, and has informed virtually all scholarly works on the goddess.

In this book, I argue that, to appreciate the place of Śītalā in Indian culture, one should study her from a trans-regional perspective. It has been posited that there exist two isoglosses: the Bengali disease-inflicting goddess, and the north-western protector of children (Wadley 1980: 35). I do not agree. The vindictive goddess of *maṅgal* poems is an exception confined to a small section of a regional literary genre. Bengalis, as other Indians, do not fear Śītalā, whom they worship as a protector and an auspicious presence.

Giving a comprehensive portrayal of Śītalā, however, is a gigantic task. The goddess has adapted variously to *āñcalik* culture. Sanskrit and vernacular texts, written and oral alike, describe her as a benevolent mother, a riverine goddess, a murderous hag, a tantric Śakti, a wise Brahman elderly woman, a sweeper, a washer-lady and a queen/princess. She has been associated with characters of the *Rāmāyaṇa* and the *Mahābhārata*, and is worshipped as a form of pan-Hindu (Kālarātrī, Gaṅgā, Sarasvatī, Parvatī, Lakṣmī, Vaiṣṇo Devī, Durgā) or regional (Masānī, Manasā, Olā Bibi, Ṣaṣṭhī, various Caṇḍīs and the seven sister) goddesses. Her titles are generally those of a protective mother.[2] Other appellatives point at royalty and auspiciousness: Bhagavatī, Ṭhākurāni, Maṅgalā (Auspicious One), Jāgatrānī (Queen of the World), Dayāmāyī (Compassionate One) and Karuṇamāyī (Merciful One). Only in the ŚMKs, she is the threatening Vasanta Rāy (Queen of the Spring, i.e. of the pox season), Rog Rāy (Queen of Fevers) and Rogeśvarī (Lord of Diseases).

Ritual culture too is not uniform. Śītalā is offered stale, cooling and refreshing vegetarian edibles, but also the blood and flesh of sacrificed animals. Her *pūjārī*s (votaries) are Brahmans but also members of low occupational classes. She is celebrated by the working class, the peasantry, middle and upper classes and royalty in open-air shrines (*thān*) and majestic temples (*mandir*). She has a standard anthropomorphic iconography, but is believed to inhabit stones, ponds, rivers, terracotta animals and various trees. She is the rain and, more generally, the waters. Devotees have *darśana* (vision) of Śītalā when worshipping her *mūrti*s and *pratimā*s (icons). Alternatively, the goddess manifests on occasion of intense meditation, austerities, in dreams and during phenomena of devotional possession.

Within such apparently chaotic landscape, Śītalā has continued to give voice to the same anxiety: protection from disease. The following song, collected by Dr Robert Pringle, Superintendent General of Vaccination in the North-western Provinces, illustrates the nature of the goddess in a historical period marked by virulent smallpox epidemics:

> Visit, oh! Seetla, this secluded dwelling; stand at the door, / And give this child the gift of health. / Much have we worshipped thee for its sake before its birth: / We have worshipped thee at Pryag (Allahabad) and Juggernauth [in Puri], / And bathed in the sacred Ganges at Hurdwar [Haridwar], / And we have made obeisance at all thy shrines. / We will paint thy face with 'roree' [H. *rorī*, red clay], and pour into thy lap sweet smelling spices. / Then go, and swing thyself happy on thine own neem tree, / That so all in this house may be happy likewise. (Pringle 1885: 740)

Lexicographers confirm the protective nature of the goddess, and report that Śītalā is *adhiṣṭhātrī* (Skt. *adhiṣṭatr̥*: presider, controller) (Nā 1245; BaŚ 2029) and, more specifically, *vasantavisphoṭakāderadhiṣṭātrī* ('She who controls the spring [fever] and the pox') (ŚKD 346, vol. 5). Śītalā is the goddess who hinders disease (H. '*rog nivarāk devī*')

(Giri et al. n.d.: 75). She is a remover and a destroyer (*haranī*) of illness, a skill she derives from her being actually and intrinsically cold (Wadley 1980: 35; Filippi 2002: 196). In particular, she controls and heals from imbalances that express themselves through unnatural states of hotness (e.g. disease, misfortune and environmental catastrophes). Interpreting her name as a euphemism, 'an attempt to ward off the goddess's fire as she rages through the Bengali countryside [...]' (Dimock 1982: 184; see also Kolenda 1982: 236) is inaccurate.[3] Though Śītalā can be angry and seek revenge, nobody in India would call her *masūrikā* or *visphoṭaka devī*. This is no pedantic remark.

The label 'smallpox goddess' – or 'disease goddess' – suggests identity with, or dependency upon, illness. In fact, Śītalā is not the deification of smallpox. Poxes exist independently, and used to be associated with the coming of the spring season (Skt. *vasanta*) (cf. RSC xciv). North Indian languages bear witness to this coincidence, as smallpox is popularly known as *vasanta roga* (spring fever). Alternatively, the disease is called with names evocative of its most evident symptoms, i.e. pustules. Smallpox is 'lentil' (H. and B. *masūr*); 'bursting' (H. *sphoṭ*; B. *sphōṭak/phuskuḍi*); 'itching' (H. *khasrā*); 'pustule' (H. *goṭī*; B. *guṭikā*); and 'pearl' (H. *moṭī*; B. *muktā*). But the symptoms of smallpox are not just the ulceration of the skin and the appearance of boils and

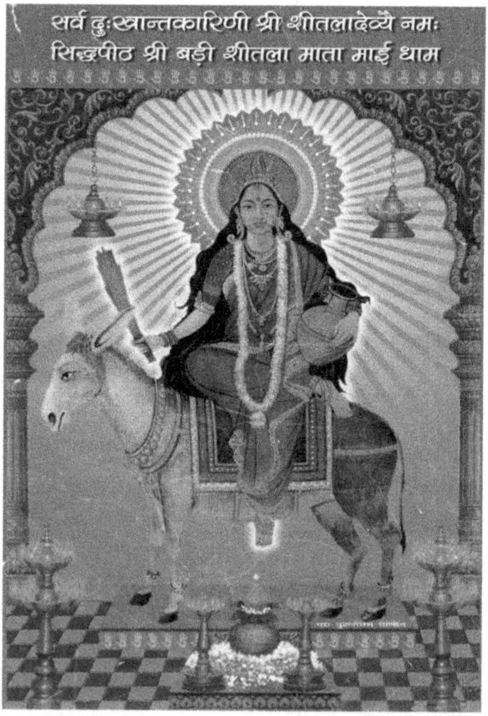

FIGURE 1.2 *Śītalā Mātā, front page of vintage calendar (author's collection). The invocation reads:* sarva duḥkhāntakāriṇī śrī śītalādevyai namaḥ *(Skt. 'Obeisance to the goddess Śītalā, the destroyer of all sufferings').*

vesicles.[4] The shivering of a smallpox victim is a powerful sign, and a visual reminder, of its cure. Fevers are thus called *ṭhaṇḍī*, *śīt*, *śītalī* or *śītalikā* (lit. 'coolness'). Such names provide not just an indication of the most obvious therapeutic course, but are evocative of the much-needed (i.e. auspicious) visitation of the Cold Lady.[5] Not by chance is the goddess called *sarvarogahāriṇī* (B. 'the destroyer of all diseases') and *vasantarogahariṇī* ('the destroyer of the spring disease' – i.e. smallpox) (Bhaṭṭācārya 1997: 150–1).

Bursts of *vasanta roga*, *visphoṭa*, *masūrikā*, etc. are associated with Śītalā Mā precisely because she is *śītalā*, 'cooling', 'soothing', 'refreshing' and therefore welcome (*maṅgalā*). This is clearly denounced in the *Śītalācālīsā* ('hymn in forty verses'): '*visphoṭak se jalat śarīrā / śītal karat harat sab pīrā //* (H. 'When the body burns with the pox, you [Śītalā] cool it down and take away all suffering').[6] In fact, most scholarship (Western and Indian alike) seems to struggle in telling Śītalā from *śītalā*. Nicholas has noted this in discrepancies between early āyurvedic texts and later commentators. In the twelfth-century commentary of Ḍalhaṇa to Suśruta 2.13, '*śītalikā* [is] the "popular designation" of *masūrikā*' (Nicholas 2003: 174). But in a sixteenth-century appendix to *Mādhavanidāna*, the pathology *śītalā* (which Nicholas spells 'Śītalā', thus equating it with the goddess) is 'based on the theory that they [poxes] are caused by the Goddess Śītalā' (ibid.; cf. Lambert 2015: 13.). A similar use is confirmed in BhPr.Ma. 60: 55. Here Śītalā Devī is not the same as *śītalā roga*. Bhāvamiśra informs us that *masūrikā* (pox) is featured by *śītalā*, a form of intermittent fever (*viṣamajvara*) associated with the presence of spirits (*bhūtādhiṣṭha*).[7] Conversely, the shivering, agitated (*ākrānta*) stage coincides with the manifestation of Śītalā (ibid.).

What has been highlighted so far indicates that the myth of the 'goddess of smallpox', more or less directly informed by the ŚMKs, has been privileged. Other Indian texts have been mentioned, but often not examined. Rites and narratives have been dismissed as folklore; a label used vis-à-vis Sanskrit/Brahmanic culture, the great Indian medical tradition (Āyurveda) and, later, Western empiricism. Finally, discourses on hygiene, health and religion in Śītalā culture have been conveniently twisted to fit functionalism, structuralism, theology and literary criticism. Let us see what Indian sources say.

The goddess Śītalā in Indian literature

The study of textual references to Śītalā is lacunose. Most analyses are derivative, and fail to exhaustively investigate Śītalā's presence in Sanskrit literature. The earliest source is unanimously indicated in an eight-part hymn, the *Śītalāṣṭakastotra*. This appears in a late āyurvedic compendium, the sixteenth-century *Bhāvaprakāśa*, authored by Bhāvamiśra. The *stotra*, however, is not original. Bhāvamiśra himself informs us that the hymn is extrapolated from *Kāśīkhaṇḍa* (c.ca thirteenth to fourteenth century), the fourth section of *Skandapurāṇa*. Beside the *Śītalāṣṭakastotra*, and its alleged purāṇic origin, we learn that Śītalā is also mentioned in the little-known *Picchilātantra*, a text coeval to Miśra's compendium (see below p. 20).

Some have tried to balance Śītalā's absence in earlier Indian literature by finding possible antecedents of the 'goddess of smallpox' in demonic females. Tiwari, for instance, suggests that 'Pūtanā with poisonous milk affecting the entire body of children is identical with Śītalā. Another spirit of identical nature with name Sīta-Pūtanā [*sic*] is worshipped to the present day as Śītalā' (1996: 455). The argument is not substantiated by any textual, ritual or iconography evidence. Both Pūtanā ('Putrid') and Śītapūtanā ('Cold Putrid') are *rakṣasī*s (a class of female demons), and are known as *grahī*s, 'graspers' responsible for negative possession and various associated diseases. White too sees in Śītapūtanā a Śītalā prototype (2003: 287, n. 156; cf. Smith 2006: 281 n. 52). He bases his observation on Filliozat's study of *Kumāratantra* (1937: 114–17; cf. Auboyer and De Mallmann 1950: 225) and on the widely advertised aggressive nature of Śītalā, especially with respect to children.

Śītapūtanā is mentioned in *Mahābhārata* (3.37.219: 25) as an ogress responsible for abortions. This is confirmed by Suśruta, who gives a series of invocations to protect children from the danger of the nine inauspicious and disease-carrying graspers (*graha*) (Utt. 27–36). The seventh *grahī* is Śītapūtanā, who is placated with an offering of *mudga* (green gram), liquor and blood.[8] Mādhava too reports on the grasp of Śītapūtanā, which results in emaciation, fits, vomiting, eye-disease (*netraroga*) and diarrhoea (MN 68: 27).[9] Śītalā, conversely, protects children. Although in Indic culture there is evidence of malignant beings who have turned into protective deities (e.g. the goddess Hārītī),[10] this is not the case. The only apparent similarity between Śītapūtanā and Śītalā is their association with coldness (√*śīta*) and water. The former resides in lakes; the latter is the fertilizing rain. Apart from that, the *grahī* and the goddess share very little. Śītapūtanā is a dangerous grasper, whereas Śītalā cures from the harm caused by graspers (SkP 5.13: 5, see below p. 9). This is quite evident even in the worship of Śītalā as an *ugra* (fierce, irate) goddess, such as in Patna (Agam Kuāṅ, see below pp. 54–4) and in the Dakṣiṇāśītalā shrine flanking the Kāl Bhairo Mandir, in Banaras. Here Śītalā shares the power of Bhairava, the *kotvāl* (H. policeman) of the city, and is worshipped to keep away *graha*s, evil spells (*jādūṭonā*) and the evil eye (*najar* < A. and F. *naẓar*). In short there is no ritual, textual and iconographic correspondence between Śītapūtanā and Śītalā.

The ill fame of Śītalā has caused other misreadings. One such case is Goudriaan's examination of the *Mañjuśrīmūlakalpa*, a circa eighth-century Buddhist *tantra* from north-eastern India. A mantra – the *mahābrahmāmantra* – is there given to get rid of Śītalā, 'the dreaded smallpox goddess', and 'dangerous spirits' (1978: 92). This information would have made it possible to locate Śītalā considerably earlier in Indian literature. In fact, Goudriaan's translation bears witness to how contemporary discourses on the 'goddess of smallpox' and her alleged dangerous nature have influenced a number of scholarly discourses. The text should read:

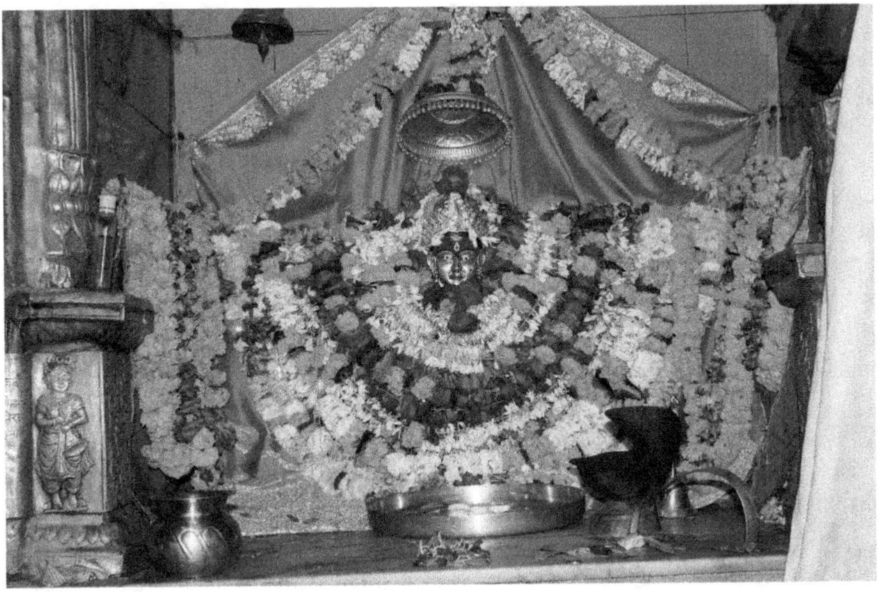

FIGURE 1.3 *Dakṣiṇāśītalā, Kāl Bhairo Mandir, Banaras (photo by author).*

> I prostrate to the all-pervading *buddhas*, whose teachings is eternal. [The mantra] says: 'O Brahmā, O perfect Brahmā, O divine glory: *svāhā*.' This *mahābrahmāmantra* was uttered so by the Bodhisattva. [All] beings (*bhūtāni*) attained peace (*śāntiṃ*) and immediately become appeased (*śītalā*).[11] (MMK 2.33.18–19)

Attempts to associate Śītalā with dangerous tantric goddesses are equally adventurous. Distinctive attributes of the Cold Lady are found in the iconography of intimidating goddesses such as Aghorā, whose *dhyānamantra* (visualization formula) is found in *Mahākālasaṃhitā* (or *Mahākālayogaśāstra*), a ritual text for the worship of Kāmakalākālī attributed to Ādinātha (Goudriaan and Gupta 1981: 79). The goddess is described as a three-red-eyed creature, dark-complexioned and living in the cremation ground. She stands on a corpse in meditation, has protruding fangs and ornaments made of human bones. She has long dishevelled hair, is naked and holds a broom and a winnowing fan (8: 283). Similarly, the broom and the winnower are found in the iconography of *yoginīs*. This has led some to speculate on parallels, or to construct a case for social critique toward higher classes (Kaimal 2013: 102, but cf. Kim 2013: 12-13). Tempting as it may be to associate Śītalā with goddesses with similar attributes, there is little evidence supporting such a thesis. Conversely, we will see how purāṇic, tantric, normative and devotional literature from at least the twelfth century unanimously agree in presenting the ass-riding Śītalā as an auspicious protector.

Purāṇas and *dharmanibandhas*

The first documented source on Śītalā in Indian literature is not, as previously argued, the *Kāśīkhaṇḍa* of *Skandapurāṇa*. The chapter on Banaras (Kāśī) of SkP is a comparatively late work and, in the published editions existing today, there is no record of a *Śītalāstotra* (Nicholas 2003: 225–6).[12] The goddess, however, appears in three separate sections of SkP: *Prabhāsakhaṇḍa* (circa twelfth century), *Vaiṣṇavakhaṇḍa* (c.ca twelfth–thirteenth century) and *Āvantyakhaṇḍa* (circa fifteenth–sixteenth century).

In *Prabhāsakhaṇḍa*, in a chapter called 'The Greatness of Śītalāgaurī', the goddess is praised as a healer and a protector of children. Her name is here explained in relation to her cooling and refreshing, that is healing, power:

> Iśvara said: [1–3] A pilgrim should visit the misery-quelling goddess stationed there itself. Earlier she was well known as Śītalā in Dvāpara Yuga. But in Kali Age she is famous as *Kali-duḥkhāntakāriṇī* (She who quells miseries in the Kali Age). If adored with ardent devotion, she will make the bodies of children cool (*Śītalā*) and free from ailments. Hence she is remembered as *Śītalā*. In order to dispel swellings (boils) in the case of children, *Masūras* should be properly measured and pondered. [4] The same is placed before Śītalā uttering, "May the children be free from ailments". Thereby there shall be suppression of *Vishpoṭa* (swelling, boils), *Carcikā* (small boils) etc. as well as *Vāta* (rheumatic complaints) etc. [5] Śrāddha should be performed there and Brāhmaṇas should be fed. [6] Camphor, flowers, muck, excellent sandalpaste, saffron and sweet scents should be offered. The food offering shall be pudding made with ghee. After dedicating it to the goddess, everything should be given to a couple. [7] On the ninth day in the bright half a splendid garland of Bilva should be offered to the goddess. Thereby the devotee shall attain all Siddhis. (SkP 7.1.135: 1–7)[13]

In the slightly later *Ayodhyāmāhātmya* of *Vaiṣṇavakhaṇḍa*, we find the description of a *śākta tīrtha* (ford) hosting a temple of Śītalā (Bakker 1986: 127). The *mandir*, located south of Faizabad, is mentioned in relation to two other goddesses: Bandīdevī,[14] protector of thieves, and Cuḍakīdevī, the one who grants *siddhi* (power and success). All the three goddesses are praised as 'removers of fear', namely fear of smallpox (Śītalā), of imprisonment (Bandī) and of risks and hazards (Cuḍakīdevī).

> The man who knows how to worship her [Śītalā] is completely liberated from all sins. One should always worship her specifically on Monday. Men carefully complete *pūjā* for the fulfilment of all aims (*artha*). [Śītalā] is worshipped by those who fear smallpox, etc. Prescribed rituals should be performed properly to have the fear of diseases, etc. vanquished. (SkP 2.8.8: 21–3)

Though this short passage offers minimal insight into the iconography and worship of Śītalā, it bears witness to the popularity of the goddess, who is here included in two *śaiva* circumambulatory pilgrimages (*parikrama*) performed on the auspicious *aṣṭamī* (eighth day) and *caturdaśī* (fourteenth day [of the waxing or waning phase of the moon]).[15]

Śītalā is then invoked in *Āvantyakhaṇḍa*, in a section called *Śītalāmāhātmya* ('The Greatness of Śītalā'). There, she is confirmed a protector of children, even though her power is not just limited to health issues. The goddess is a holistic healer. She removes demerit ('sins') and is functional to liberation (*mokṣa*). Finally, and significantly, the goddess protects from the evil influence of graspers:

> Sanatkumāra[16] said: I will now describe the excellent Markaṭeśvara. [1] There is a famous *tīrtha* there, which fulfils all desires (*sarvakāmapradāyakam*). When bathing in that *tīrtha*, a man is rewarded with the merit equivalent to (the gift) of a hundred cows. To destroy poxes (*visphoṭa*) and for the sake of children (*bālānāñcaiva kāraṇe*), [2] a devotee takes lentils (*masūra*) by measures and grinds them. Due to the power of Śītalā, children become free from the disease. [3] O excellent Brāhmaṇa, neither sin nor poverty afflicts those men who devoutly visit Śītalā, the destroyer of sins. [4] Nor need they fear disease (*rogabhayaṃ*) or the affliction of graspers (*grahapīḍā*). [5] (SkP 5.1.13: 1–5)[17]

The grandeur of Śītalā is further exalted in *Nāradapurāṇa (or Nāradīyapurāṇa)*, a heterogeneous and lengthy text named after the sage Nārada and conventionally listed among the eighteen *mahāpurāṇas*.[18] In the first part (*pūrvabhāga*), we find instructions about the worship of Śītalā in a list of ritual fasts (*vrata*)[19] to be observed on the eighth day (*aṣṭamī*) of every lunar phase (*pakṣa*):[20]

> One should worship Śītalā on the eighth day of the second fortnight of the month of Phālguna (*phālgunāparapakṣe*) with all sorts of food prepared, according to the rules, on the previous seventh day. [94] O Śītalā! You are the mother of the world, you are the father of the world. Śītalā you are nurturer of the world, I bow to you. [95] I bow to the goddess Śītalā, seated on the ass, naked, holding the broom and the pot, who destroys the pox (*visphoṭaka*). [96] Śītalā Devī gives relief from *visphoṭaka* to those who stand in water and repeat: 'Śītalā, Śītalā.' [97]. O twice-born! He who worships Śītalā with these mantras, by the mercy of goddess Śītalā, will be serene for a year. [98] (NāP 1.117: 94–98)

In the second part (*uttarabhāga*) of NāP, there is further confirmation of Śītalā's power in relation to sacred fords:

> If a man worships Śītalā Devī in the Dark Forest,[21] he should not fear *visphoṭaka*. (NāP 2.78: 12)

Finally, Śītalā is traditionally associated with *Bhaviṣyapurāṇa*. This depends on a narrative (*kathā*), and the related fast (*vrata*), mentioned in the *Vratarāja* (eighteenth century) of Viśvanātha, who ascribes it to BhaP. All editions known to me do not confirm this. In fact, Śītalā is virtually absent from BhaP – a text otherwise replete with instructions on *vratas*.[22] The goddess is briefly mentioned in relation to fertility in *pratisargaparva* (4.3: 54), and a Śītalāsthāna is identified near Kanauj (3.24: 1–36).

The apotheosis of Śītalā is found in *Śītalāṣṭakastotra*. The hymn appears in its entirety in two sixteenth-century sources: the *Picchilātantra*, to which I will return later, and a medical compendium, the *Bhāvaprakāśa*. The *stotra* says that the only cure for smallpox is repeating the name of Śītalā with firm devotion. This is a rare occurrence in medical literature. *Bhakti* is not one of the virtues of the physician. In Āyurveda, medical science (*vaidyakaśāstrajñāna*) is the only requirement of the *vaidya*. Devotion is rather explained as 'extreme diligence in the treatment of disorders' (Wujastyk 2012: 100). Alternatively, it is empathy toward the patient. Śītalā is irrelevant to *vaidya*s, but exceptional circumstances require exceptional measures.

Indian medical literature is vague about smallpox. Caraka and Suśruta mention diseases whose symptoms are skin eruptions. These, however, do not appear to be contagious in nature, and are not discussed as life-threatening conditions (CaS. Sū. 26: 102; CaS.Cik. 12: 90, 93; SuS.Ni. 17 and 37). Vāgbhaṭa, in his *Aṣṭāṅgahṛdayasaṃhitā*, indicates *visphoṭa* and *masūrikā* as *kṣudraroga* (minor ailments). Conversely the eighth-century *Nidāna* of Mādhavakara discusses the very same diseases as serious conditions which may cause death (MN. 53: 11; 54: 30–31). It seems thus likely that smallpox was not known in South Asia before the fifth century CE, whereas the strand known between the sixth and seventh centuries was not as deadly as the one that plagued the subcontinent in the following centuries. Regardless of the nature and the seriousness of *visphoṭa*, the disease is associated with a deity (Śītalā) only in BhPr. The *stotra* celebrating Śītalā and her protective power against *visphoṭa* is believed to have been composed by Śiva for the wellbeing of mankind:

> For this prayer, Mahādeva is the *ṛṣi*, *anuṣṭubh* is the metre (*chanda*), Śītalā is the goddess. The purpose of chanting it is to get relief from troubles with *śītalā*.[23]
>
> Skanda said: 'O lord of lords, please teach me the auspicious hymn of Śītalā which wards off the fear of poxes.' [70] Lord Īśvara speaks: 'I bow to the goddess Śītalā, seated on the ass, naked, holding the broom and the pot, wearing a *śūrpa* (winnower) on the head. [71] I bow to the goddess Śītalā who destroys the fear of all diseases. Upon approaching [her], one is no longer scared by smallpox. [72] He who says "Śītalā, Śītalā" is immediately relieved by the burning feeling and the dreadful fear of poxes. [73] A man who worships you with determination standing in the water should not fear the dreaded pox in his house. [74] O Śītalā, when a man is scorched by fever, he becomes foul smelling, and his sight is ruined. Then he regards you as the living medicine. [75] O Śītalā, take away the dreaded disease from inside human beings. You are the one who sprinkles nectar on those suffering

> from *visphoṭaka*, [76] goitre (*galagaṇḍa*) and malignant possession (*graharoga*). Men get cured by merely [meditating] upon you, o Śītalā. [77] There are neither mantras nor remedies to cure the diseases caused by sin. You, O Śītalā, are the mother (*dhātrī*). There is nobody like you amongst the gods. [78] O goddess, you have a navel cord like a lotus stem, and stay in the middle of the heart. Whoever mediates on you should not fear death.' [79] The house (family) of a person who chants this eight-part hymn of Śītalā will not fear the dreaded pox. [80] This should be read and heard with devotion for getting cured of other side-effects of the disease and for restoration of health. [81] This *Śītalāṣṭaka*[*stotra*] should not be given to anyone. It is worth-giving only to one who has devotion (*bhakti*) and faith (*śraddhā*). [82] (BhPr.Ma. 60: 70–82)

Alternative versions I heard in many temples include a few extra verses:

> Śītalā you are the mother of the world, you are the father of the world. Śītalā you are the nurturer of the world, I bow to you. [82][24] Rāsabha [Brayer], Gardabha [Crier], Khara [Ass], Vaiśākhanandana [That which grows fat during Vaiśākha], [83] Śītalāvāhana [Śītalā' mount], Dūrvākandanikṛntana [Destroyer – eater – of heaps of *dūrva* grass]. [84] The house and children of he who reads these names of the ass in front of Śītalā will never [suffer] the pox. [85] This *Śītalāṣṭaka*[*stotra*] should not be given to anyone, but it is worth-giving only to one with absolute faith and devotion. [86] So ends the *Śītalāṣṭakastotra* from *Skandapurāṇa*.

As short as purāṇic passages may be, they confirm that the worship of Śītalā in her current form was already established by the twelfth-thirteenth century. This is echoed in law digests (*dharmanibandhas*) regulating, among other things, women's rituals fasts (*vrata*), meritorious acts rewarded with protection extended to the whole family. *Vrata* manuals are easily available at cheap prices at markets or around temples, they are generally printed in local vernacular, although it is not unusual to find bilingual versions (Sanskrit-vernacular). They give detailed ritual instructions revolving around fasting (the *vrata* proper) but also include narratives (*kathā*) and a series of hymns (*stotra*), eulogies (*vijaya*) or songs (*gīti*) testifying the goddess's glory. The narrative element is of great importance for it provides, by means of an exemplary story, a way to memorize the various ritual actions and to associate them with meaningful events in the cycle of the goddess. Although Śītalā's presence in such literature is quite limited, her *vratas* continue to enjoy popularity across North India. These are:

- *Śītalāṣaṣṭhīvrata* (Śītalā's sixth), on the sixth day of the bright half (*śukla pakṣa*) of the month of Kārtika. In Bengal this is observed on Māgha.
- *Śītalāsaptamīvrata* (Śītalā's seventh), on the seventh day of the dark half (*kṛṣṇa pakṣa*) of the month of Śrāvaṇa.[25]

- *Śītalāṣṭamīvrata* (Śītalā's eighth), on the eighth day of the dark half of the months of Caitra, Vaiśākha, Jyeṣṭha, Āṣāḍha and Śrāvaṇa (but cf. NāP 1.117: 94–98).[26]

The observance of scheduled fasts varies to a great degree, depending on regional traditions. A typical ritual I observed in the Rajasthani region delimited by Bikamer, Jaisalmer and Jodhpur, is the presentation of offerings to donkeys on *Śītalāṣṭamī*.[27] The ritual, observed by women (often accompanied by their children), takes place on Caitra *aṣṭamī*. Animals are fed with fried food,[28] sprinkled with water, marked with *sindūr* and covered with colourful red-and-golden drapes. (Some carry colourful bags with presents, but this seems a recent innovation.) The ritual is meant to invite the goddess who, in exchange, will protect children.

The general custom for women observing the fast is to avoid domestic chores. Being the *vrata* a 'cooling' event, nothing is cooked. Women bathe in cold water, or stay in the water of rivers or ponds in meditation, and offer the goddess *naivedya* (a dish made of raw fruits and vegetables mixed with uncooked rice, milk and curd), leftovers or other stale edibles. A Hindi *Śītalāṣaṣṭhīvrata* (see below p. 13–14) concludes thus:

> Nowadays, on occasion of the annual worship, people cook the food (*bhoga*) to be offered to the goddess the night before, and they offer it to her early next morning. They consume some of this *prasād* along with their own family, and then they cook fresh food and eat it while it is still hot, which is a wrong thing to do. Consuming food cooked the day before and avoiding hot substances helps cool down the heat inside the body, which in turn cures many diseases. If one does so, she will be free from diseases for a whole year. This practice will also destroy the fear of painful diseases such as poxes.

Ritual instruction tends to be quite detailed, although devotees use them with some liberty. See for instance the list of items for *pūjā* in a Hindi version of a *Śītalāsaptamīvratakathā* (Appendix A):

> [...] vermilion powder (*rolī*), red-yellow wrist thread (*maulī*), incense (*dhūp*), lamps (*dīp*), camphor (*karpūr*), yogurt (*dahī*), rice (*bhāt/cāval*) or *cūḍā*,[29] cucumber (*kakaṛī phāl*),[30] rainwater (*dhār*),[31] betel leaves (*pān*), cloves (*lauṅg*), sandalwood (*candan*), a sacred thread (*yajñopavīt*), *itra* (natural perfume), tools used by married women (*suhāg kā sāmān*),[32] seven kitchen utensils (*sāt vartan*), clothes (*vastra*), fee for the Brahmins (*dakṣiṇā*), coconut (*nāriyaṇ*), seasonal fruits (*ṛtu phāl*), sweets (*miṣṭhānna*), a thread with seven knots (*sāt gāṇṭha dhāgā*), etc. (ŚVK 14)

A more detailed example is found in the two *vratakathās* (Appendices B and C) reported in the *Vratarāja*, a *dharmanibandha* of the Banarsi scholar Viśvanātha.[33]

Ritual instructions (*vidhi*) are usually followed by long narratives. In the case of VR, Viśvanātha indicates as his source SkP and BhaP. A shorter version of the latter, along with a brief *stotra*, is found in the *Vratārka*,[34] an earlier an equally authoritative *nibandha* composed toward the end of the seventeenth century in Banaras by Śaṅkarabhaṭṭa (1937: 217–23). This author too does not reference his source, although the material is very similar to ŚAS.

The *vratakathā* genre – beside its practical outputs – recapitulates core Hindu concepts of *bhakti*. Stories about fasting promote exemplary ritual, moral and devotional conduct for women and, at the same time, they bear witness to the enculturation of the *caturarthas*, namely *dharma* (duty, morality), *kāma* (pleasure), *artha* (wealth) and *mokṣa* (liberation) (see below, *Śrī Ādi Śītalā Stotram*, p. 18–19). This is particularly explicit in the purposed rationale of rituals, and in the narrative elements. For instance, the *Śītalāsaptamīvratakathā* that Viśvanātha ascribes to *Bhaviṣyapurāṇa* (Appendix C) tells the story of the pious princess Śubhakārī (the daughter of King Indradyumna of Hastināpura)[35] and shows the way of the ideal woman, or *pativratā* (Skt. 'devoted to the husband'). The text says that women worship Śītalā and observe the *vrata* to be blessed with a good husband and to be spared by poverty and the social drama that is widowhood.

The observance of *Śītalāvratas* is not just limited to the three scheduled fasts mentioned above. In fact, *vrata* manuals can be used to give authority to, and to establish the ritual agenda of, other festivals. I observed this in Banaras, with the merging of the *Śītalāṣaṣṭhīvrata* with the annual *Chaṭhpūjā*.

The *pūjā* – which falls on the sixth day of the bright half of Kārtik – is actually intended for the worship of Sūrya, the Sun. Women fast (including abstention from water) for up to 48 hours, present elaborate offerings and spend prolonged periods of time standing in the water of a river or pond. On perfection of the *vrata*, Sūrya rewards them with good health for their sons, daughters and husbands, and keeps disease away. In Banaras, special instructions are given for the worship of Śītalā in the *Mā̃ ke chāṭh pūjan kā vidhān*, a set of rules presented as *Śītalāṣaṣṭhīvrata*:

> The sixth day of the dark half of the month of Māgh: this day is famous in Bengal for the worship of the goddess Śītalā. There lived a rich man (*dhanī*) in a village. His wife used to duly observe the fast for the goddess Śītalā on the sixth day of the dark half of the month of Māgh. In the evening, after worship, she used to offer the goddess *bhoga* made of cooled rice mixed in yogurt, and to consume some after distributing it as *prasād*. One day, she was worshipping the goddess on the sixth day as per the rule when she was summoned to her parents'. In haste, she did not let the rice cool down. She mixed it with yogurt, offered it to the goddess, ate it as *prasād* and left for her parents' place. When she had gone some distance from her own house, she saw under a *nīm* tree [margosa] an old woman with the body covered with blisters (*phaphola*). She was moaning in pain. When she heard the woman's lament, she came closer. She asked her who had reduced her to such

> a state. The old woman said that the wife of a landowner in her neighbourhood had done so. As soon as she heard this, the landowner's wife came to her senses and begged forgiveness: 'Mother, I am that despicable woman whose behaviour has caused you this terrible condition! Please tell me what mistake on my part has reduced you so, and how can I make it up.' The Mother in the form of that old woman said: 'Daughter, in your haste to go home you did not let the rice cool down. You hastily mixed yogurt in it, offered it to me as *bhoga* and ate it. This is what made me suffer. Now hear what to do: bring yogurt and smear it all over my body, bathe me with cold water, and fan me with *nīm* leaves. Only this will take away my suffering. But remember: if you give me even the smallest hot substance when you worship me during the *vrata* and then eat it yourself, it will cause me the same pain as in this incident.' Hearing this, she [the landowner's wife] begged Mātā's forgiveness and went back home. She told this story to her husband [and] asked him to build a temple to the Mother near the *nīm* tree and to dig a well. In this way she could repent for her mistake during her daily worship by serving and offering *bhoga* to the Mother. The landowner praised his wife and began the construction works. He said that this will protect the people of his village from diseases and bring good fortune. (ŚVK 15–16)[36]

The *pūjārīs* of the Śrī Dakṣiṇī Ādi Śītalā Mandir on the Śītalā Ghāṭ of Banaras explained to me they included a 'Bengali *pūjā*' in the calendar of the goddess as a sign of respect to the local Bengali community, one of the largest and wealthiest presences in the city.[37]

Another similar case is the *vārṣik annakūṭ* ('annual [offering of the] heap of grain').[38] Originally a way to celebrate the victorious deeds of Kṛṣṇa in Vṛndāvana, and known as *Govardanapūjā*, the festival is a *śṛṅgār mahotsav*, a feast of beauty and love. In Benares it is associated with the goddess Annapurṇā ('[She who is] full of rice', i.e. the Food Giver). The festival is held every year in the main Śītalā Mandir on the first day of the light fortnight of Kārtika, and lasts three days. Tickets are sold for a fee of ₹ 101 (around 98 pence).[39] The food (*bhoga*) – rice, pulses, fruits, sweets decorated with flowers – is arranged in heaps resembling mountains in front of Śītalā's altar. (I have been informed that 64 different types of edibles are used.) The many visitors bring quite a lot of wealth to the temple. This permits regular refurbishment, the purchase of decorations (lights, flags, incense, garlands, perfume, etc.), new clothes and jewels for the goddess and the hiring of professional performers (singers and musicians). Pilgrims from surrounding areas visit the city on account of the *annakūṭ*, and many come from other states (mainly Bengalis and Biharis, but also 'Madrasis' – as people from the south are called). The festival requires fasting on its second day, an observance followed by women only.

Local women help with the preparation of food as part of their *vrata*. While busy with peeling vegetables and other chores, *kathās* (unrelated to Śītalā) are told and usually there is some singing in the form of devotional *bhajan*. The celebration serves not just to invite the auspicious and protective presence of Śītalā, or to display individual devotion. The *annakūṭ* is a family festival. As a place for well-wishing, it serves as an arena for reunions and merriment, but also as a way to mix and meet with others, a welcome occasion for those with limited means of action and expression (e.g. women and teenagers).

As per the instructions given in *vrata* manuals, singing is core to these festive occasions. In a moment when normal social barriers fade away, men and women of all ages and from all backgrounds join to loudly sing hymns such as the *vijaya stuti*, in which Śītalā is associated with pan-Hindu goddesses everybody is familiar with. One does not need to know Sanskrit to sing a *vijaya*. If the lyrics are not known, devotees join in and repeat together the invocation to the goddess: *namo śītalā kaṣṭa haranī bhavānī* ('Obeisance to Goddess Śītalā, who destroys [all] pains'):

namo ādi māyā umā sr̥ṣṭhikārī, namo śāradā ambikā īśapyārī /
namo kālikā īśvarī vākavānī, namo śītalā kaṣṭa haranī bhavānī //
namo candravadanī girā mr̥ganayanī, namo sundarī mohanī koka vayanī /
namo haṃsagamanī sati rūpa khānī, namo śītalā kaṣṭa haranī bhavānī //
namo siṃhanī kālikā joga māyā, namo tāranī jālipā veda gāyā /
namo ambikā mohanī rūpa khānī, namo śītalā kaṣṭa haranī bhavānī //
namo ambikā caṇḍikā khaḍgadhārī, namo śāradā devī mahiṣāpacārī /
namo saṅkaṭā kālikā īśarānī, namo śītalā kaṣṭa haranī bhavānī //
namo mātu ambā umā jyoti rūpī, namo devī durgā sukalyāṇakārī /
namo caubhujī śakti girajā bhavānī, namo śītalā kaṣṭa haranī bhavānī //
namo gaurī girijā namo śaila bālā, namo sarasvatī śaṅkarī devī jvālā /
namo ambikā caṇḍikā sarvajñanī, namo śītalā kaṣṭa haranī bhavānī //
namo śambhū māyā umā bhadrakālī, namo devī dāyā karo merī ālī /
namo jagadambāgirā devī vānī, namo śītalā kaṣṭa haranī bhavānī //
namo devī vindhyā girā siddha karaṇī, namo jogamāyā sadā viśvabharaṇī /
namo dāsa icchā vinaya vegi vāṇī, namo śītalā kaṣṭa haranī bhavānī //

The *Śītalācālīsā* (hymn in 40 verses) is also extremely popular:

> Couplet: Victory, victory, victory to Mother Śītalā. The heart of the one who meditates upon you becomes pure and cool, [and] intelligence, strength and knowledge are enhanced. O Śītalā, your abode is everywhere; your coolness (*śītala*) is your splendour. Let me swing in your shade, O protecting mother.

Quatrain: Victory to the goddess Śītalā! Victory to the mother, who is a goldmine of qualities. [Your] power is on every house. It is your ornament, like the growing Harvest Moon. When the body burns with the pox, you cool it down and take away all suffering. Mother Śītalā is your auspicious name. You protect everybody in times of trouble. You are Śākambhari ('Bearer of the greens'), Śaṅkarī ('Auspicious') and Bhavānī ('Giver of life'). You are the protector of children's lives and the giver of happiness. A broom and a pitcher of water in your hands, your head is fulgent like the radiance of the sun. The sixty-four *yoginī*s sing together. They play the *vīṇa* (a large lute), the *tāla* (cymbals) and the *mṛdaṅga* (double-sided drum) for you. Bhaironāth shows you his dance. Śeṣa and Śiva cannot grasp you completely. Blessed are you, Great Queen Mother. Gods, humans and sages praise your glory. An extremely powerful demon (*daitya*) by the name of Visphoṭak [Pox], in the form of a flame, with overwhelming strength, entered every household and no one was able to give protection. [Taking] the form of disease, he devoured children. A huge cry for help filled the world. When no one was able to avert this crisis, the Mother took a wondrous form. Carrying in her hands a broom and a winnowing basket, she caught Visphoṭak. She hit him with a club (*mūsal*) all along. [So] he pleaded with her in all possible ways: 'Mother, I did not know how to tell right from wrong! Mother, I won't go to anyone's house now. I will only stay in those households that are unclean/impure (*apavitra*).' When people recite the worship of the Mother, they are blessed and all their suffering will be destroyed. The burning body will become cool (*śītala*). The terrible fear of poxes will be driven away. By worshipping Śrī Śītalā, one will be blessed with good fortune (*kalyāṇa*). The Lord speaks the truth when he says so. Brother, if in somebody's place there is fear of the pox, one should worship the goddess – this is the only solution. One should consecrate a pitcher (*kalaśa*) to Śītalā, and invite a Brahman (*dvija*) to recite the texts (*pāṭh*) according to the rules. Śītalā, you are the mother of the world. You are the father of the world, you alone grant happiness. You are the mother of the world, [and] the one who bestows joys. I bow to you, O goddess Śītalā. I bow to you, the destroyer of sufferance and the one who brings happiness. I bow to you, the One who grants liberation to the world. I bow to you, who are worshipped in the three worlds. [I bow] to the One who uproots suffering and poverty. Śrī Śītalā is known as: Śoḍhalā, Mahalā, Ruṇakī, Hyuṇakī and Mātu Mandalā [= Maṇḍalā]. You are naked [and] splendid while riding [your vehicle] with five names: Rāsabha ('Brayer'), Khara ('Ass'), Vaiśākhanandana ('That which grows fat during Vaiśākha), Gardabha ('Cryer') and Dūrvākandanikṛntana ('Destroyer [i.e. eater] of heaps of *dūrva* grass'). If these [names] are remembered along with Mother Śītalā, all suffering will be gone. Neither mantra nor medicine can cure swellings, goitre, etc. There is no other means of curing [the pox] but the worship of the Mother. Whoever seeks the protective shelter of the Mother, will certainly obtain what s/he wants, and will be freed from fear. The leper (*koṛhī*) has a pure body, the blind sees in all directions with his eyes, barren (*bandhya*) women beget sons, and the poor from birth becomes rich. I have seen the dumb creating poetry [and] singing the praises of Mother Śītalā. No one should doubt that it is only the Mother who reigns supreme in the world. So speaks Rāmsundar Prabhudāsā [sic]. My residence is in Tivārīpur, east of the riverbank of Prayāg [Allahabad], at a remote place on the bank of the Ganges. It has been some time since I have been calling [the Mother], since I have been waiting for the Mother's grace. I am lying at your doorstep, hoping to see you. Protect me, Mother Śītalā![40]

Another popular devotional hymn is the *ārti* song, regularly recited during daily *pūjā*:

Refrain (*ṭek*): Victory to Mother Śītalā, victory to Mother Śītalā.
[She is] the Primordial Light, the Queen, the Giver of all the fruits [of action].
You are splendid on [your] gem-studded throne, the white royal umbrella over your head.
Ṛddhi (Prosperity) and Siddhi (Accomplishment) fan you with a flywhisk, the whole world sings about your lovely form.
Ref.
Viṣṇu [and] Śiva, the bearers of this world, are at your service.
Vedas and *purāṇa*s describe you, [but] cannot measure [your greatness].
Ref.
Indra plays the *mṛdaṅga* for your pleasure, and Candra plays the *vīṇā* with his own hands for you.
Sūraj (Sūrya) plays the *tāl* (cymbal) and sage Nārada sings for you.
Ref.
The bells, the conch-shell, the *beṇu*[-pipe] and the *sahanāī* (a kind of oboe) play in a delightful way.
Devotees perform your *ārti* overjoyed at seeing you again and again.
Ref.
You have the form of Brahman, [you are] a boon-giver and the knower of the three ages.
You give happiness to your devotees just like a mother, a father and a brother.
Ref.
Whoever meditates upon you brings home love and devotion, will get all wishes fulfilled and will be saved from rebirth.
Ref.
(ŚC 15)

The praise concludes with a mantra for the liberation from the torment caused by fevers and poxes (*visphoṭaka* or, in Hindi, *cecak*): *aum hrīṃ śrīṃ śītalāyae namaḥ*.

An alternative printed version, which I found at the main temple of Śītalā in Banaras, presents a different opening: 'Victory to the Siddhapīṭha of the Elder Mother Śītalā', a statement aiming to celebrate and confirm the authority of the temple. The conclusion is also different:

> Whoever suffering from disease [x2] comes under your protective shelter, Mother, comes under your protective shelter. The leper gets a pure body, the blind gets eyesight, a barren woman gets a son [x2] and the poor becomes rich. Victory to Mother Śītalā. Those who do not worship you deeply regret not doing so, Mother, deeply regret it. You are the one who cools the world [x2]. You are the saviour of the world. You are Satī. You have neither beginning nor end. [You are] the preserver of all, Mother, the preserver of all [x2]. Your servant stands with his hands joined in supplication [x2]. Listen to me, Mother, listen to me: Give me your devotion, O giver

> of all happiness, O Mother, [you are] the giver of all happiness. Victory to Mother Śītalā! (ŚVK 31)

In this composition, as well as in other similar texts, Śītalā's much-advertised association with poxes and fevers, and the idea she might inflict disease, is missing. This is no isolated pattern. See for instance this Hindi *vijaya* intended for the worship of Śītalā as Śrī (i.e. Lakṣmī):

> Victory to Mother Śītalā! Victory to Mother Śītalā! Protect us forever. We [are] your babies, [and we] are under your protective shelter. [1] You are naked, an ass is your vehicle, your form is that of cold (*śīta rūpiṇī*) and you are the giver of happiness. You carry in one hand nectar-like pure water and in the other a shining broom. You are the destroyer of smallpox; you are compassionate and have a bright laughter. If one chants your name every day, you will destroy all his pains. You eat cold food (*śitala bhojan*) such as yogurt mixed with grains, and you grant boons and auspiciousness to gods and humans. [2] You are happy with a simple offering of water. If one gives you leaves of *bel* (wood-apple), you will remove all the obstacles. You give strength to your devotee. By your grace, the conquerors of the world Nandana [Kṛṣṇa], the son of Nanda, Raghunanda [Rāma], the son of Raghu, and other great devotees partake of your bliss. You are the devotion of the *Bhāgavata [Purāṇa]*, you are Śakti, you are all ingenuities. You are the devotees' craving for the feet of Hara [Śiva], you are knowledge (*jñana*) and liberation (*mukti*). I beg of you with my hands joined so that I may be the best one in this world. May I speak the virtuous language of saints, and may I be devoted to noble deeds. You alone are the destroyer of the disasters that strike everybody. In this world you alone are protection (*varmādā*), noble deeds (*śubh karmadā*) and righteousness (*dharmadā*). [3] (ŚVK 21–22)

The permeability of gods in Hinduism is well-known. Śītalā is no exception. Not only is her healing power associated with Vaiṣṇavite goddesses; hymns like the following *Śrīādiśītalāstotram*, which echoes the popular Śrī Durgā Saptaślokī ('Seven verses of Durgā') from *Devīmāhātmya*, show how Śītalā is safely assimilated into *śākta* devotional contexts:

> O Śītalā, you are the mother of the world and the father of the world. Śītalā, you are the nurturer of the world. I bow to you [1]. I bow to [your] six names: Śītalā, Śīḍhalā, Mahalā, Maṇḍalā, Ruḍakī and Guḍakī. [2] [I bow to the names of the ass]: Rāsabha [Brayer], Gardabha [Crier], Khara [Ass], Vaiśākhanandana [That which grows fat during Vaiśākha], [83] Śītalāvāhana [Mount of Śītalā], and Dūrvākandanikṛntana [Destroyer – eater – of heaps of *dūrva* grass]. [3] Auṃ: 'O you who are blessed with every felicity, [you] auspicious one [who] accomplishes every aim (*artha*); O protector, O three-eyed Gaurī, praise be to you, Nārāyaṇī.'[41] [4] There is no doubt

> that you, with your *prasād,* free human beings from all the obstacles and bless them with money and food, and with children. [5] Auṃ: 'O you who are busy protecting those who suffer and are helpless, and who come to seek refuge in you; O you who take away everyone's suffering, O Nārāyaṇī, praise be to you.'[42] [6] Auṃ: 'O you who are the true form of everything, queen of everything, endowed with the energy (*śakti*) of all things; protect us from all fears, O Goddess. Praise be to you, O goddess Durgā.'[43] [7] Auṃ: 'When you are pleased, you destroy all diseases, when you are angry, you destroy all desires wished. There are no dangers for those who surrender to you. Having sought refuge with you, they can give refuge to others.'[44] [8] Auṃ: 'Let the pacification of all the obstacles of the three worlds [and] the destruction of our enemies be accomplished by you.' [9][45] (ŚVK 19)

The goddess celebrated in purāṇic literature, but also in *dharmanibandhas* and *vratakathās*, is emphatically praised as a protector.[46] Changes in her otherwise protective nature depend on the interpolation of textual material associated with other, *ugra*, goddesses, as in the case shown above. As per her much-advertised low origin, there is no mention of Śītalā's association with impure social groups. The goddess is principally a giver of fertility and one who heals children from infectious disease that manifests with boils on the skin (*visphoṭa*). In short, Śītalā is a great goddess who cleanses sins and gives liberation.

Tantric and āgamic literature

Śītalā makes her appearance in tantric literature comparatively late. The few texts mentioning her do not shed any light on her origin, although some offer unprecedented details of ritual practice (*sādhana*) and a unique perspective on the nature of Śītalā as a remover of impurity as well as a goddess associated with impure professions. All sources I have been able to consult confirm the description of purāṇic texts: Śītalā is a protector who heals 'boils,' (*vi*)*sphoṭā*. The aggressive, infecting element lacks in tantric manuals (*āgamas*).

Meditative formulas (*dhyānamantras*) for the visualization of the goddess and ritual instructions first appear around the sixteenth century and, more convincingly, in the next two centuries. Prior to that, the name Śītalā appears in the *Agnikāryapaddhati,* a post-twelfth-century Kaula *āgama* from Kashmir on fire sacrifice. Śītalā is mentioned as the fiftieth goddess to be invoked in a list of 65 *yoginīs*.[47] Yet apart from her name, there is no useful element to ascertain her nature and specialism. It is thus hazardous to assess the likelihood of the presence of the goddess within Kaula circles.

Similarly problematic is a passage in the *Khecarīvidyā* of Ādinātha (prior to the fifteenth century), an important *haṭhayoga* text instructing *yogins* on the practice of *khecarīmudrā*.[48] In its second *paṭala*, a description is given of the points (*kalā*) in which the nectar of immortality is stored. One of these is called 'Śītalā':

> Below the nostrils and above the lips is the great place [called] the Royal Tooth. There, O goddess, is a pair of *kalās*, Pūrṇāmṛtā and Śītalā. Holding the breath, [the yogin] should touch [them] with the tip of [his] tongue. A sweet, cool fluid is produced there, O goddess. Focusing his mind there, the ascetic should drink [the fluid] for three months. He becomes ageless and undying, free from all disease. (*Khecarīvidyā* 2.30)[49]

It is hard to establish whether the name *śītalā* is that of a *kalā* featured by coldness or if it is in some way reminiscent of the Cold Lady (Śītalā). It is nonetheless interesting that the *śītalākalā*, by means of its cooling properties, has the power to vanquish all diseases, just like the goddess.

The first unambiguous reference to Śītalā in tantric literature is found in *Picchilātantra*.[50] This information is first given in 1917 by Sarkar (1972: 258) and in 1939 by Bhaṭṭācārya (BMKI 886; cf. Bhattacharyya 1952: 56). Many have subsequently indicated in PiT, along with SkP, the earliest reference to Śītalā, even though – to my knowledge – none has managed to examine the latter.[51] *Picchilātantra*, which is the only ritual manual for the worship of Śītalā, is mentioned in the 1577 *Śrītattvacintāmaṇi* (15: 107; 16: 616) of Pūrṇānanda, in the *Sarvollāsatantra* (12: 9; 16: 9; 16: 16; 39: 8) of Sarvavidyāsiddha Sarvānandanātha (sixteenth century), in the *Tantrasāra* of Kr̥ṣṇānanda 'Āgamavāgīśa' Bhaṭṭācārya (late sixteenth/early seventeenth century), in the *Āgamatattvavilāsa* of Raghunātha Tarkavāgīśa (1687) and in Rāmatoṣaṇa Vidyālaṃkāra's *Prāṇatoṣinī* (circa 1820).[52] This permits us to safely locate *Picchilātantra* no later than 1577. If, however, we maintain that Sarvānandanātha obtained *siddhi* circa 1426 (Woodroffe 2009: 237; Banerji 2003: 113), then *Picchilātantra* is relatively earlier, i.e. early fifteenth century, and therefore it predates *Bhāvaprakāśa* in reporting the *Śītalāṣṭakastotra*.

Gopīnāth Kavirāj, in his *Tāntrika Sāhitya* (1972: 371), gives a short summary of the contents of *Picchilātantra*. Written in Sanskrit, but in Bengali script, the text deals with *yantras*, mantras and ritual instructions to worship Kālī. Kavirāj does not mention Śītalā. Bhaṭṭācārya (BMKI 887) quotes Śiva's eulogy (*stava*), which corresponds to ŚAS 71–74, and then the *Śītalādhyānamantra*:

> *śvetāṅgīṃ rāsabhasthāṃ karayugalavilasammārjanī pūrṇakumbham/*
> *mārjanyā pūrṇakumbhādamṛtamayajalaṃ tāpaśāntaiḥ kṣipantīṃ//*
> *dig vastrāṃ mūrdhniśūrpāṃ kanakamaṇigaṇairbhūṣitāṅgīṃ trinetrām/*
> *visphoṭakādugratāpa praśamanakarī śītalāṃ tvāṃ bhajāmi //*[53]

Śītalā then appears in the *Devīnāmavilāsa* (circa 1666) of the Kashmiri philosopher Sāhibakaula (b. 1636). The work is a *stotrakāvya*, a poetical composition in *kāvya* style on the thousand names of the goddess:

> In the sacred fords of Kashmir (*kaśmīratīrtheṣu*), on ice or on the moon, in the heart of the *sādhu*, eternal success has been attained. May she who is celebrated

> as Śītalā be benevolent; she destroys the heat of wrath and is responsible for the knowledge of the self (*krodhoṣmahantrī nijabodhakartrī*). (8: 92)

The *Merutantra* (32: 285-91), an eighteenth-century heterogeneous text, gives an emphatic rendition of Śītalā, and offers interesting details about her worship as a goddess who protects from 'boils' (*sphoṭā*):

> The sacred monosyllable [*auṃ*] and then the nine syllables: '*māyā ramā śītalāyai hr̥d.*' [Of this mantra] the silent seer is Upamanyu, the metre is *br̥hatī*, the goddess is Śītalā. [285] It is made of six parts, six syllables and two seed mantras of Lakṣmī. Let's then meditate on the goddess Śītalā, [who sits] on an ass, sky-clad [286], holding a broom and a winnower, [who is] worshipped with red flowers and ice, on whose head is a bundle of sesame oil-dirty clothes tied together (*tailādimala saṃyuktavastrapoṭaliśīrṣikām*) [287]. Let a sacrifice of mixed grains (*kodrava*) and red lentils (*masurā*) be offered to the goddess inside the triangle whose corners are occupied by an earthen tray; in the city of the earth (*bhūpure*)[54] [the sacrifice is offered] to the eight Bhairavas. [288] The mantra must be repeated ten thousand times. After offering oblations of rice and milk to each one of the ten parts [of the *yantra*] [and] after the water libation, he who repeats the mantra becomes perfected. [289] The one who stands in the water up to the navel [and] repeats the mantra a thousand times is set free from eruptions (*sphoṭā*) that are destroyed instantly [290]. In the lineage (*vaṃśa*) of the one who has mastered this mantra there is no fever (*śītalā*); in the house where there are the consecrated ashes (*bhasman*), there is no [pox]. [291]

A short meditating mantra is mentioned in the *Śrītattvanidhi*, a treatise on iconography composed by Kr̥ṣṇarāja Oḍeyar III (1799–1868), Mahārāja of Mysore:

> Now the visualization of Śītalā Devī (in the practice of Śītalā [as per] *Rudrayāmalatantra*).[55] Let us meditate on Śītalā Devī [who sits] on an ass and is sky-clad, holding a broom and a vessel, on whose head is a winnower. (1908: 24)

A later tantric ritual compendium, the *Puraścaryārṇava*, compiled by the Maharāj of Nepal Pratāpasiṃha Sāha (1751–77), has a whole section on Śītalā. This, however, seems to borrow from previous tantric literature, including MT:

> And now the mantra of Śītalā as per the *Merutantra*. I will now explain she who is the washer of the clothes of Maheśa [Śiva] (*maheśaya vastraprakṣālikā*) [80] and is known [with the name of] Śītalā, [the one of] the red lentil [*masurā*], the Lord of the flattened rice (*cipiṭeśvarī*): the sacred monosyllable and then the nine syllables: '*māyā ramā śītalāyai hr̥d.*' [81] While in the *Yāmalatantra*[56] it is uttered the mantra (*manu*) of the eight syllable: '*māyā śrīśītalā*' with the dative stem (*ṅentā*) ending

> with *hṛd* (heart) [*māyā śrīśītalāyai hṛd*], in the *Merutantra* the silent seer (*muni*) is Upamanyu, the metre is *bṛhatī*, the goddess is Śītalā; [the mantra is] divided in six parts, with six syllables and the seed mantras of the protecting Lakṣmī. [82] And now the visualization (in the *Yāmala* and other [texts]). I prostrate to the goddess Śītalā, who sits on an ass, sky-clad holding a broom and a vessel, on whose head is a winnower. [83] In the *Merutantra*: 'one should then meditate on the goddess Śītalā, [who sits] on an ass, sky-clad, holding a broom and a winnower, [who is] worshipped with red flowers and ice [84], on whose head is a bundle of sesame oil-dirty cloths tied together. Let a sacrifice of mixed grains (*kodrava*) and red lentils (*masurā*) be offered to the goddess inside the triangle whose corners are occupied by an earthen tray while in in the city of the earth (*bhūpure*) [let the sacrifice be] to the eight Bhairavas' [85]. Now the *puraścaraṇa* [the acts leading to the completion of ritual]: the mantra should be repeated ten thousand times. After offering oblations of rice and milk to each one of the ten parts [86], after the water libation, he who repeats the mantra becomes perfected. The one who, standing in the water up to the navel, repeats the mantra a thousand times [87] is set free from eruptions that are destroyed instantly. In the lineage of the one who has mastered this mantra there is no pox fever. [88]; in the house where there are the consecrated ashes, there is no [pox]. The mantra of such a man is presented right there. Now, therefore, I will reveal the supreme mantra of her [Śītalā's] consort: [89] The seed mantra of grace (*prāsādabīja*, i.e. *auṃ*), the 'to the one who pervades the sky' (*vyomavyāpine*), and then *svāhā* (*dviṭha*). [*auṃ vyomavyāpine svāhā*]: this is the mantra of the eleven waves (syllables). The *nyāsa*,[57] the visualization, the oblation, etc. [90] are equivalent to the *prāsādabīja* [-mantra]. Its preparatory rite (*puraskṛti*) is five thousand repetitions. Offerings of butter should be presented to the ten parts [of the *yantra*] and then a water oblation should follow (91). So [ends] the section on Śītalā. [12: 80–91]

This section, or a similar version from *Rudrayāmalatantra*, is acknowledged in the *Râs Mâlâ* (1856) of Alexander Kinloch Forbes, a civil servant of the East India Company. Forbes, who became an expert of Gujarati language, literature and culture, reports on *śītalāṣaṣṭhī* and the practice of local Brahmans to read from 'Roodrayâmul' an opening invocation aiming at inviting the goddess to have children cured of smallpox. Stale edibles (grass and wheat cakes) are then offered to donkeys (1856: 327) (see above p. 12). Although Forbes does not report the opening hymn from *Rudrayāmalatantra*, we learn that the goddess is thought to belong to 'the Chundâl caste' (ibid.), just as *Merutantra* and *Puraścaryārṇava* suggest.

One more reference to the Cold Lady is found in the *Dīkṣāprakāśa*, an early nineteenth-century *Śaivasiddhānta* text of Maithila Paṇḍit Śrī Jīvanāth Śarma (1935: 26), where a mantra is given:

> *Auṃ hrīṃ śrīṃ*. Salutation to Śītalā. Let's repeat [this mantra] a thousand times and make a water oblation. The one who, standing in the water up to the navel, repeats the mantra a thousand times is set free from the eruptions (*sphoṭā*) that are destroyed instantly.

The presence of Śītalā in tantric literature, though sporadic, eventually reveals previously unacknowledged features. Texts composed around the eighteenth century, while retaining invocations derived from the ŚAS, bear witness to a complex ritualism. Both *Merutantra* and *Puraścaryārṇava*, and possibly earlier material excerpted from a *Rudrayāmalatantra*, make it possible to argue that Śītalā worship had infiltrated tantric *śaiva* and *śākta* milieus and, between the sixteenth and eighteenth centuries, it developed into a complex *sādhana*. Ritual practice includes mantric utterance and the construction of complex *yantras* for the visualization of the goddess. The ritualist is here called a *mantrī*, he who utters formulae, and apparently is a householder who acts of behalf of his family.[58] Unlike hymns extrapolated from purāṇic sources, tantric manuals lack the devotional component. The approach is strictly a ritual one. The outspoken aim is to vanquish (the fear of) boils (*sphoṭā*) and fevers (*śītala*).

An element of novelty is the description of Śītalā as *vastraprakṣālikā* – she who washes the clothes of Śiva-Maheśvara.[59] The description of the goddess who, like a laundress, holds on her head a heap of dirty clothes smeared with sesame oil (*taila*) fascinates, although it is problematic to assess. The image evokes women from low occupation classes, and tantric texts are replete with descriptions of *sādhana saṅginīs* (female ritual companion) specifically chosen from impure classes or *ādivāsī* groups. The figure of the *rajakī* ('washer-woman' – but also a woman on the third day of her menstrual cycle) is indicated as Śakti in various *śākta* and tantric sources (*Devīpurāṇa* 9: 32–35; *Kubjikāmatatantra* 25; *Kulārṇavatantra* 7: 42–45; *Tantrasadbhāva* 15: 88 and 127ff). Śītalā, however, is never discussed as *sādhana saṅginī*. She is alien to this sort of ritualism and its culture. I am thus inclined to read the passage as symbolic of the role of 'low caste women' (sweepers, washer-women) as practical agents of purification. Śītalā is thus confirmed as a goddess of hygiene.

The Bengali *Śītalāmaṅgalkāvyas*

References to Śītalā in Sanskrit literature concur in describing a benign goddess whose specialism is the protection from smallpox in particular, and diseases in general. The only consistent exception to this trend is found in the *Śītalāmaṅgalkāvyas*. *Maṅgalkāvyas* have been defined as 'eulogistic poetry' (Dimock 1962: 308), 'poetry of blessing' (1976: 75, 82 n. 1),[60] and 'epic of the low castes' (Bhattacharyya 2000). Written from the end of the fifteenth century, and devised for on-stage recitation, they celebrate *āñcalik* deities such as Dharmarāj, Manasā, Caṇḍī and Ṣaṣṭhī, and their struggle to be accepted and worshipped by humans and gods (Zbavitel 1976: 159). But the gods of *maṅgalkāvyas* are vengeful, and often cruel. They are worshipped out of fear (BMKI 6–11). Although their stories celebrate courage and devotion, their success depends upon vivid representations of the suffering of the oppressed at the hands of the corrupted. Graphic and horrific descriptions of battles, ordeals and death are common. This is particularly evident in the case of ŚMKs.

Unlike other *maṅgal* poems, ŚMKs are later, shorter and less articulated in structure and linguistic register. Known authors are: Kavi Vallabha (nom de plume of Daivakīnanda; early seventeenth century); Kr̥ṣṇarām Dās (late seventeenth century); Dvija Harideva, Kavi Jagannāth, Mānikrām Gāṅgulī,[61] Śaṅkar and Nityānanda Cakravartī (who all wrote in the second half of the eighteenth century); Rāmnārāyaṇ Bhaṭṭācārya (late nineteenth century); and Nīlkāṇṭa Bandhyopādhyāy (early twentieth century) (BMKI 195–202; Mukhopadhyay 1994: 85–103; Nicholas 2003: 107–8). The majority of these works are little known to the Bengali public. It is not so for Nityānanda's poem, a text that has been reprinted in many versions and that continues to enjoy much popularity by means of theatrical representations of its most successful sections (*pālā*) (cf. Nicholas 2003: 211). The plot revolves around the following points:

1. Miraculous birth: Śītalā arises from the cold embers of a fire oblation.
2. Exclusion 1: the gods do not acknowledge her divine status.
3. Revenge 1: Śītalā infects the gods with all sorts of diseases.
4. Relocation: Śītalā decides to settle on earth, where human beings are respectful to gods and goddesses.
5. Exclusion 2: Śītalā is rejected by (powerful) humans, who refuse to worship her.
6. Revenge 2: Śītalā infects the land and brings disease, death and destruction upon everybody. When she is promised devotion, Śītalā heals her victims/devotees.
7. Redemption: when the worship of Śītalā is established at all levels, the goddess returns among the gods.

Some elements are unique to this particular genre. First, unlike purāṇic and tantric literature, ŚMKs are not ritual texts. Distinguished Bengali practices such as animal sacrifice (*balidān*), but also devotional exploits involving austerities such as *daṇḍīkāṭā* and *vāṇ phõṛā*,[62] or invited possession (*bhar*) are not given any attention. Second, Śītalā is portrayed as ambiguous and highly unstable. She is rough, violent, mysterious and passionate. Only when she is pleased with human and divine behaviour does she calm down. Third, there is no reference whatsoever to healing practices of any sort (i.e. medical, ritual and devotional).[63] The world described in ŚMKs is a dark dimension where the only remedy for disease (or chaos) is surrendering to a greater power – or at least this is what *maṅgal* poets tell us. Since an examination of this genre will be conducted in Chapter 4, I will here limit myself to the physical and behavioural peculiarities of what I call the *maṅgal*-Śītalā.

First and foremost, the goddess is prone to fury. She is violent, aggressive and fearful. She is never sky-clad (*digambara*), and she is not predominantly an ass-riding goddess. In fact, she is deceitful. Śītalā may appear as a beautiful and decently dressed young woman. Alternatively, she disguises herself as an old and wretched (widowed) Brahman woman or, in theatrical *pālās*, a witch-like crone dressed in ragged clothes and sporting matted hair (see below p. 122). Unlike the Śītalā worshipped across North Indian regions, in ŚMKs the goddess is associated with intimidating gods and unsettling attendants. Śītalā, at the apex of her fury, is described at the head of armies of diseases, plagues or demonic presences. Her most loyal companions are:

Jvarāsura: the fever demon (also known as Jvarapātra). Described as an ugly, three-headed and unruly creature, Jvarāsura is born out of Śiva's perspiration, or from Rudra's breath.[64] He takes the role of Śītalā's deputy, general or advisor (*pātra*).[65] He is the leader of poxes, fevers, plagues and other diseases. Anthropomorphic images of Jvarāsura are very common in Śītalā's temples or shrines across Bengal. The god is dark blue-complexioned, three-headed, with long black matted hair, and holds tridents. Jvarāsura is believed to attack those who disrespect his mistress, or are guilty of misdeeds. There is neither special worship nor temples dedicated to Jvarāsura alone, who is always associated and worshipped with Śītalā.[66] The *dhyānamantra* of Jvarāsura is found in PiT (see below pp. 186–7).[67]

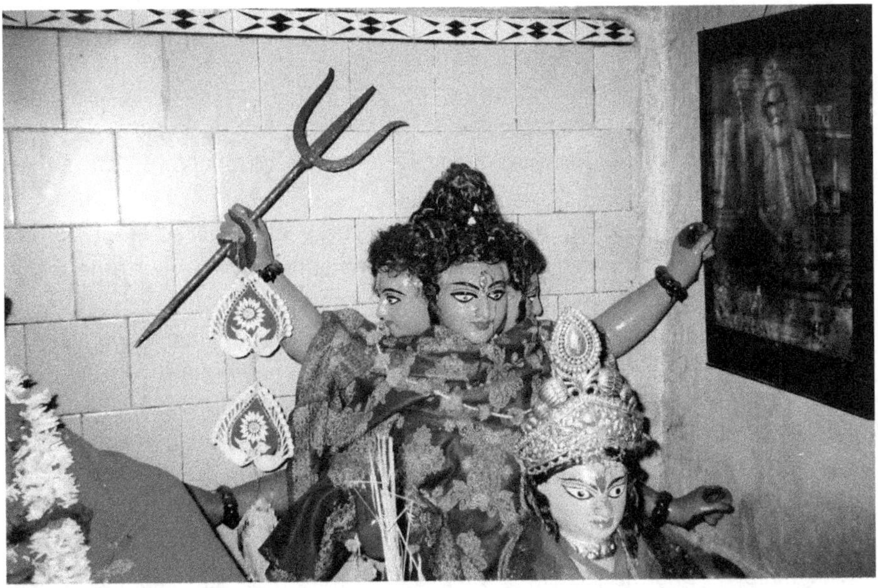

FIGURE 1.4 *Jvarāsura, Śītalā Mandir, Kolkata (photo by author).*

Vasanta Rāy: the Lord of Spring (i.e. the season of smallpox). Basu discusses him as a medieval god of the *Śītalāmaṅgalkāvya* (1405BS: 99). In KD.ŚMK, he is the son (*putra*) of Śītalā, whereas in the shorter poem of Harideva (in Maṇḍal 1960), he acts as a counsellor, along with Jvarāsura, of the goddess. In Nityānanada, as well as his epigones, 'Vasanta Rāy' becomes a title of Śītalā. Vasanta Rāy originally emerged as a separate character in the eighteenth century, a time of dramatic growth of smallpox epidemics, and was later incorporated in the *maṅgal* version of Śītalā.[68] This seems confirmed by Basu, who says there are no temples dedicated to this deity, but managed to find a *dhyānamantra* in Sanskrit: 'Naked and beautiful, with big eyes, scary and surrounded by flocks of disease; with large lips, matted locks and broom in a hand, I sing to you, Vasanta Rāy!' The image is highly evocative of Śītalā, and it would not be a surprise if this had been fashioned after the ghoulish rendering of the goddess in Nityānanda's *pālās*.

Raktāvatī ('Bloody'), also known as Raktāvatīkā or Raktāpriyā: the goddess of blood infections and blood diseases. She is generally portrayed as a malign presence, like Jvarāsura. She preys on children (*śiśusaṃhārakāriṇī*) and was associated with haemorrhagic smallpox, a fatal form of smallpox also known as the black pox.[69] Raktāvatī is represented as a charming young lady with long matted hair. In one of the temples where she is presented offerings,[70] the goddess's *pratimā* is installed in a separate shrine along with Śani (Saturn), Kālī, Manasā, Jvarāsura, Jogināth Bābā and a *śivaliṅga*. On the right, at the centre of the temple, there is a large Śītalā *mūrti*. Raktāvatī is given worship by women who ask for protection for their children.[71] Bengal is to my knowledge the only Indian region with a goddess specifically associated with 'bad blood' (*khārāp rakta/khun*), blood-oozing fevers and blood-borne diseases. Raktāvatī too is believed to have a *vāhana*. She rides an ass, like Śītalā, or, alternatively, a tiger. In Bakkhali (South 24-Parganas) and contiguous villages, Raktāvatī is consistently described as a scary blue-complexioned lady, bare-breasted, with long black dreadlocks, her loins covered with a tiger-skin and riding a tiger. The *dhyānamantra* of Raktāvatī, along with instructions for her worship, is given in PiT (see below p. 187).

Other gods can be associated with Śītalā on occasion of public representations of *maṅgal* episodes, even though their presence is sporadic in ŚMKs. Among these:

Olāi Caṇḍī or Olā Bibi: the 'Lady of the Descendant Flux'. Olā is worshipped by Hindus and Muslims as a protector from diarrhoea, vomit, dysentery and cholera. A very popular goddess in West Bengal, she is occasionally found with her twin sister Jholā (or Uṭhā).[72] Her annual festival coincides with Dolpūrṇimā (Holi). Animal sacrifices are still performed to honour Olā Bibi/Olāi Caṇḍī, although the practice is in decline. Regardless her specialism, the goddess is worshipped by (mostly Hindu) women as a protector and a giver of fertility (Hora 1933; Nicholas 2003; Ferrari 2015).

Dharmarāj (or Dharma Ṭhākur): a sun god whose wrath causes blindness, vitiligo, leprosy and sterility. Dharmarāj has been absorbed into the Bengali Śiva. He is sporadically indicated as Śītalā's husband but his marital status, and his relationship with Śītalā, is not confirmed in *maṅgal* literature. Dharmarāj is worshipped as a solar deity who presides over the fertility cycle of the earth. His festival on the vernal equinox culminates in the *gājan* festival, a major celebration in Bengal (Nicholas 2009; Ferrari 2010a). The apex of the *gājan* is the marriage of Dharmarāj with Devī, an event that ensures wellbeing and good crops. Dharmarāj has his own corpus of texts: the more ancient *Dharmamaṅgalkāvyas*.

Pañcānan: the Five-Faced One, a vernacular form of Śiva. Blue-skinned or dark-complexioned, Pañcānan is worshipped mostly by women who wish to conceive. Besides granting fertility, he is invoked as a protector of children and a healer.

Gheṇṭu (Gheṇṭudevatā or Gheṇṭākarṇa): the god protecting against itches, furuncles, pimples and other skin diseases (occasionally, leprosy). He is worshipped in the form of a small dark earthenware pot by women, usually at the end of Phālgun. Gheṇṭu is offered pulses and rice along with medicinal plants renowned for their cooling effects on the skin (e.g. *Clerodendrum infortunatum*, B. *gheṇṭu*) and antiviral properties (e.g. *Cynodon dactylon*, B. *dūb* or *dūrvā*). At the end of the ceremony, mothers sing happy songs in his honour whereas children are expected to break the pots used for *pūjā*. Broken pieces used to be carried as amulets or heated on the fire and then applied to the skin to relieve pustules, sores or itching furuncles (Crooke 1978: 137, I). These rituals are now rare, although *Gheṇṭupūjā* is still mentioned in liturgical manuals (see below p. 186; cf. Anderson 1988: 75).

Bhakti gīti

A systematic study of devotional songs on Śītalā is simply unrealistic. Umbrella terms like *bhakti gīti* or *maṅgal gān* encompass an enormous and heterogeneous corpus of songs in a myriad of languages and dialects. In this section, I will present an insight of Hindi and Bhojpuri *sohar* and *devī pacrās*. My familiarity with both is primarily derived from fieldwork conducted over the years in Uttar Pradesh, Haryana and Bihar.

Sohar are essentially women's songs of praise and welcoming (Skt. *śobhā*, 'splendour', 'grace', 'wish', 'desire'). The number of participants taking part in singing sessions varies from a few units to larger cohorts (up to 30 people). Bigger parties are rare. A group leader usually directs the performance, a routine that is not necessarily public. The leader acts as a coordinator, and she often sings a few solo lines that are then repeated by the chorus.[73] The melody is very simple and the use of instruments is limited to drums (*ḍholak*), cymbals (*mañjra*) and bells. Clapping hands is customary. As per the melody:

> [its] range is usually less than an octave, with melodic activity concentrated within a tetrachord. The skip of a third is most prevalent within a single melodic line, as

> well as in joining the verse to the refrain (and vice versa), although skips of a fourth are also common. The melodic form is basically ABA or AB throughout the song. (Tiwari 1988: 270)

The lyrics resonate with local variants of purāṇic motifs or *vratakathā*. Alternatively, they borrow from personal experience, or highlight elements of *āñcalik* culture. *Sohar* are the core of an immense and ever-changing tradition, and offer a unique insight into women's lives and family rituals. Traditional motifs and lyrics are transmitted from one generation to another.[74] Lyrics are not impermeable to change. During singing sessions, a singer may improvise and add lines that mirror recent personal experience. Though repetitive in terms of melody and rhythm, the message conveyed by *sohar*s is an emotionally charged one. Stories of goddesses reflect the everyday suffering, or worries, blighting the life of a woman. The underlying message, however, is an extraordinary sense of empowerment. Devotees describe their performance as a service (*sevā*), and the strength derived from it generates hope and solidarity. While singing their love for Śītalā, women of different ages, background and social status learn how to cope with daily hardships, and to strengthen their position in the society as members of the *strījāti*. The singing of *sohar* gives participants a break from a daily routine consisting of labour, domestic chores and other responsibilities in a socially accepted way. The arena in which sessions take place is a safe environment to address tensions, and to resolve issues among peers, including the goddess. Communal singing is therefore a way to pay homage to a very akin power, and to learn to cope with suffering. It is thus unsurprising that regular meet-ups have turned into women's self-help groups, or collaborations with local NGOs.[75]

When female devotees (*mahilā bhakta*s) meet up and sing for Śītalā, they ask for protection and forgiveness, and see in Śītalā a mother who, like them, knows about suffering (Junghare 1975: 301). In a Hindi *sohar* I recorded in November 2012 in Adalpura (Mirzapur district, UP), devotees, sitting in a circle and clapping their hands rhythmically, each sang a short verse in which they confessed wrongdoing. The session lasted almost one hour and at one point it reached high levels of emotional tension, with some women in tears incapable of continuing singing. There was no mention whatsoever of the role of Śītalā in relation to disease. The goddess here is a forgiving protector of mothers. Here follows the refrain:

> Eh Mother, forgive me!
> Please, bless my family again, Mother
> Eh Mother, forgive me!
> Please come again to my house, Mother
> Eh Mother, forgive me!
> I'm coming to beg you, my Mother
> Eh Mother, forgive me!
> I am coming to cleanse your feet, Mother

Eh Mother, forgive me!
I'll pay my respects, my Mother
Eh Mother, forgive me!
I will do your service and make my life better
Eh Mother, forgive me!
Eh Mother, forgive me![76]

Another *sohar* emphasizes the specificity of Śītalā as a healing and rescuing goddess:

Ref: Hug me, mother, embrace me.
I'm losing my life, please help me!
Hug me, mother, embrace me.
O mother, those who truly love you are the lucky ones.
So I'll worship at your feet.
Ref.
I bow my head and present offerings to the Mother.
You are so good, so please hug me.
Ref.
My boat is sinking just like my life
is in trouble. So please, bring my boat ashore.
Ref.
You are my Mother, I am your son,
please cast your sight on me too
because I'm losing my life.
Ref. [x2][77]

In the following Bhojpuri *sohar*, Śītalā is portrayed as a compassionate mother who gives shelter and mercy. The song transpires sorrow, as for some reason Śītalā is unresponsive to the cry of her devotees:

Ref: O Mother, I need the dust of your feet,
I'm thirsty, Mother, I need to meet you.
O Mother, I need the dust of your feet.
Am I fallen in disgrace that you don't want to meet me?
Those who make mistakes won't do it anymore,
if they are blessed with the dust of your feet.
Day and night you are blossoming and giving mercy.
When I'll get this flower, my life will be perfect.
Ref.
O Mother, I have faith in your vision. [x2]
It is so dark that sometimes I don't find the way.
If you show me the light,

my life will be changed.
Ref.
O Mother, your blessing is like the monsoon. [x2]
If you show me your love
my life will be changed. [x2]
Ref.[78]

A similar anxiety is expressed in a Bhojpuri song collected in 1961 by Hari Upadhyaya, who observes how these songs used to be sung by women at the bedside of their sick children:

In whose courtyard are the Danawa and Maduawa [two cereals]?
O Devi ji, in whose courtyard is the Neem tree
O Giver of offspring, where have you been delayed?
O devotee, in the courtyard of the Mali [gardener],[79] there are the Danawa and Maduawa.
And O devotee, in the courtyard of my worshipper is the Neem tree.
O my Joginia [*yoginī*] mother, where have you been delayed?
O traveller, you are my brother,
O Brother, did you see Sitala going on this road?
My Joginia mother is angry with me.
O yes, I saw her in the Hazipur Hata [market].
O Brother, she chews betel leaves
If I would have known that Sitala chews many betel leaves;
I would have settled down a betel-seller for my mother.
If I would have known that she wears garlands,
For mother (Sitala), I would have had settled down a Mali.
O, for the sake of Devi ji.
(*Śītalā kā gīta*, in Upadhyaya 1967: 86–8)

The lyrics have been passed on, along with many others (500, according to the author), by a single informant, an elderly Brahman woman called Devī. Described as 'of old age' in 1961, Devī explains that when she was young, Śītalā was celebrated as 'the wife of Allāh:'[80]

O Allah, *jauriya* [a sweet] has been cooked at my parents' house.
O Allah, its fragrance reaches at my in-laws' home.
O Allah, how can I go to my parents' house?
O Allah, I will pick up a cow-dung cake,
O Allah, I will go there to ask for the fire.
O Allah, upon my arrival, the sister-in-law gives me fire from her hearth.
O Allah, the sister-in-law teases me.

O Allah, upon hearing this much the seven sisters go swiftly on the road.
O Allah, brother Bhayarv [Bhairava] mounts a horse.
O Allah, I find sister Śītalā angry with me.
O Allah, sister Śītalā should return home.
(*Śītalā kā gīta*, in Upadhyaya 1967: 89–91)

Singing *sohar* is not ritual healing, although it may accompany health-seeking *manautī* (H. promises, vows). A merely devotional performance, it is simply a cry for help in attracting the welcoming presence of the goddess who is worshipped as *sarvaduḥkhāntakāriṇī* (Skt. 'remover of all sufferings') (See Fig. 1.2, p. 4).

Another popular genre in the landscape of devotional songs is the *devī pacrā*. The origin of these songs seems connected with folk healing. The Hindi word *pacrā* – alternatively spelled *pacṛā* – indicates worries, trouble and concern. Navaljī says that *pacṛā*s are the songs that folk healers (*ojhā*s) used to recite in front of goddesses (Nā 763).[81] More plausibly, these songs are popular melodies that tell stories of goddesses in strophes of five (*pāñc*) verses. *Devī pacrā*s include foundational songs where the mythical origins of a particular site (*thān*) of the goddess are celebrated. A good example is the popular *Sītlā ghāṭ pe Kāśī meñ* ('In Kāśī [Banaras] at the Śītalā Ghāṭ'), a major Bhojpuri hit in the Varanasi region:

Ref: In Kāśī at the Śītalā Ghāṭ
I'll go and bow my head
In Kāśī at the Śītalā Ghāṭ [x2]
Seated on the lap of the Mother [x2]
I will spend *navarātrī*.
Ref.
Each of the nine days has a different beauty [i.e. goddess]
I'll go and light a lamp [x2]
And under the shadow of Mother Śītalā [x2]
I'll strengthen my devotional mood.
Ref.
Mother Śītalā is the Mother of the Universe
She brings happiness to the world [x2]
If anything should happen in this world [x2]
I will show my feelings to the Mother.
Ref.
Following the rhythm of Śiva's *ḍamaru* (a small two-headed drum)
I'll sing the songs of the Mother [x2]
And I'll bath in the Ganges [x2]
After offering her a yellow sari.
Ref.
At the Durgā Mandir in Durgākuṇḍ

I'll go for *darśan* [x2]
I will follow Śītalā [x2]
And again I'll meditate in the temple of Śītalā.
Ref.
In [the temple of] Mother Annapūrṇā and in Saṅkaṭmocan [Hanumān's temple][82]
I'll offer *prasād* [x4]
As long as I'll continue to breathe [x2]
I'll sing this *devī pacrā*.
Ref. [x2]
(*Bāṛī Śer par Savār*, Track 4)

The greatness of the goddess is further magnified in a *pacrā* included in the *Dasāśvamedhamāhātmya* (ŚVK 17):

Ref. O remover of pain (*duḥkha haranī*)
O remover of misfortune (*saṅkaṭ haranī*)
Protect me, mother, your *līlā* is infinite.
You are the primal power
[You are] The goddess who always protects
Victory to Mother Durgā and Bhadrakālī.
Ref.
During *navarātrī* I will call you
You are splendid in your nine forms
I meditate on you and have faith in you, Mother
O Śītalā, Queen of the world.
Ref.
Brahmā and Viṣṇu praise you
Nārada, Sārada and Śeṣa worship you
Śiva and Indra meditate upon you
The fourteenth most auspicious day of the light half of Caitra [i.e. Hanumān Jayanti] is the best moment to ask Śiva for *prasād*
O mother of the world, giver of fortune, listen to my cry.
Ref.
We are all your children in this world
You are everybody's protector.
Ref.
You are the always protecting Vindhyāvāsinī,[83] the mother of the world
O mother, your *līlā* is infinite.
Ref.
Upon hearing the sound of *ḍol*, *nagāṛā* and bells, all pains are vanquished
The river Ganges flows in front of you, O my Mother, give me salvation.
Ref.

Sūrya and Candra worship you; gods, men and sages get happiness
You bring fortune to the wretched and distressed one.
Ref.
O remover of pains, O source of joy, listen to my prayer.
Ref.
At the Śītalā Ghāṭ, by Rudra's pond is your abode
Everybody comes with hope that you will fulfil every desire they ask
You benefactor and granter of gifts, forgive me, my Queen!
I am wretched and distressed, Mother Goddess: listen to my prayer.
Ref.

See also a *pacrā* to Śītalā in the form of Pārvatī (cf. BhaP 3.4.3: 54) from the repertoire of Hindus in Suriname:

Had I known, mother Pārvatī (Śītalā), that you would come by this route –
Mother, I would have had a pond dug on the way (so that) you would have come taking dips (in it).
Had I known, mother Śitalā, that you would come by this route –
Mother, I would have had a garden grown on the way so you would have come in the cool (shades).
Had I known, mother Śitalā, that you would come by this route –
Mother, I would have settled a shopkeeper on the way and taking cloves (from him) I would have made an offering (thereof to you).
Had I known, mother Śitalā, O mother Pārvatī, that you would come –
Mother, I would have settled a cowherd on the way and taking yoghurt (from him) I would have made an offering (thereof to you).
Had I known, all seven mothers, you would come by this route –
I would have settled a hunter on the way and taking the killed (creature from him) I would have made an offering (thereof to you).
Had I known, mother Pārvatī, O mother Śitalā, that you would come by this route –
I would have settled a pāsī [low class labourer] on the way and taking thatch (from him) I would have made an offering (thereof to you).
(in Arya 1968: 119–20)

Contemporary *devī pacrās* as well as *maṅgal gītis* confirm the gentle, caring and loving nature of the goddess. Though Śītalā, like other goddesses, can be offended, there is no consistent evidence she is a disease-inflicting presence. In fact, devotional songs, while continuing to promote the myth of the protective mother, are projecting a new Śītalā in the global market. This contemporary version of the goddess, as I discuss in Chapter 5, shows how Śītalā is changing in response to upward mobility and globalization, and how she responds to new trends and values.

Concluding remarks

The chapter has shown that Śītalā's presence in Indian literature is attested from at least the twelfth century. Hymns and ritual instructions are scattered across a number of genres, including *purāṇa*s, *dharmanibandha*s, *tantra*s and one medical compendium. Eulogies and ritual sections are accompanied by stories (*kathā*) that promote the stature of Śītalā among human and divine beings. The fact that more or less the same material is presented in various texts should not lessen the role of Śītalā in Indian culture. Rather to the contrary, it bears witness to her mobility and success among all strata of the Indian population. On the basis of the texts here examined, Śītalā:

- rides an ass
- is naked and white-complexioned
- holds a broom and a pitcher full of fresh (nectar-like, i.e. healing) water
- is crowned with a winnower
- has three eyes
- heals from 'boils' and the fear of pustular diseases
- heals children
- is called Śītalā because of her cooling power.

In *vratakathā*s, Śītalā serves as an example for the *pativratā* model, whereas in tantric ritual texts a unique description emerges. The goddess, who is worshipped by means of complex ritualism involving mantra and *yantra*, is described in at least two important and widely used manuals as:

- holding on her head a bundle of dirty clothes tied together (*tailādimalasaṃyuktavastrapoṭaliśīrṣikā*)
- the washer of the clothes of Śiva (*maheśasya vastraprakṣālikā*)

The only genre that tells stories of a dangerous, infecting goddess is the Bengali *maṅgalkāvya* tradition. Śītalā is there an ambiguous goddess, one who spreads contagious diseases, particularly various forms of smallpox and plagues, in retaliation for any form of disrespect, but also at her whim. Bearing in mind the considerable difference between the Śītalā of Bengali poems and the goddess worshipped widely across north India, we now move to the examination of Śītalā's iconography.

Notes

1 Sometimes the goddess is rendered as a four-armed goddess holding a pitcher, a broom, a lotus and a conch. Alternatively, the fourth hand may rest on the donkey's head (Caudhurī 2000: 236–7).

2 Auboyer and De Mallmann (1950: 226) report: Mātā, Mātājī, Ujalī Mātā ('White Mother'), Mātā Daī ('Midwife Mother'), Jag Rāṇī and Jagdamma ('Mother of the World') and Mahā Māi ('Great Mother'). Regional variants of Choṭi Mā (Small/Younger Mother) or Baṛī Mā (Big/Elder Mother) are also found (Lambert 2015: 12–3).

3 Similar interpretations are given by Arnold (1993: 123); Babb (1975: 130–1); Neog (1994: 52); Stewart (1995: 389), Nicholas (2003: 230 n. 16) and Lambert (2015: 13).

4 Blindness resulting from corneal ulcerations and severe forms of arthritis are seldom mentioned in the myth of smallpox.

5 This explains the Hindi expression *māiyā nikal āī* ('the mother has come out'; cf. Lambert 2015: 13–4) to indicate the rigors featuring the first bout of fever.

6 Tod (1920: 1304) observes that when a patient is affected by '*sitala*, or smallpox', it is the custom to invoke the protection of 'Sitala Mata'. Historical records confirm this: when, in 1726, Abhai Singh, the Prince of Marwar, is summoned to Delhi, he is infected with smallpox. Upon receiving the news, 'the nation called on Jagrani [Śītalā] to shield him from evil' (Tod 1920: 1038). I thus confute the notion that *mātā* (or equivalent) is a deflector of smallpox (Junghare 1975: 298; Kolenda 1982: 229; Mull 2000: 303).

7 Miśra classifies seven types of *śītalā*: *bṛhatsphoṭa-*, *kodravā-*, *pāṇisahā-*, *sarṣapikā-*, *rājikā-*, *koṭha-*, and *carmaja-śītalā*.

8 The *grahī* Pūtanā is referred to as cold ('*śītalā*') in KKG (91). Nārāyaṇa, in *Tantrasārasaṅgraha* (11: 33) (fifteenth- to sixteenth-century), called the seventh *grahī* 'Śītalā.' These are the only occurrences in which the two characters overlap significantly.

9 The grasper responsible for a disease causing skin ulcers and boils (*sphoṭa*) and burning fever (*jvarī dāhī*) is Revatīgraha (MN 68: 24).

10 Hārītī too has been discussed in several instances as the Buddhist counterpart of Śītalā. See: Auboyer and De Mallmann 1950: 225; Bhaṭṭācārya 1997: 152–3; Maity 1989: 112; Caudhurī 2000: 246; White 2003: 63, but cf. Bhattacharya's scepticism (1952: 58–9). A similar problem exists for discourses on Śītalā and the southern goddess Māriyammaṉ, which I discuss in Chapter 4.

11 *namaḥ samantabuddhānām apratihataśāsānām // tadyathā / auṃ brahma subrahma brahmavarcase śāntiṃ kuru svāhā // eṣa mantro mahābrahmā bodhisattvena bhāṣitaḥ /śāntiṃ prajagmurbhūtāni tatkṣaṇādeva śītalā* // MMK. 2.33. 18–19.

12 A critical edition of the text is being prepared under the direction of Professor Hans Bakker (University of Groningen), who informed me that this is 'completely different from the printed *Skanda Purāṇa* that consists of *khaṇḍas*'. The hymn to Śītalā is wanting in the material so far examined (email communication, 20/02/2014).

13 Translated by G. V. Tagare. The *tīrtha* of Śītalā is also mentioned in SkP 7.1.134: 1.

14 A small shrine to Bandīdevī is found in Banaras at the back of the Śītalā Mandir in Dāsāśvamedha Ghāṭ (cf. KKh 70: 47–8).

15 The enculturation of Śītalā in the worship of major deities is confirmed by Bakker, who notes that inside the temple of Śītalā is hosted an eleventh- to twelfth-century *mūrti* of Viṣṇu (possibly belonging to an earlier site) (Bakker 1986: 306).

16 The name Sanatkumāra appears in several purāṇic dialogues. Traditionally four Kumāras (Skt. child, son; prince; heir) were born from the mind of Brahmā. Sanatkumāra is functional to the transmission of knowledge to sages, or in conversations with gods.

17 Based on the translation of Tagare (1999: 57).

18 Although there are chapters in NāP that can be dated between the ninth and the eleventh centuries, the passages below are with all probability later (post-thirteenth century) (Tiwari 1996: 456; Hazra 1987: 132).

19 The *vrata* and their narrative elements (*kathā*) are women-only rituals. See McGee 1991; Pearson 1996; McDaniel 2003.

20 The *Śītalāṣṭamī* is not mentioned in the passages from SkP. It may be thus inferred that this ritual was not known (or was not popular) before the sixteenth century. This is further confirmed by its appearance in post-sixteenth-century *dharmanibandha*s (see below p. 11ff.).

21 The *Kālavanatīrtha*, in the kingdom of Avanti.

22 See BhaP 1.17 ff. Also see: BhaP *uttaraparvan* (the fourth and last part), where hundreds of *vrata*s are listed.

23 Alt. version: 'Mahādeva is the *ṛṣi*, *anuṣṭubh* is the metre, Śītalā is the goddess, Lakṣmī is the seed, Bhavānī is the power. The purpose of chanting it is to get relieved from all sorts of poxes (*visphoṭaka*) and disorders.'

24 This verse is found in NāP 1.117: 97.

25 Cf. VR 310. The *vrata* used to be performed across all months of the hot season: Jyeṣṭha, Āṣāḍha, Śrāvaṇa and Bhādrapada. Tod confirms the custom of worshipping Śītalā as the protector of children on this *saptamī* (1920: 664). See also the explanation of the *vrata* and its rules according to Paṇḍit Vaibhavanāth Śarmā, astrologer of the Royal Family of Varanasi (Śarmā 2012). Pearson, writing some 20 years ago, noted that *Śītalāsaptamīvrata* was observed by a tiny percentage of her informants. She ascribes this to the eradication of smallpox (1996: 93). In my experience, the *vrata* is still popular. My informants, also from Banaras, indicate as the rationale of the ritual the power of the goddess to protect their children.

26 In West Bengal and Odisha there are no fixed dates for this *vrata* (but cf. Wadley 1980: 43; Nicholas 2003: 19–27). A list of monthly observances from Vaiśakha to Caitra is given in Chaudhurī 2000: 239–40.

27 Informants confirmed this rite was customary but it is now growing obsolete. It is also found in Gujarat, I was informed. According to *Kṛtyatattva* (462), a *dharmanibandha* composed by Raghunandana in the sixteenth century, donkeys used to be donated on *Śītalāṣṭamī* (Kane 1958: V, 428). Feeding donkeys is also reported by Crooke at the end of the nineteenth century (1978: 18).

28 Most devotees nowadays offer random items such as fruit, vegetables and sweets. It is however significant that the donkey, a 'hot' animal, is traditionally fed hot food, whereas Śītalā, a cold goddess, is presented with stale or cold edibles (see my analysis of the ass *vāhana* below, pp. 67–74; cf. PiT below p. 187).

29 Rice boiled, pounded and roasted.

30 *Cucumis utilissimus*.

31 *Dhār*, a manifestation of the power of the goddess, is believed to have healing qualities.

32 Bangles, *bindī* (a red dot used by married women on their forehead), *sindūr* (vermilion applied by Hindu wives on their hair parting) and *āltā* (lac dye used by married women on their feet).

33 Viśvanātha borrows extensively from earlier *dharmanibandha*s, principally Hemādri's *Caturvargacintāmani* (late thirteenth century), *Nirṇayasindhu* of Kamalakārabhaṭṭa (early seventeenth century) and *Vratārka* of Śaṅkarabhaṭṭa (late seventeenth century). All these digests derive their material principally from various purāṇic sources.

34 Kane (1958: V, 428) also indicates the nineteenth-century *Ahalyākāmadhenu* of Keśava Prasād Dvivedi.

35 The narrative links Śītalā to an illustrious mythical lineage. Hastināpura is the capital of the Kuru dynasty whose story is told in the *Mahābhārata*. In the *purāṇa*s, the city is associated with the Lunar Dynasty (Somavaṃśa) and the reign of the great king Bhārata. Indradyumna is Bhārata's son and reigned over the Avanti region. On Śītalā's shrine is in Avanti region, see NāP 2.78: 12.

36 For an alternative version of the *Śītalāṣaṣṭhīvratakathā*, see Wadley 1980: 45–6.

37 Some local informants provided a different exegesis. With a mixture of irony, malice and realism, I was promptly, and colourfully, informed of the greediness of *pūjārī*s always ready to take advantage of religious festivals.

38 The festival started to be celebrated regularly from the beginning of the twentieth century. Vidyarthi, who wrote at the end of the 1970s, notes that only five temples in Varanasi actively celebrated the *vārṣik annakūṭ* (2005: 68). As per my experience, most temples dedicated to goddesses celebrate this now popular festival in various fashions.

39 The number 101 is an auspicious one. Devotees can also give ₹ 1,001 or 10,001. In fact, any offering is welcome. We learn from Vidyarthi that in 1972 'the minimum rate for a ticket was one rupee' (2005: 69).

40 There are no records of Rāmsundar Prabhudās in the literature I consulted, nor is he mentioned in *bhakti* anthologies.

41 DM 11: 9.

42 DM 11: 12.

43 DM 11: 24.

44 DM 11: 28.

45 DM 11: 39.

46 An exception to this trend is found in a Gujarati *kathā* associated with *Śītalāsaptamī* reported by Wadley (1980: 48–51) and Gopalan (1978: 120–3). Gopalan summarizes a further Gujarati tale. There it is shown that expensive rituals (and feeding Brahmins) are useless against infections. In fact, basic hygienic rules taught by Śītalā are the best protection.

47 Similarly, the *Ācāradinakara* (1923: 207) – a text composed in 1412 by the Jain *śvetāmbara* teacher Vardamāna Sūri – mentions Śītalā in a list of 64 goddesses.

48 The practitioner is supposed to pass his own tongue above the palate and drink the nectar of immortality (*amṛta*) that drips from the top of the skull. Successful completion of this practice grants immortality, the power to endure prolonged mediation and other superhuman skills.

49 Translated by James Mallinson (2007: 214).

50 From the adjective *picchila,* Skt. 'slimy'. The term also indicates the mucilaginous paste obtained from *Basella Rubra*, or red vine spinach (H. *po*; B. *pui*). This paste is used to heal skin lesions, skin ulcers and burns.

51 Tiwari, for instance, suggests that *Picchilātantra* is a section of SkP (1996: 456). PiT is not found in a published form. The complete manuscript is recorded with the number G4649 at the Asiatic Society of Bengal, Kolkata (but cf. Goudriaan and Gupta [1981: 117] who indicate No. 5991). Nobody in the manuscript department at Asiatic Society was able to trace it, and it has been suggested that it is now lost. All successive inquiries have been truncated, or ignored. I have been fortunate enough to find a contemporary *pūjāpaddhati* (in Sanskrit but Bengali script) which indicates that instructions for the worship of Śītalā are taken from PiT (Appendix D).

52 *Sargakāṇḍa* (p. 3), *Dharmakāṇḍa* (pp. 190, 235, 254), *Kamyākaṇḍa* (p. 532) and more extensively in the *Jñānakāṇḍa* (pp. 736–7, 742, 942, 1010).

53 The text corresponds to the *dhyānamantra* in SPP 317 (see below p. 186). Cf. Nirmalānanda 1413BS: 197.

54 The perimeter of the *yantra*.

55 Texts like *Rudrayāmalatantra* are indicated in many late *tantra*s as original sources, thus serving the purpose of conferring authority to later compositions. 'The most famous case of this group is the *Rudrayāmalatantra* which covers a host of ascriptions by usually small texts, especially *pañcāṅgas* (collections of fragments on the worship of a deity) or parts of them' (Goudriaan and Gupta 1981: 24). In fact, there are serious doubts about its actual existence: 'The text which is most often credited with being the *Rudrayāmala* proper, the *Uttaratantra*, is certainly much later than the period in which the old Yāmala literature flourished' (ibid: 47). In the *Uttaratantra* there is no evidence of a Śītalā mantra. In fact, the goddess is not even mentioned.

56 Presumably, the *Rudrayāmalatantra* mentioned above in *Merutantra*.

57 The act of touching parts of one's body while uttering a mantra. The ritual is meant to summon the presence of a deity.

58 *sādhito yena mantro'yaṃ tasya vaṃśe na śītalā* (*Merutantra* 32: 291 and *Puraścaryārṇava* 12: 88).

59 The only reference to this aspect of Śītalā is found in Pāṇḍey Ārya 2037 VS: 88.

60 *Maṅgalkāvyas* are not properly poems. They contain long prose sections and do not adhere to the classic (Sanskrit) *kāvya* style.

61 Best known for his *Dharmamaṅgalkāvya*, a lengthier and more articulate work, Mānikrām Gāṅgulī is conventionally located around 1750. Bhaṭṭācārya has proposed a much early date, mid-fifteenth century (1998: 703–5).

62 The former is a votive practice in which a devotee measures up with her body the distance of a pilgrimage. The latter entails the piercing of the flesh on the arms, but also the tongue and cheeks, with small arrows.

63 In MG.ŚMK 9: 219, Danvantari gives *chob* to victims of smallpox infected by Śītalā. This may be tincture (B. *chopa; choba*) or simply his healing touch (*chupa*). Nicholas asks whether this may be inoculation (2003: 163).

64 Mukharji (2013: 271) mentions an unpublished 1916 writing of an eminent Bengali *kavirāja*, Vrājavallabh Rāy, who quotes the *dhyānamantra* of Jvārasura: '*jvārastripādastriśirah ṣaḍbhujo navalocanaḥ bhasmapraharaṇo raudraḥ kālāntakayamopamaḥ* [Jvara, born of Rudra, has three feet and three heads, [six arms] and nine eyes. Showering ashes, he resembles Time (as god of death, i.e. Yama)]' (transliteration mine). See also ibid. 280, where Jvarāsura is born 'from the rage of Siva [sic] at being insulted by his father-in-law by not being offered the customary sacrificial gifts'. In the *Jvarāsurer Janma* of NC.ŚMK, the demon was born from the sweat of the forehead of Śiva. His unruly behaviour caused the wrath of the gods, who summoned Viṣṇu. With his *cakra*, Viṣṇu-Nārayaṇa cut the body of Jvarāsura in three parts. Peace was temporarily restored. But Brahmā, to please her daughter (Śītalā), decided to revive the demon, whose three-parted body had already started to grow heads, arms and legs.

65 Bang (1973: 90) reports that, around Tamluk, Jvarāsura is regarded as the son of Śītalā, and the goddess is an emanation of Kālī.

66 But cf. Maity (1988: 87), who mentions the worship of Jvarā and his twin sister Jvarī. I never found shrines to Jvara-Jvarī, nor were my informants able to confirm this.

67 For a critical study of Jvarāsura see Mukharji 2013. In particular, Mukharji shows that Jvarāsura is not – as argued by many – a figure limited to Bengali folklore and modernity. While tracing his origins and antecedents in medical compendia and in the epics, as well as in the myths that informed them, Mukharji challenges functionalist approaches and historical analyses that privileged the 'folk/classical divide' in South Asian studies, including medical culture. In Bengal, Jvarāsura is not just the companion of Śītalā. Basu (1405BS: 73) notes he is also the attendant of Dharmarāj and Pañcanānda. This is precisely the case in the Śītalā Mandir in 45, S.N. Banerjee Road, Kolkata, where a big blue *mūrti* of the Fever Demon is surrounded by three equestrian statues of Śītalās, Pañcānanda, Manasā, Caṇḍī (aniconic) and Dharmarāj (aniconic). (see Figure 1.4).

68 This is reminiscent of the birth of Olā Bibi in the same period (see Ferrari 2015).

69 This rare form of smallpox (circa 2 per cent of the infections) does not cause ulceration. Instead there is subcutaneous bleeding which makes the skin almost black, as if the flesh had been burnt.

70 Śītalā Mandir, 30/1 Raja Mahindra Road, Belgachia (Kolkata). The *sevāit*, Śrī Śambhu Cakravartī, confirmed to me that there is no such thing as a worship of Raktāvatī independent from Śītalā.

71 Since Raktāvatī is difficult to discern – she has no special sign or tool – only local women know her identity. In general, she is not one of the best well-known goddesses in contemporary West Bengal, especially in urban centres where representations of *pālā*s are increasingly rare.

72 In Bengali *olāuṭhā* is colloquially used to indicate cholera. It refers to the ascending (*uṭhā*) movement of vomit and the descending (*olā*) flux of diarrhoea.

73 Welcoming songs may follow a refrain–stanza–refrain style, or simply repeat the last few words of each line (cf. Tiwari 1988: 269).

74 Oral transmission is not the only mean. Most matrons nowadays carry in their large jute bags, or handbags, notebooks with dozens of songs along with *vrata* manuals, various *paddhati*s and *pūjā* items (incense, flowers, bells, sweets, candles, etc.). Notebooks are regularly updated and passed on to younger generations.

75 One such case is the Shitala Mata Self Help Group of Banswara, Rajasthan. A consortium of women has established a collaboration with GAIN (Global Alliance for Improved Nutrition), the World Food Project and the Government of Rajasthan, to produce food supplements for starving children and pregnant mothers (GAIN 2012).

76 *e maīyā māph karīñ*, recorded in Adalpura, Baṛī Śītalā Mandir (21 November 2012).

77 *gale se lagā lo, mā*, recorded in Banaras, Śītalā Mandir, Dāsāśvamedha Ghāṭ (November 2009).

78 *Maiyā tere caraṇõ kī dhūl lo nil jāe*, recorded in Adalpura, Baṛī Śītalā Mandir (October 2012).

79 On *mālin*s see below p. 133–4.

80 Upadhyaya reports that only the intervention of members of the Arya Samaj prevented villagers from persevering in this kind of belief (1967: 89). In his *Satyārtha Prakāśa* (1875), Swami Dayananda Saraswati, founder of the Arya Samaj, expresses harsh criticism toward 'folk gods' such as Śītalā and Bhairava, those who believe in them, ritualists and folk healers (Saraswati n.d.: 24). I witnessed a similar situation in contemporary Bangladesh, where Islamists are trying, often with the use of force, to eradicate folk tales such as stories of Olā Bibi and her relation with God (Allah) (Ferrari 2015: 38). Cf. also Śītalā as a 'Muslim goddess' – called Turkini – in Crooke 1978: 126–7, I.

81 Though there is no reason to doubt Navaljī, I never heard of this use of *devī pacrās*, nor did my informants.

82 Hanumān is here celebrated as the one who removes trouble, pain and suffering (*saṅkaṭ*).

83 The 'Dweller of the Vindhya Range', a form of Durgā, whose main temple is located on the bank of the Ganges in Vindhyācal, Mirzapur District (UP). A *mūrti* of the goddess in enshrined in the main Śītalā Mandir of Banaras.

2

Visions of the goddess: The iconography of Śītalā

Indian texts show general consensus in describing Śītalā as a pale naked woman sitting side-saddle on an ass. The goddess's tools – winnower, broom and a pitcher full of water – confirm her cold nature, and are functional to her healing skills. It is thus surprising that alternative narratives have reversed this scheme. Śītala is described as *ugra* (irate), or prone to retaliation. Her pitcher contains poisonous pulses. The broom serves to spread infected germs around. The ass is a strong beast of burden that carries the goddess with her heavy load of (infected) pulses. The winnower too transmits infection: when the goddess shakes her head, she disseminates infectious viruses.

In this chapter, I examine the iconography of Śītalā bearing in mind how the goddess is worshipped (a mother goddess), rather than how she has been fantasized (a disease goddess). My investigations include: a) aniconic *mūrti*s (stone slabs and rocks); b) non-anthropomorphic (zoomorphic and phytomorphic) icons; and c) anthropomorphic images (equestrian and cephalomorphic images). The task is complicated by the fact that Śītalā is often worshipped in conjunction with other Śītalās (in different shapes), or as the eldest of a group of seven sister goddesses. In the latter case, she can be: a) the chief deity; b) the embodiment of all seven sisters; c) one of a group in which each has different powers. Finally, when discussing Śītalā's iconography – but not only – one should keep in mind that the presence of the goddess is flexible. Śītalā can assume the form, and inhabit the *mūrti*s, of other goddesses.

Aniconic *mūrtis*

In 2006, while travelling across Bihar from Varanasi toward rural districts of West Bengal, I was impressed by the way in which Bihari women observe *śītalāṣṭamīvrata* in the absence of temples, shrines and even *mūrti*s. The offering of stale edibles is preceded by the installation of the goddess. A random stone is selected to host Śītalā. The stone is then laid under a tree, wrapped in a red cloth and presented with a series of items. I noticed *kumkum* (< Skt. *kuṅkuma*, powder made from saffron or turmeric) small plastic combs, incense, flowers, milk, yogurt, henna, small mirrors and a few coins. (One is free to offer any item that is supposed to make the goddess happy.) After the stone is prepared to receive the goddess, the woman who coordinates the ritual ties a *kalāvā* (a red cotton thread, also called *mauli*) to a branch of the tree, thus binding the party to the goddess. Only then does singing and story-telling begin.

This is not an isolated incident. Śītalā is awakened and installed in countless temples and shrines across India in the form of *patthar pratimā* or *śilā*, a roundish dark stone, or a series of rocks.[1] These may be enshrined, or function as temporary ritual supports. Roundish stone slabs are more common, and their stories are often similar. In most instances, they are found by devotees after a dream vision in which the goddess reveals her whereabouts. The message is usually followed by the request to build a temple, or to install the *mūrti* in a pre-existing *mandir* – thus generating conflict between factions of devotees, or social classes. Stone slabs are believed to be self-generated (*svayambhū*) and they are usually found in deep water, or hidden in groves and jungles. Once enshrined, the *śilā* is smeared with *kumkum* powder and may be surmounted with a small gold-plated or metal crown. (The crown is explained as a marker of higher, royal, status.) In times of environmental or community crises (e.g. epidemics or droughts), the *śilā* is believed to perspire, that is to boil with rage. When this is the case, ritual specialists try to lower the temperature of the 'lord of the place' by sprinkling cold water on it, winnowing it and presenting various items, including the (not traditionally cold) blood and flesh of sacrificed animals.[2]

When represented aniconically, Śītalā is often found in groups of goddesses variously called seven sisters (*sāt bhagiṇī*), seven ladies (*sāt bibi*), seven virgins (*sāt kanyā*), seven mothers (*sāt mā*) or seven Caṇḍīs (*sāt caṇḍī*). Seven sister shrines, a common sight in India, host not just stones. The goddesses may be rendered as wooden posts, pitchers, coconuts or head-shaped icons. Such shrines (*thān*) are dedicated to guardian goddesses (male deities are rare) and worshipped as the local lords (*ṭhākur*). The seven sisters are capricious, hungry, prone to rage and vindictive. Like the *maṅgal*-Śītalā, whose features their worship might have informed, *śilā*s protect and heal, yet if not properly honoured they can be harmful. The earliest and most systematic evidence of this pattern emerges from nineteenth-century ethnographic sketches.

Writing at the end of the nineteenth century on Punjab, Crooke says the seven sisters are called: 'Śītalā, Masānī, Basanti, Mahā Mal, Polamde, Lamkanijā and Agwanī' (Crooke 1978: vol. 1: 225).[3] Rose informs us that in Ambala (Haryana), Mātaṅgī (one of the ten *mahāvidyas*) was worshipped as a protector of children from smallpox. She gives the names of eight sister goddesses: 'Ranká, Ghranká, Melá, Mandlá, Sítala, Siḍala, Durgá and Shankara Deví' (Rose 1919: 354). In Haridwar (UP), the seven sisters are named: Śītalā, Sedalā, Ruṇukī, Jhunukī, Mihilā, Merhalā and Mandilā (ibid.: 226).

Alternatively, they have been listed as: Śītalā, Phūlmati, Camariyā, Durgā Kālī, Mahā Kālī, Bhadrā Kālī and Kālikā Bhavānī (ibid.: 129). Bang confirms that the variants are countless, and that the sisters may be nine, or more (1973: 85).[4] In Banaras, Śītalā is worshipped in her principal temple at Śītalā Ghāṭ, adjacent to Dāsāśvamedha Ghāṭ, as the *sāt śītalā* even though the goddess is one: Dakṣiṇī Ādi Śītalā. In a small yet popular temple in the village of Deo Chandpur, around 57 kilometres north of Banaras, is a small Śītalā Devī Mandir where devotees worship five *mūrti*s as the *sāt śītalā*. This seems to be confirmed by devotional texts like the *Śītalācālīsā* (see above pp. 18–19) and the *Śrīādiśītalāstotram* (see above pp. 15–16) that indicate the goddess is worshipped by the names of: Śītalā, Śoḍhalā, Mahalā, Ruṇakī, Hyuṇakī and Mātu Maṇḍalā.

In their ethnography of a north Indian village in the proximity of Delhi, Shanti Nagar (a pseudonym), Freed and Freed have reported that the goddesses are: Śītalā (smallpox), 'Kalka (ki) Mata, also named Masani Mata, goddess of the cremation grounds', 'Khamera Mata, the goddess of measles', 'Khasra Mata, the goddess of itches, scabies, eczema, and similar maladies of the skin', 'Marsal Mata, the goddess of mumps', 'Phul ki Mata (the Flower Mother), the goddess of boils and other similar large skin eruptions', 'Kanti Mata or Moti Mata or Moti Jhara, the goddess of typhoid'. An eighth goddess is occasionally worshipped: 'Chaurahewali Mata, Crossroads Mother Goddess' (Freed and Freed 1988: 124–5; cf. Kolenda 1982: 228). In West Bengal shrines to the seven sisters are very common. Even when *mandir*s are erected, the *ṭhākur*s continue to enjoy great popularity, especially on occasion of scheduled *vrata*s. Such is the case for an urban temple in the Dum Dum area of Kolkata where, after an initial struggle, I was able to find sufficient consensus[5] on the names of the *sāt bibi*s (seven ladies): Olā Bibi (the Lady of the Descendent [Flux], i.e. diarrhoea), Jholā Bibi (the Lady of Loose [Bowel Movements]), Uṭhā Bibi (the Lady of the Ascendant [Flux], i.e. vomit), Caṇḍī Bibi (a variant of Durgā), Masān Bibi (the Lady of Whooping Cough, see below), Bāhārī Bibi (the Beautiful Lady), and Jhāṇṭā Bibi. The last *bibi* is the 'Lady of the Broom' (B. *jhāṇṭā* or *jheṇṭā*), that is Śītalā. A similar set of deities is found in the Śrī Olāi Caṇḍī Mātā Ṭhākurāni Mandir off Khudiram Bose Road, Belgachia, Kolkata. The *mandir* is an extremely popular one, and supposedly quite old (circa 420 years). The seven sisters are: Olā, Jholā, Manasā, Śītalā, Ṣaṣṭhī and two Caṇḍīs. They are placed at the feet of anthropomorphic images of Manasā, Śītalā, Ṣaṣṭhī, Caṇḍī and Bābā Pañcānan (Ferrari 2015: 39–40).[6] Writing at the end of the nineteenth century, Risley reports that Śītalā is one of the seven sisters who are known as 'Motiya, Matari, Pakauriya, Masurika, Chamariya, Khudwa and Pansa' (1891: 61, II). In Maharashtra (Nagpur district), Junghare notes that: 'Mata-May [Śītalā] is believed to have six sisters, one brother, and fourteen cousins, all of whom symbolize various diseases. The seven sisters symbolize seven different kinds of small-pox and their brother, Bhiwsan, symbolizes gowar [M. *govar*], germ measles. Chicken-pox is thought of as their distant cousin' (1975: 302). Whether in isolation or in groups of sister goddesses, *śilā*s identified with Śītalā are consistently considered ancient seats of the goddess, and by virtue of that, they are both powerful and dangerous.[7]

Ethnographic vignette 1: Śrī Mātā Śītalā Devī Mandir, Gurgaon (Haryana)

The highly popular Śītalā Mandir of Gurgaon is a major centre of worship in north India with a long history as a healing site.[8] Located in Sector 6, Atul Kataria Marg, in a neighbourhood known as Masani village, the *mandir* is advertised as a *śāktipīṭha*, and is alternatively known as Masānī Mā Mandir. Its annual celebration, a major spring fair, falls in mid-Caitra and is known as Masānī Melā. Śītalā is worshipped here for her power to protect children, to bless newlyweds with offspring and to ward off diseases.[9] Most pilgrims are small to medium-sized working- and middle-class family groups. There is a significant presence of Indian tourists too. The temple is currently open to everybody, and there are no restrictions on age, gender or class.[10] The majority of pilgrims are Hindus, but I had the chance to meet Sikhs and few mixed Hindu/Muslim families from Delhi.

The Gurgaon Mandir is surrounded by a large garden, a (dried) pool (*kuṇḍa*) with *ghāṭs* (steps), a canteen for pilgrims (*bhojnālāya*), a series of smaller shrines run by *śaiva sādhus* and astrologers, and a shaving pavilion (*muṇḍan khānā*). The large rectangular two-storeyed concrete building used as *muṇḍan khānā* is a must-go for mothers. Women queue in small groups to have their babies' heads shaved. For a fee of ₹ 51 (around 61 pence), one of the local barbers completes the procedure. Barbers are also available for piercing ears and noses. The whole performance is a devotional as well as a social act.[11] Head-shaving is considered an important inclusive moment, and a way to ensure long life for the children.[12] The event is recorded with cameras and camera-phones. The atmosphere is warm and welcoming. Children play together all around the place (even on the altar), women chat and rest, families unpack their tiffins and enjoy a relaxing lunch or snack in the shade. After head-shaving, it is customary for women and children to trace auspicious swastikas with their fingers on the walls, and to impress their children's handprints around the altar. The children's hair is brought outside by temple workers and left on a wooden structure. There is Śītalā's basket, a large bin where the hair is gathered and proudly displayed as a sign of devotion.

Unlike around the *garbhagṛha* (innermost sanctum) in the *mandir*, where action follows a seemingly ritualized fashion, the *muṇḍan khānā* allows for informal gatherings and narrative exchange. Groups of women from different parts of the region meet and bond. Invited on several occasions to join picnics or to drink a *cāy*, I had the opportunity to closely observe how the festive occasion of *muṇḍan* favours the dissemination of prophylactic measures and hygienic norms. Women exchange recipes to counter exanthemata, coughs, rashes, fevers and other minor ailments. The way in which such information is passed is not one regulated by any particular structure. The informal atmosphere makes it possible for women from the most disparate social backgrounds to express anxieties and share remedies (*ilāj*), some

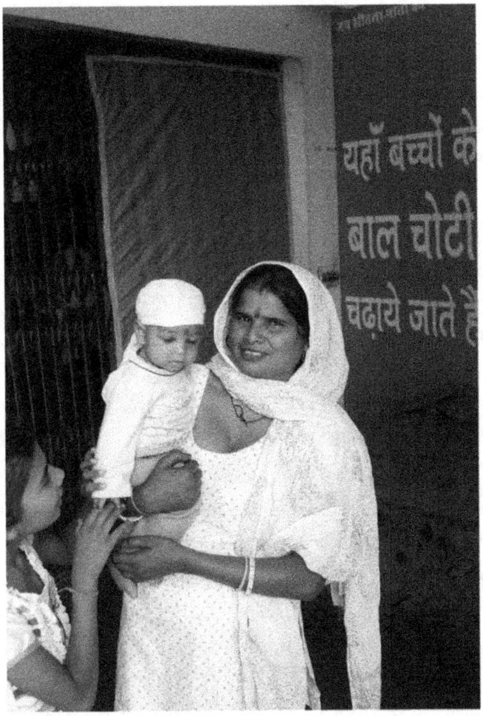

FIGURE 2.1 *Punjabi mother with child,* muṇḍan khānā, *Śrī Mātā Śītalā Devī Mandir, Gurgaon (photo by author).*

of which are proudly presented as belonging to the family for generations. Healing narratives consist of instructions to prepare simplified versions of āyurvedic remedies. These are then associated with family histories (often pointing to miraculous effects). Such remedies are used as a panacea for most childhood diseases (*baccõ kī bīmārī*). Naturally, women inform each other of the best doctors or pediatric clinics in the area.

The Gurgaon *mandir* is not just a place where mothers seek the protection of the goddess. It is also a socially acceptable arena for youngsters to elude the strict surveillance of parents. During conversations with regular devotees, I learnt that many couples around the pool area were not newlyweds but *lovers*.[13] This elicited critical discourses on 'love sickness' (*prem kī bīmārī*), a condition that for many is the inevitable consequence of the clash between tradition and the new India. Yet while most turn a blind eye, some parents are not afraid to show their concern. On one occasion, I observed a sixteen-year-old girl authoritatively brought forward by her mother and paternal aunt in front of Śītalā's *mūrti* so that she might be healed of her infatuation with a boy living in their neighbourhood. The girl refused to marry into the family chosen by her father, was belligerent and wanted to continue her education along with her *boyfriend*. The elder lady (the aunt) made it abundantly clear she was bringing dishonour on the family. A *bhagat* (healer) in their neighbourhood suggested visiting Śītalā Mā at Gurgaon.

The temple bears witness to the fluidity of goddess worship not just in ritual and devotional terms, but also from an iconographical point of view. Before the construction of the temple, which was erected in this form toward the end of the nineteenth century, the location was already known as a healing site where various mythical narratives intersect.

In the first story, the *mandir* is associated with the Masani village, a neighbourhood of *bhaṅgī*s (sweepers) whose shrine was dedicated to the seven mothers (*sāt mā*). The memory of three goddesses and their names now seems lost. Along with Śītalā, who emerged as the lord of the place, three more goddesses are still worshipped. The first one was mentioned to me by only a tiny percentage of local informants. Her name is goddess (Bhagavatī) Lalitā Mā. Unfortunately I could not find any consistent information about her specialism (if any), individual features and ritual requirements. In fact, Lalitā is often used as a title of Mahādevī,[14] or an alternative name of Śītalā.

The second goddess is Masānī Mā. Like Śītalā, Masānī is used as a collective name to indicate the seven sister goddesses. Masānī Devī was brought to Gurgaon in the second half of the seventeenth century by a rich *jāṭ* (member of an agriculturalist community) from Keshopur (east of Delhi) known as 'Siṅgh'. The goddess appeared to him in a dream and granted him the power to heal with the mud of the miraculous pond now enclosed in the temple perimeter. Masānī is believed to be the little sister of Śītalā, and her helper.[15] The two names, however, are used interchangeably and for many they are the same goddess. Though now a benevolent protector, Masānī has an ominous origin. The word *masān*, in Hindi, indicates the place of cremation (Skt. *śmaśāna*). In north Indian folklore, the cremation ground is home to Masān and his twin sister Masānī, two demons who prey on children and are often associated with vampirism (cf. Sax 2009: 83–91). Masānī is believed to be a *ḍākinī* (witch) or a *piśācinī* (flesh-eating demon) who rises from funeral pyres. She attacks children and afflicts them with burning fevers and excruciating coughs. *Masānī*s, I was informed, are the spirits of women who died in childbirth and seek revenge on children, the cause of their untimely passing. In the current parlance, *masān* is whooping cough (cf. Rose 1919: 352–3). Despite the association with death and children's diseases, the worship of Masānī in north India is fairly widespread. Unlike her male counterpart who is consistently described as a dangerous predator, Masānī is now a protector of children and a healer in vast areas across north India, Pakistan and Nepal.

The third goddess associated with the Gurgaon *śaktipīṭha* is Caurāhā Mātā ('Crossroad Mother') or Cauk Mātā ('Market-place Mother'), the protector of the *bhaṅgī*s. Due to her association with an impure *jāti*, her shrine is found outside the perimeter of the temple, although sweepers (and other low classes) are now allowed into the main site of worship. The shrine to Caurāhā Mātā is found near the crossing that leads to the temple's entry and close to the market surrounding the area. Because of the popularity of Śītalā, Caurāhā Mātā's worship remains confined to a fringe of the local populace. Pilgrims on their way to the main temple continue to leave food offerings and flowers on the small shrine, although most are unaware of the nature and origins of the goddess.

As per the main temple, Śītalā Mātā is a majestic and powerful Śakti whose golden image (actually a gold-polished alloy of eight metals) attracts hordes of devotees. In contrast to the Masānī-visitation narrative, the origin of the temple is discussed as dependent upon Śītalā's association with political and charismatic power. According to local oral histories, Mahārāj Javāhar Siṃha (d. 1768) of Bharatpur (Rajasthan) was on his way to Delhi to attack Najīb Khān, the city administrator who was held responsible for the death of his father, Mahārāj Surāj Māl (1707–63), leader of the *jāṭ* clans. In the proximity of Gurgaon, the army stopped to rest and to let the animals drink from a nearby pond. This was the *Śītalākuṇḍa*, the abode of the goddess of the place. After drinking, horses, camels, elephants and cattle refused to proceed. The Mahārāj summoned an astrologer (other versions indicate a *jādūgar*, H. 'magician') who informed the king that the goddess Śītalā was furious. Neither did the king offer oblations nor did he request permission to pass. Javāhar Siṃha asked for forgiveness, performed *pūjā* and vowed to build a great *mandir* should he return victorious. After

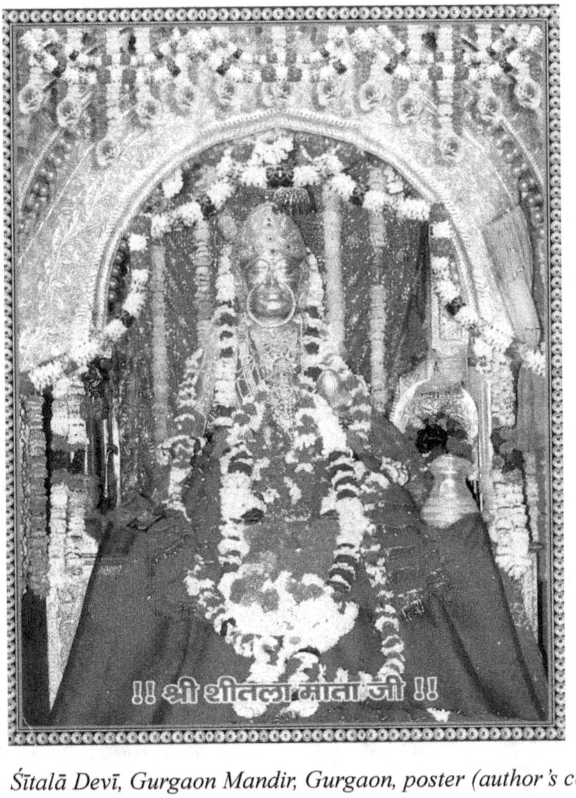

FIGURE 2.2 *Śītalā Devī, Gurgaon Mandir, Gurgaon, poster (author's collection).*

his successful expedition to Delhi, Javāhar Siṃha returned to Gurgaon and built a huge Śītalā Mandir in front of the pond. A golden *pratimā* of the goddess was then installed.[16]

The icon of Śītalā lacks the distinctive features recorded in the textual sources examined in the previous chapter. The *mūrti* sits on a large silver throne, has two eyes and her forehead is dotted with a red gem (i.e. the goddess's third eye). Śītalā wears a tiara-like crown, two big earrings and sports a huge nose ring that passes through both her nostrils and falls on her chest. The ornament is quite unusual in Śītalā's iconography. It is typical of north-western married women and, depending on the material, it indicates social status. (This may be due to the Rajasthani background of Javāhar Siṃha.) The goddess holds a golden lotus and is covered with garlands, food offerings and heavy red drapes. Standing on her lap is a miniature goddess that most devotees consider to be either another form of Śītalā or her attendant/sister, Masānī. Some women believe the statuette simply represent Śītalā's baby, a fact they see as a confirmation of her motherly nature.

A further myth provides an explanation of this smaller figurine, and in so doing it points once more to mobility, polymorphism and transformation in Śītalā worship. The source of the story I heard several times from many proud devotees and Gurgaon residents, including the *paṇḍit*s of the temple, is the *Mahābhārata*. The little goddess is a form of Kṛpī, twin sister of Kṛpa and wife of Droṇa (or Droṇācarya) (MBh 1.121: 11–15), the *guru* of both the Pāṇḍava brothers and their opponents (and cousins), the Kauravas. For his merits, Droṇācarya received some land from King Dhṛtarāṣṭra of Hastināpur. There he settled and built an ashram. The place became a village known as *guru grāma*, the guru's village (H. *guru gāṅv* > Gurgaon). Kṛpī is a marginal character in the *Mahāhārata* and is mostly mentioned because of her being related by marriage to Droṇa. She is praised as a model of a self-controlled *dharma* abiding woman (MBh 1.121: 12), and is known for her calm and gentle (*śītala*) attitude. The *Mahābhārata* bears no witness to such story.[17] What we known is that Kṛpi – after the death of her husband (cf. MBh 11.23: 34–42) – is praised by Gāndhārī,[18] who calls her a *brahmacāriṇī* (MBh 11.23: 36), a person who can control the heat of passions. This may be a feeble link to Śītalā, whose healing action depends upon taming heat, and therefore suggests control over *karma*. Besides this somehow adventurous exegesis, there circulates in Gurgaon an interesting narrative about Kṛpi the healer.

Known to the local populace as Gurumātā and praised for her virtuous patience, Kṛpī became a semi-divine figure after her death. Her *pratimā* was enshrined in the premises of the ashram, close to a pond whose waters were believed to be miraculous in preventing diseases and favouring conception. Centuries later, all the temples of the area were destroyed by Muslim invaders. One night, a sweeper from the Masani village was visited by Śītalā in a dream. The goddess told him that Kṛpi – in the form of a stone slab – was lying at the bottom of the pond. The *bhaṅgī* found the icon and built a shrine. Śītalā gave him the power to heal, and from henceforth Kṛpi is worshipped as a manifestation of Śītalā, one of the seven sisters of the local *bhaṅgī* community. *Bhaṅgī pūjārī*s still administer the site lying outside the *mandir*

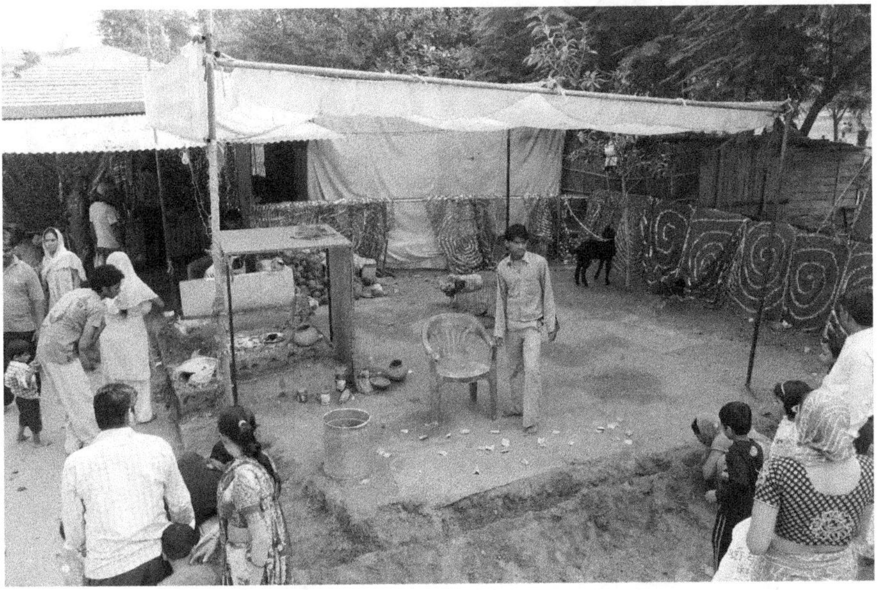

FIGURE 2.3 Śītalākuṇḍa, *Gurgaon Mandir, Gurgaon (photo by author).*

main structure. Devotees, upon leaving the temple, gather in front of the area where the original pond used to be, and dig some earth with their hands. This is then used to build a small heap that delimits the external perimeter of the *kuṇḍa*. A symbolic offering (usually a few rupees) is left on the wet sandy soil, or placed at the feet of a small *mūrti* of the goddess. In exchange, Śītalā/Kr̥pi/Masānī fulfils all desires.[19]

The water pitcher

The water pitcher (B. *kalsa/kalsi*; H. *kalsā/kalsī* < Skt. *kalaśa*; alt. H. and B. *ghaṭ* < Skt. *ghaṭa*) is not just one of Śītalā's tools. Tin, brass and clay pots of all dimensions are believed to be filled with the power of the goddess. When incorporated in temple worship, the *pitcher* – unlike stone slabs that are self-generated – requires a ceremony of 'installation' (H. and B. *ghaṭ sthāpana*). The presence of a Brahman is needed, although it is not unusual for male and female ritualists from a variety of classes to conduct the ceremony. The *pūjārī* is supposed to awaken the goddess, to let her descend and take a seat. (The *kalaśa* is called 'throne,' *siṃhāsana*.) Before being installed on an altar or in a shrine, usually at the feet of more elaborate *mūrti*s, the pitcher is filled with cold *gaṅgājal* ('Ganges' water', irrespective of its provenance). Alternatively, a mixture of curd, milk, ghee, sugar and honey called *pañcāmr̥ta* ('five nectars') is used. The pitcher is then topped with mango or *nīm* leaves (*Azadirachta indica*, referred to as *harā pattā*,

H. 'green leaves') and a coconut. A red-and-yellow cotton thread (*mauli*) is tied around the coconut. The *pūjārī* draws with the ring finger of the right hand stylized human figurines and auspicious swastikas on the sides of the pitcher. Welcoming mantras are recited and offerings presented. These include cold items such as fenugreek (H. and B. *methī*), aniseed (*B. mauri; H. sauṁph*), liquorice (*B. yaṣṭimadhu; H. yaṣṭikā*), white sandal (H. and B. *śvetacandan*), jasmine, *bāsā* (H. and B. *Justicia gendarussa*), and branches of *Calotropis gigantean (*H. *āk;* B. *ākanda), Aegle marmelos* (H. and B. *bel*), *Shorea robusta* (H. and B. *sāl*) and *Gmelina arborea* (H. *gamhaṛ*, B. *gāmār*). Cooling fruits and vegetables are offered too: limes, coconuts, bananas and cucumbers.

The pitcher, a well-known symbol of fertility, is evocative of the power of Śītalā to release cold healing water. Bhatti (2000: 153–6), however, reports a more ominous use of Śītalā's *ghaṭ*. Such vessels, we are informed, represent the human body. They are broken at the intersection of four roads when a corpse is brought to the cremation ground, and the broken pieces are used to carry human ashes. Bhatti argues the ewer is symbolic of the mother who gives life but also takes it away (ibid.: 155). Such a reading – which borrows vastly from German psychologist Erich Neumann's theories – is not confirmed in any oral and textual source I know of. Śītalā is a goddess extraneous to funeral rites (*śrāddha*). Bhatti's description of Śītalā in Punjabi folk culture differs substantially from most reports and studies. Although many sources insist on the paradigm of the ambiguous mother, there are some features that seem unique to Bhatti's work. Among these: Śītalā has a 'hideous face', 'her teeth are projecting', 'her ears are large as winnowing fan [sic]', her 'mouth is wide open', and 'she has a snake as a whip' (ibid.: 142).[20] This iconography is one missing from the body of written and oral texts on Śītalā. As per the worship of Śītalā in Punjab, my experience is quite limited but I never encountered such iconographical features.[21] Punjabis from the Hindu and Sikh communities across north India and in Britain are equally unaware of this 'demonic' rendering of Mā Śītalā.

The broom and the winnower

The brush is the tool used by the goddess to wipe away the germs of contagion, and impurity in general. For women, Śītalā is an example of a good mother and housewife. The goddess teaches the importance of domestic chores associated with hygienic norms. Textual sources in Sanskrit call the brush *mārjana*, a generic name indicating a broom. In vernacular literature, however, this is unanimously called *jhāṛū*. In almost all visual representations, including early statues (circa ninth to twelfth centuries), the goddess holds a short brush for domestic work, a tool called in Hindi *buhārī* (or *buhāranī*). The *jhāṛū* proper is a bigger instrument with a longer handle and long and harder bristles. It is used for sweeping the ground on the outside. The *jhāṛū* is the kind of tool used by sweepers, such as the *bhaṅgī*s. This may indicate the association of

Śītalā with low social classes who specialize in cleaning. Textual sources , however, do not confirm this.

The agricultural background of the goddess, and her presence in peasant culture, clearly emerges in relation to her last distinctive tool, the *śūrpa*. Like the broom, the winnower (variously called a fan, tray or basket) is a cleansing implement, and a women's tool of labour. The *śūrpa* is U-shaped with an external frame of cane stretching a mat. It is held in both hands, and the arch stays next to the body. Winnowing trays are uneven, with a pronounced depth at the back that gradually flattens toward the front. With rhythmic movements, women throw a mixture of cereals (but also rice or pulses) in the air so that the breeze blows away lighter elements such as chaff, dirt and other residues. Unlike vignettes of Śītalā as a volitional goddess who spreads contagion by shaking the *śūrpa* on her head (Junghare 1975; BMJ 1980), the winnower is a protective implement in the hands of a mother who uses it to purify food and to throw cold air at children afflicted with high temperatures.[22] The *śūrpa* is also a ritual implement used by folk healers (including *ādivāsī* 'shamans') to invoke various goddesses, to facilitate possession and to negotiate health on behalf of their customers. Another ritual use of the *śūrpa* I had the chance to observe (especially in Bihar or among Bihari women in Uttar Pradesh or West Bengal) is the practice of the *jhulāi* (H. and Bhp. 'swinging'). When somebody is ill, or when an auspicious ceremony is taking place, women beat big winnowers to ward off the evil eye (*najar*) (see below p. 108, n.16).

Cephalomorphic *mūrtis*

Images of Śītalā in the form of big heads (*māthā*) are fairly widespread across north India. As in the case of stones and pitchers, this iconographic rendering too is not exclusive to the Cold Lady. Further, the lack of specific attributes (broom, winnower and the donkey) makes it quite difficult to tell Śītalā from other goddesses. The dimensions of cephalomorphic icons vary. The majority of those I observed are around 30 centimetres in height. Substantially larger images can be found, though. Heads are usually made of wood, clay or metal alloys. Not being self-generated, these images require the skills of professional craftsmen and ritualists (*pūjārī*s). Once the material has been reduced to the desired form, the image-maker paints it with bright colours, usually yellow, orange or red.[23] After applying the colour, the artist – whose performance is *de facto* a ritual and who works along with a *pūjārī* – draws all remaining facial features: big eyes, eyebrows, nostrils, and black hair parted in the centre (wigs are also used). Finally Śītalā's head is crowned, earrings and nose-rings are applied and, while the craftsman draws the pupils (*cakṣurdāna*), the ritual specialist infuses the goddess with breath in a ceremony called *prāṇapratiṣṭhā*. Then a *sindūr* mark is traced on her forehead. Upon completion of the rite, the head is placed in the shrine on a special seat, a throne or a palanquin. Alternatively, the icon is put on a frame and wrapped in a sari so as to suggest a human-shaped body. Unlike aniconic *mūrti*s, the key feature of cephalomorphic icons is their capacity to attract gaze by staring at devotees.

Ethnographic vignette 2: The Agam Kuāṅ, Patna (Bihar)

The Agam Kuāṅ (H. 'bottomless well') is located in Kumhrar Road, Ranipur, in the city of Patna. The complex is located on the site of a prison where the great king Aśoka (ruled ca. 268–233 BCE) of the Maurya dynasty, before his conversion to Buddhism, used to torture his enemies and, often, throw them down the well (Waddell 1903: 44). The *kuāṅ* is a triangular brick construction enclosed in a circular structure whose basis has a diameter of circa 6 metres. The perimeter of the site is delimited by a series of eight arched windows, and painted in red. Aside the Agam Kuāṅ – now a popular site visited by many as a wishing well – there is a small but popular Śītalā Mandir. The place is known as a centre of worship of the *saptā matṛkā*s (seven mothers), here rendered as seven *piṇḍa*s (roundish stones) covered with red *kumkum* powder and lined up. Two guardian deities, Bairõ (Bhairava) and Caṇḍī, flank the seven sisters. On a separate shrine, in the *sancta sanctorum*, is Śītalā. Her *mūrti* is a big dark stone with two wide white sclerae with big black pupils painted on its surface. The *māthā* is crowned with a tall tiara; it is marked with *ṭīkā* and draped with heavy garlands. The *pratimā* combines elements of the self-generated *śilā* with the iconography of the *māthā*. On the right of the goddess is a standing *mūrti* of Gaurī, and on the left is Aṅgār Mātā ('Mother Burning Charcoal'), a local goddess. Tridents are on both sides, and on the tiles of the wall behind the goddesses there are (recent) images of Lakṣmī and Sarasvatī. The temple is family-run by *mālin* (gardener) *pūjārī*s. According to their story, the *pratimā* was found in the lush garden separating the Agam Kuāṅ from the nearby Tulsi Mandi village (Sadikpur) by an ancestor of the present *gotra* during his duty.

The Agam Kuāṅ area is an ancient Buddhist site that at some point in the nineteenth century – possibly as a result of an increase in smallpox epidemics – became a centre for the worship of Mātā Māī (Śītalā). Offerings used to be thrown in the well on the eighth day (*aṣṭamī*) of every *pakṣa*, and with more emphasis during the month of Āṣāḍha, for protection against smallpox. Between 1879 and 1880, Alexander Cunningham, then director of the Archaeological Survey of India, reports on a fragment (presumably a pillar) of Mauryan epoch (c.ca second century BCE). The block, surrounded by stone tablets possibly belonging to the same structure, represents two large-breasted *matṛkā*s worshipped as Mātā Māī, i.e. Śītalā, for protection against smallpox (British Library 2009). This should not surprise. The goddess is multiform, and her presence simultaneous. Śītalā appropriates symbols, as well as the liturgy, of other goddesses. She is unproblematically worshipped in any form, including the *mūrtis* assigned to other deities, whenever there is need. Meister has briefly discussed this in his study of the Ambikeśvara temple in Rajasthan (1991: 192–6). On a doorway panel of this *mandir*, it is possible to recognize a Garuḍa-like male figure and, to its right, a couple in *maithuna* (Skt. 'union'). The latter, c.ca eighth century, has been worshipped for the past century as Śītalā.[24] Though the worship of Śītalā at or around Ambikeśvara is unattested, what matters here is the fluidity, and diachronic mobility, of the goddess and her representation.

> Iconicity and symbolism are not precisely the same thing. The visual formula *is* what it means (its iconic value), but *what* it means may vary according to use and tradition (its symbolism). The development of iconic formulas guaranteed the *identity* of the image with its meaning, without restricting further evolution of meaning or transformation of myth. (Meister 1986: 245)

I observed this pattern in the Baṛī Śītalā Mandir of Adalpura (see below pp. 114–19). Outside the temple, on the path leading to the *ghāṭ* on the Ganges, there is a series of *pipāl* trees. Under one such plant, there is a stone panel belonging to a pre-existing structure which Singh and Rana date back to the late Gāhaḍavāla dynasty (twelfth century) (2002: 272). The panel shows a standing couple. The figure on the left holds a small pitcher and both exhibit an elaborate hairdo, or a crown.[25] Around it, there are some (badly damaged) fragments showing various human figurines. The block is worshipped as a *thān* of the goddess, who is addressed as Baṛī Mā (H. 'Elder Mother').

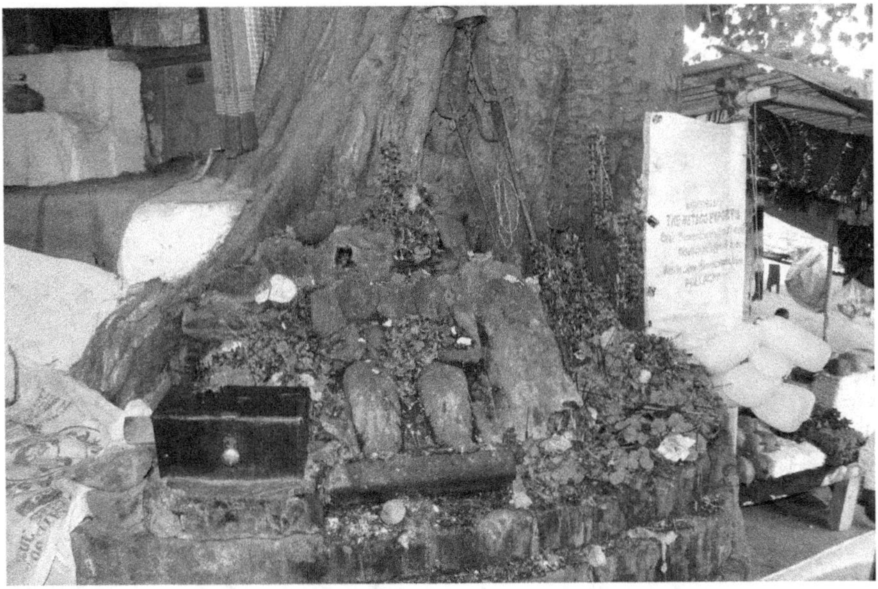

FIGURE 2.4 *Standing couple, black stone, Baṛī Śītalā Dhām, Adalpura (photo by author).*

Similar panels are scattered inside the temple, in the *garbhāgṛha*, and on the outer walls. None resembles Śītalā as we know her today, but they are all presented offerings as Śītalā. (Some are covered with gold-plated masks to evocate the goddess.)

Back to the Agam Kuāṅ, just like the two *matṛkās* identified by Cunningham, the seven mothers inside the temple today share the power of Śītalā. Mothers continue to gather here every other Tuesday (H. *maṅgalvār*) from the entire region, and pray to the goddess to protect their children (cf. Waddell 1903: 45–6) from childhood illnesses (mainly chickenpox) or the dreaded evil eye (H. *najarī, najar*). On the Āṣāḍha *Śītalāṣṭamī*, a large *melā* (H. festival) is held. Womens observe the vow in their bridal garments, and couples join communal worship to ask Śītalā for the gift of a healthy son.

Ethnographic vignette 3: The Choṭa Mā Yātrā, Salkia (West Bengal)

Unlike the Śītalā *mūrti* in Patna discussed above, most *māthā*-icons of Śītalā are portable. They are paraded or brought to visit other deities, including other forms of Śītalā, on occasions of special celebrations. One such case is the *snānyātrā* (B. 'bathing procession'), a pageant held every year on the full moon (*pūrṇimā*) of the light fortnight (*śukla pakṣa*) of Māgh to honour Śītalā as 'Younger Mother'.[26]

Pilgrims start to reach Salkia in the early hours of the pageant, or the evening before. They arrive from the two sides of the city, by boat or ferry on the *ghāṭ*s (Banda Ghat, Chattu Babu Ghat, Chaulpatti Ghat, Hoogly Dock Ghat or Golabari Ghat), or from the two main roads from outside the district (the Durgapur Expressway and the Surat-Hazira Bypass). The walk (B. *calan*) of the pilgrims is controlled by the local police and volunteers from various temple committees. The centre of Salkia is closed to traffic and devotees are required to follow two separate routes; one leads to the *ghāṭ*s, where the bathing takes place, from the outskirts of the city, the other moves in the opposite direction.

Attracting thousands of devotees, the festival is the occasion to celebrate Śītalā as a loving and benevolent protective mother. Śītalā, however, has many forms. The most authoritative – and the Lord of the Place – is indisputably Choṭa Mā (Small/Younger Mother). The temple of Choṭa Mā is actually a small family shrine located on the ground floor in 13/1, Upendranath Mitra Lane. The *snānyātrā* is the busiest moment of the year for the temple. Not only is Choṭa Mā, who is never removed, visited by thousands of pilgrims on their way to the *ghāṭ* on the Hoogly River where communal bathing takes place, but also all Śītalās from Salkia and the surrounding areas are brought in procession on richly decorated palanquins (*pālki*) in front of Choṭa Mā. This has a twofold meaning. It confirms the authority of Choṭa Mā over the territory, and it provides an arena for intense outpourings of devotion and displays of power.

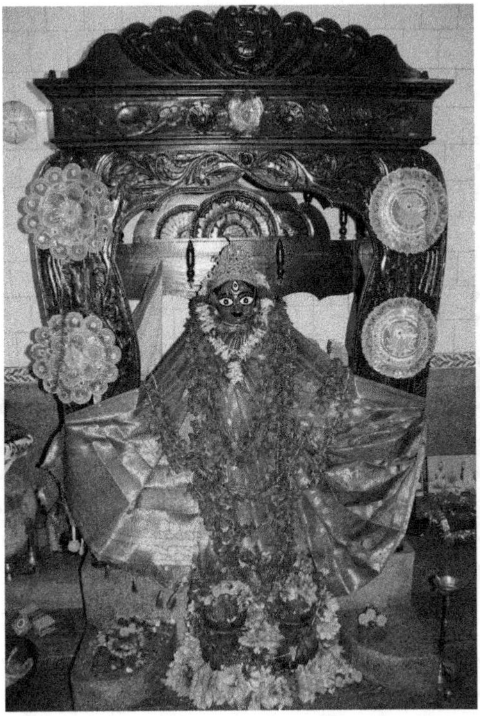

FIGURE 2.5 *Choṭa Mā, Śrī Śrī Choṭa Śītalā Mātā Mandir, Salkia (photo by author).*

Shri Pradip Chatterjee, the current *sevāit*,[27] showed me a register with the names and provenance of the 64 Śītalās who were paraded in 2010. The following year the list was updated to 65, a number confirmed in 2012 and 2013.[28] The apex of the parade coincides with the visit of the three biggest Śītalās of Salkia, each mounted on an elaborate palanquin. They are Baṛo Mā (big/old mother),[29] Mejo Mā (second-born mother)[30] and Sejo Mā (third-born mother).[31] All the *mūrti*s, including Choṭa Mā, are cephalomorphic. Although they vary in dimensions, they are structurally similar. Icons are wooden oval-shaped and neatly polished. They are painted in red or orange, with three large eyes and a series of golden-plated jewels (nose-rings, earrings, tiaras, necklaces, etc.). Choṭa Mā stands alone on her altar, whereas Baṛo Mā is surrounded by anthropomorphic images of Śani, Pañcānan and Manasā; Mejo Mā is flanked on her right by Śani (anthropomorphic) and at her feet is Dharmarāj (aniconic); at the feet of Sejo Mā are Jvarāsur (anthropomorphic), Śani (anthropomorphic), Dharmarāj (aniconic) and a *śivaliṅga*.[32]

The annual pageant is an occasion to make pilgrims aware of the greatness of each mother. Palanquins are prepared and the *pratimā*s are accommodated with great pomp. The various Śītalās are territorial goddesses and each represents a neighbourhood. Competition is visible. Temple committees work hard to make all the arrangements, as they want to offer the best show possible. This includes

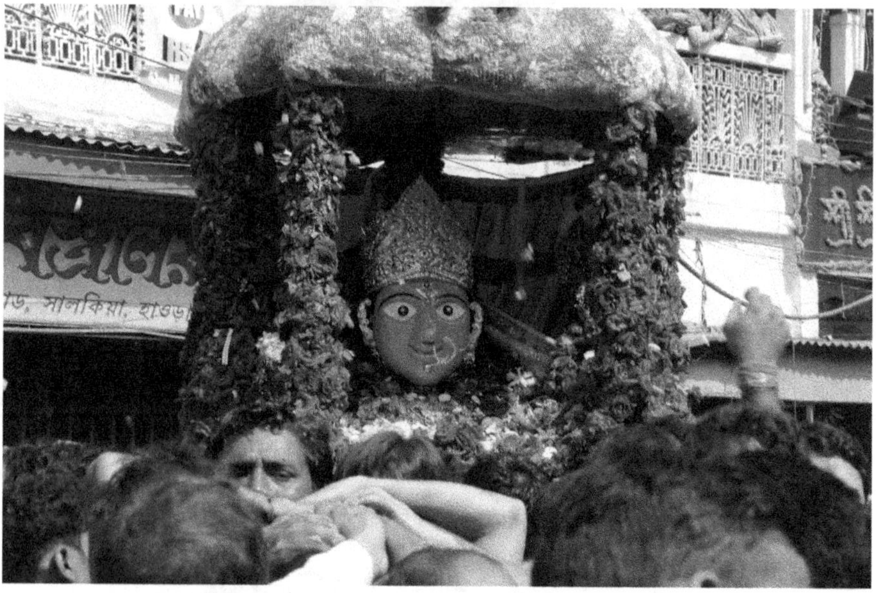

FIGURE 2.6 *Baṛo Mā on palanquin, Choṭa Mā Yātrā, Salkia (photo by Jayanta Roy).*

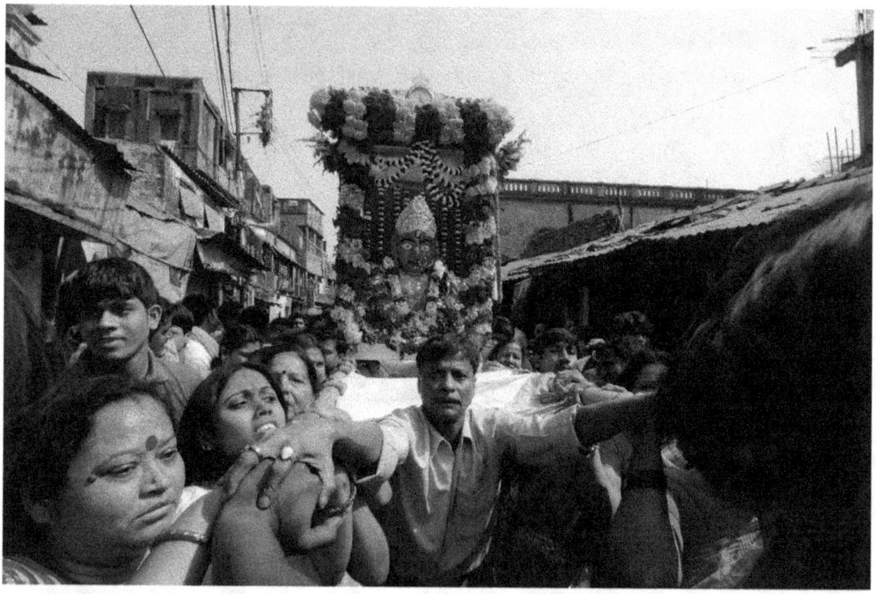

FIGURE 2.7 *Mejo Mā on palanquin, Choṭa Mā Yātrā, Salkia (photo by Jayanta Roy).*

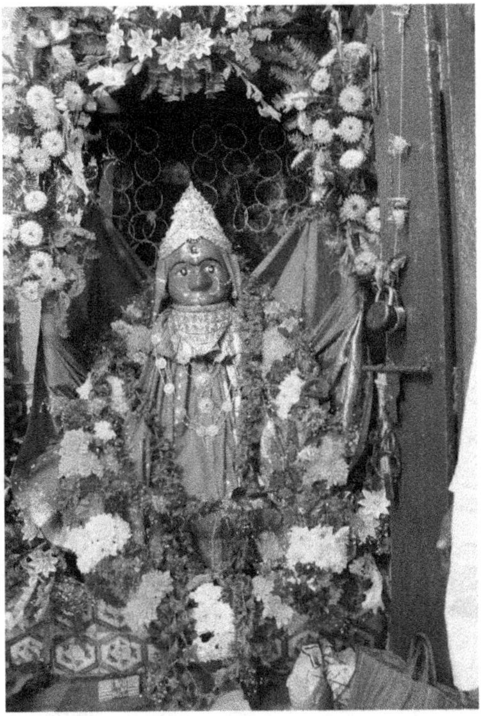

FIGURE 2.8 *Sejo Mā, Śrī Śrī Śītalā Mātār Mandir, Salkia (photo by Jayanta Roy).*

paying for drummers, musicians, insignia, uniforms (or T-shirts with the name of the goddess), new clothes and jewels for Mā, and various forms of advertising. At the end of the procession, after paying homage to Choṭa Mā and bathing in the Hoogly, each goddess is brought back and ceremonially installed anew, and thanked for another year of blessings and protection. The only temple where further rituals are performed is the Baṛo Mā Mandir, where a great animal sacrifice (*balidān*) is performed the following day (see below pp. 88–93).

Zoomorphic and phytomorphic *mūrtis*

A smaller percentage of Śītalā shrines host clay statuettes in the form of animals such as horses and elephants. I observed this principally in the West Bengali districts of Bankura and, to a lesser degree, Medinipur and Birbhum (but cf. Mukhopadhyay 1994: 38). These shrines – known as *grāmyer thān* (B. 'village [sacred] places') – are usually found under, or in the immediate proximities of, trees that are associated with the goddess, notably *nīm* (*Azadirachta indica*) but also *baval* (*Prosopis juliflora*) and *ākanda* (*Calotropis gigantean*). Along with terracotta animals, one can find agricultural tools such as ploughs, spades, winnowers or the husking pedal (*ḍheñki*),[33] all objects bearing witness to the fertility power of Śītalā. Clay horses and elephants are offered in advance of a vow, and are worshipped as sites of the goddess's power.[34] Upon completion of the vow, the clay animals are destroyed, and devotees arrange an elaborate thanking *pūjā*. Clay animals are not strictly identified with Śītalā. Icons unproblematically symbolize a plethora of gods and goddesses. The same series of horses and elephants may host, at the same time, Śītalā, Manasā, Ṣaṣṭhī, Lakṣmī, Caṇḍī, Śiva, Dharmarāj, Iṭu, Arka, etc.

Śītalā is associated with animals symbolizing the waters.[35] Clay elephants, for instance, are traditionally presented to the goddess as a votive offering in order to find a good husband, or on a wedding day. The auspicious nature of the elephant, and its power to avert the evil eye and to remove obstacles, is further witnessed by its association with Lakṣmī, goddess of prosperity, fortune and wealth, in the form of Gajalakṣmī, and Gaṇeśa Vighneśvara ('Remover of Obstacles'). The horse, conversely, is a known symbol of fertility but is traditionally associated with sun gods. This comes as no surprise, since Śītalā is variously portrayed as sister, daughter or companion of solar deities such as Iṭu, Arka and, more often, Dharmarāj (also called Jamrāj, i.e. Yama, or Sūrja/Surāj, i.e. Sūrya). The god is a radiant king riding a (white) horse, or standing on a royal chariot pulled by white horses. Śītalā's pairing with sun gods, attested as early as the ninth century (see below p. 59), probably reflects the concerns of societies depending on agriculture, and therefore on a good balance between rain and sun. Of the two elements, Śītalā is the mitigating presence whereas the Sun is, from Vedic times (cf. RV 8.91: 1–7), held responsible for skin diseases (acne, poxes, leprosy, vitiligo, etc.) and the blindness that may derive from them.

A similar logic applies to phytomorphic icons. Branches of trees with cooling properties continue to be a regular offering in many of Śītalā's shrines, temples or domestic altars. Leaves or branches of *nīm* – a known ingredient in āyurvedic pharmacopeia and widely used for skin diseases – are a welcome gift to a naturally cold goddess like Śītalā. At the same time, devotees expect that the refreshing, healing and fertilizing power of the goddess, embodied in the plant, is returned as blessing *prasād*. Shrubs of *ākanda* too are said to host the goddess and, in Gujarat, the thorny *baval* (Gopalan 1978: 120). Both plants, which have refreshing properties, serve for the preparation of remedies against cutaneous diseases.

The practice of offering cool leaves and branches, and of worshipping them as aspects/gifts of Śītalā, has always been quite widespread across north India at the point it was instrumental in the struggle against smallpox in colonial times and during the WHO Smallpox Eradication Program (SEP). The presence of *nīm* branches outside houses or huts was a visual indicator of the presence of smallpox victims, thus facilitating medical intervention and quarantine. Today, when children suffer from chickenpox or fevers, the auspicious 'green leaves' of *nīm* are still strategically positioned on doors or windows, and continue to be used to sprinkle water on the *mūrti* of Śītalā to invite her healing power.

Equestrian *mūrtis*

The only iconography of the goddess that is consistently found in Indian textual sources is the ass-riding Śītalā. Archaeological evidence lets us establish with some precision the appearance of equestrian statues of the goddess as early as the second half of the ninth century. The earliest image is found in an exterior niche of the Sun temple in Maḍhkeda (near Tikamgarh, in the homonymous district of Madhya Pradesh). Śītalā is naked and rides an ass in the upright position. Her head is surrounded by a halo; she has two arms and holds with her left hand what looks like a broom. The goddess's facial features are eroded, but she sports large earrings, and large firm breasts.

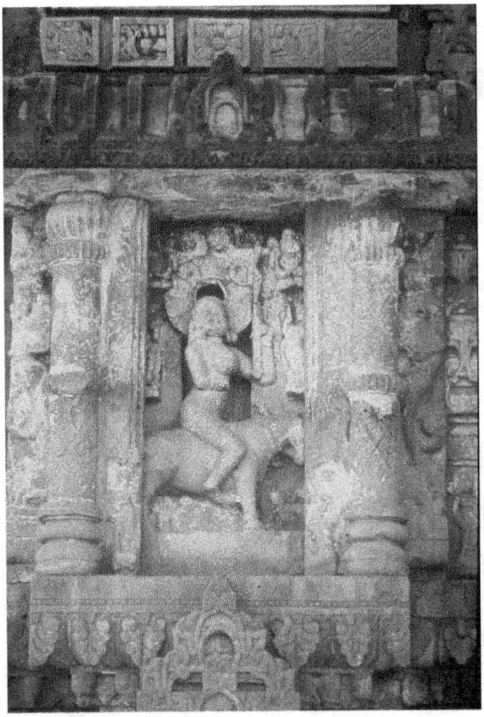

FIGURE 2.9 *Śītalā, figure in Kapili niche, north, Sūrya Mandir, Maḍhkeda (Madhya Pradesh), ninth century (courtesy and copyright of Michael W. Meister).*

Other early statues are found in western India. An equestrian sculpture from Osiañ (Rajasthan) has been identified in the Saccikamātā (or Sacciyamātā) temple, originally a small shrine to the goddess Kṣemaṅkarī ('Maker of Prosperity/Safety') built early in the eighth century. In the second half of the twelfth century, the shrine was converted into a larger temple hosting in its sanctuary an image of Durgā Mahiṣāsuramardiṇī (Slayer of the Buffalo Demon). Now a major Jain temple, the Saccikamātā Mandir bears witness to the transformative nature of South Asian goddesses (Meister 1998: 115). A *saṃvat* 1234 (1178 CE) inscription mentions the *śrīsaccikādevīprasāda*, 'an ornament with five *pratima* (visible-image) forms of the Goddess', that is Caṇḍikā, Śītalā, Saccikādevī, Kṣemaṅkarī and Kṣetrapāla (ibid.: 116; Nahar 1983: 198). The equestrian statue of Śītalā fills the central niche on the north wall of the sanctuary, where the Mahiṣāsuramardiṇī is found (Meister 1998: 116; cf. Tiwari 1996: 452; Nagar 1988: 129–30). The statue of Śītalā is badly damaged and a serious examination of its features is difficult. The goddess is naked and has large breasts. She is four-armed; with two hands she holds a *śūrpa* above the head, a third hand is in *abhayamudrā* (gesture of protection). The fourth hand is missing. The goddess sits in *lalitāsana* (side-saddle, with a pendent foot) on an equid that has been interpreted as an ass.

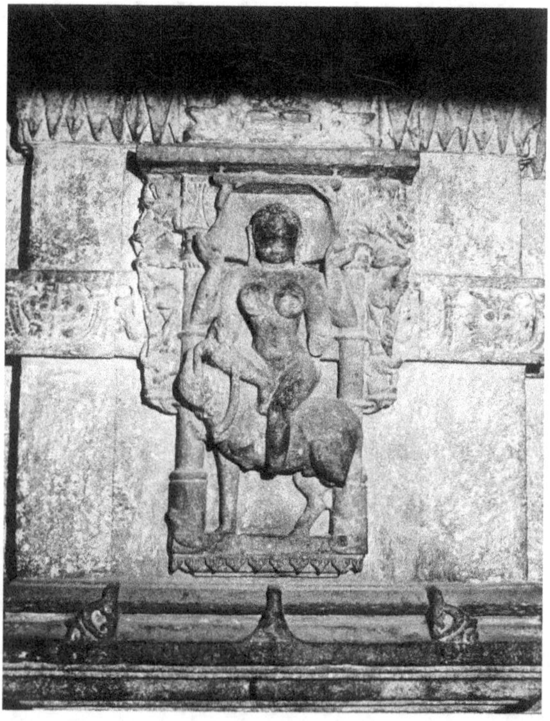

FIGURE 2.10 *Śītalā, sandstone, detail of the exterior, Saccikamātā Mandir, Osiañ (Rajasthan), c.ca twelfth century (courtesy of American Institute of Indian Studies).*

The *śūrpa* and the *vāhana* seem to confirm the inscription, thus making it possible to identify the *pratimā* with Śītalā.

A similar image is found in the Sūrya-Kuṇḍa at Moḍherā (Mahesana district, Gujarat), a sun temple complex erected around 1025 (Lobo 1982: 130; Brown 1965: 120; Dhaky 1961: 28).[36] The *mandir* is associated with the first years of the kingdom of Bhīma I (1024–66), a ruler of the Solaṅkī dynasty. The statue of Śītalā may be justified by the fact that around 1010, Vallabharāja, the title given to Bhīma's predecessors, died of smallpox fever (*śīlī-roga*; *śītalā*).[37] The goddess is in *lalitāsana* and is unusually represented with twelve arms, of which only six survive. With two hands Śītalā holds a *śūrpa* on her head. The other hands sport a trident (*triśūla*), a pitcher (*kalaśa*) and a small drum (*ḍamaru*). The fourth hand is in *varadamudrā*, a sign of welcoming and benevolence. As with other images in the area, she is plump, naked and rides a (seriously damaged) equid identified as an ass.

Other images have been carved according to this pattern roughly between the tenth and twelfth centuries in north-western India. In his list, Tiwari (1996: 457–9) mentions an early twelfth-century statue from Sejakpur (Gujarat), an image from the Nīlakāṇṭeśvara Mandir in Arthūṇā (Banswara, Rajasthan) and a twelfth-century statue from the Jasmalnāth Mahādev Mandir of Asoda (Gujarat).

Along with larger *pratimā*s, small statuettes belonging to the same period have been found. One such specimen is a sandstone equestrian image from Gandhisagar (Mandasore, Madhya Pradesh), presently located in the Archaeological Museum in Yashwantrao Holkar Chattri's monument in Bhanpura (Madhya Pradesh). Initially dated c.ca 800–899 CE, it seems more prudent to locate it between the twelfth and fourteenth centuries. The statuette is seriously damaged and the identification with Śītalā, whose face is completely ruined, is tentative. The *vāhana* seems to be an ass and the goddess, naked in *lalitāsana*, holds what may be a broom. On her head there is a crown that could have been a winnowing tray. She is flanked by two smaller figures (attendants?), one of whom looks emaciated. The second statuette, now conserved at the Allahabad Museum, is equally difficult to locate historically. A time span ranging from the eighth to the fourteenth century has been proposed, though an earlier attempt suggested c.ca 900–999 CE. The goddess sits upright on either a small horse or an ass. She is two-armed, naked, large-breasted, has a beaded necklace, holds (what seems) a broom and on her head is an object resembling a winnowing basket. At her feet is a human figure making the *namaskāra* (salutation) gesture. Two (badly damaged) human females, also with large breasts, accompany Śītalā. They are located on the upper right and upper left corners of the panel, and they seem to hold swords and small shields.[38]

A rather different iconography is found on two eleventh-century (Pāla period) Parṇaśavarī steles from the Dhaka district (Bangladesh).[39] The goddess Parṇaśavarī ('Leaves-clad Śavara woman')[40] is a well-known healing goddess in Indian Buddhism, and is still worshipped as a protector in Tibetan Buddhism with the name Lo ma gyon ma (Tib. 'Leaf-Clad Mountain-Dweller'). In the two Dhaka

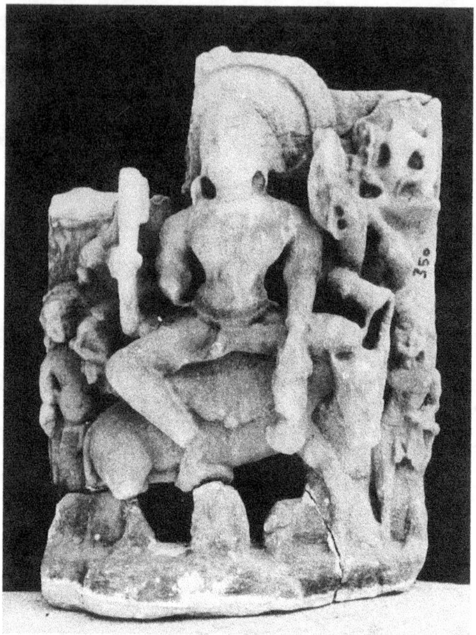

FIGURE 2.11 *Śītalā, buff sandstone standing figure, 58 x 49 cm, Gandhisagar (Madhya Pradesh), c.ca fourteenth century (courtesy of American Institute of Indian Studies).*

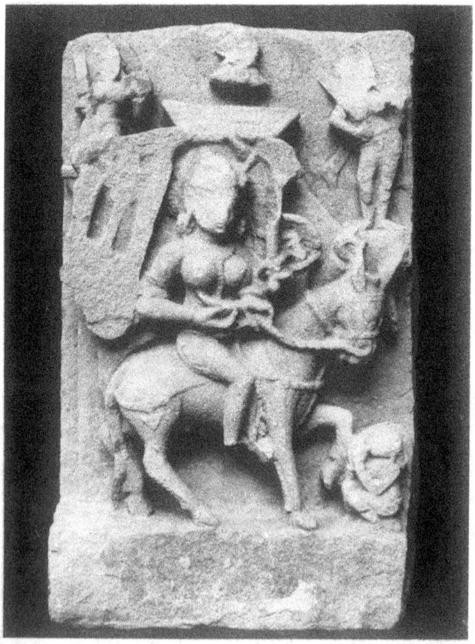

FIGURE 2.12 *Śītalā riding an ass, greyish sandstone standing figure, 54.5 x 37 cm, Allahabad Museum, c.ca fourteenth century (courtesy of American Institute of Indian Studies).*

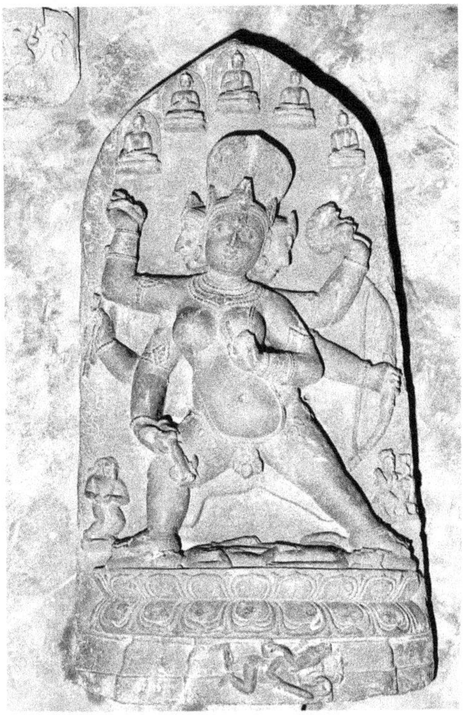

FIGURE 2.13 *Parṇaśavarī, Equestrian stone, eleventh century, Vikrampur, Dhaka district, E67.319, Department of History and Classical Art, National Museum of Bangladesh, Dacca. (Photograph by John C. Huntington Courtesy of The Huntington Photographic Archive at The Ohio State University)*

steles, Parṇaśavarī is three-headed, bare-breasted and pot-bellied. She has six arms. On her right side, she holds a thunderbolt, a hatchet and an arrow. On the left side, her first hand is in *tarjanīmudrā* (a warding-off evil posture), while with the second and third hands the goddess holds a bunch of (medicinal) leaves and a bow. A girdle of leaves surrounds her loins. She stands over two prostrated male figures lying on a lotus-shaped pedestal with their heads in the opposite directions. Both men are pitted with circular marks, in all possibility smallpox ulcers. Below the lotus is Gaṇeśa holding a shield and a sword. He seems to be flying away, possibly after a fight with Parṇaśavarī. A horse-headed miniature figure, identified by Bhattasali (1929: 60) with Hayagrīva ('Horse-necked' One), is shown at the bottom right of Parṇaśavarī. On the opposite side, is Śītalā. The figurine conforms to the standard description of the goddess: she is naked, rides an ass (astride), and holds a broom in her right hand and a winnowing basket in her left. Her appearance, however, is dramatically different from coeval plump statues found in north-western temples. In these representations, Śītalā looks old, skeletal and emaciated.

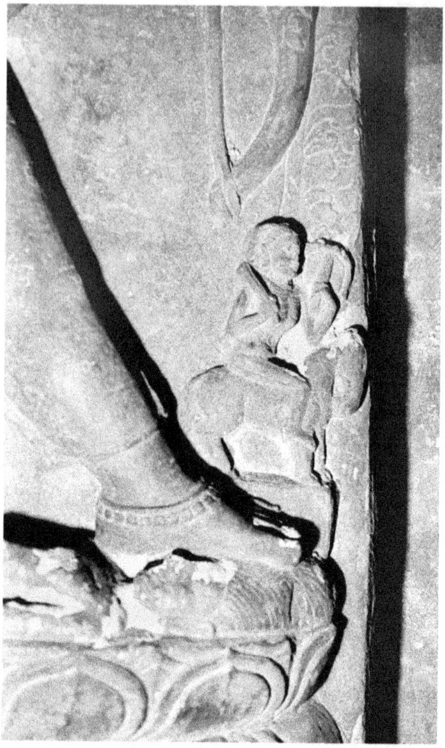

FIGURE 2.14 *Detail: Śītala, from Parṇaśavarī stele, black stone, h. 121.92, eleventh century, Vajrayogini, Munshiganj, Dhaka district, E.67.031, Department of History and Classical Art, National Museum of Bangladesh, Dacca (Photograph by John C. Huntington Courtesy of The Huntington Photographic Archive at The Ohio State University)*

The scenes on the two Dhaka steles have been variously interpreted. Bhattasali (1929: 61) and Bhattacharyya (1989: 119) have suggested both Śītalā and Hayagrīva are leaving to avoid the wrath of Parṇaśavarī – thus pointing at sectarian hatred between Buddhists and Hindus, a theory they derive from the image of an apparently defeated Gaṇeśa. This is not convincing. In one stele (E67.319), Hayagrīva is not leaving, but approaching Parṇaśavarī. The dimension and position (above the lotus and at Parṇaśavarī's feet) of the two deities on both steles indicate that Hayagrīva and Śītalā are subordinate but not necessarily opposed to Parṇaśavarī. They may be her attendants:

> Śītalā and Hayagrīva – both curers of fevers and other epidemics – are cast here as emissaries working in concert with Parṇaśavarī to banish pestilential threats to human well-being. This interpretation is consonant with the long-standing artistic practice, traceable to the earliest Buddhist art, of portraying Hindu divinities as attendants of Buddhist figures. (Shaw 2006: 196)

This interpretation reflects Śītalā's specialization in (assisting into) healing from *visphoṭa*, a disease evoked by the two men lying at Parṇaśavarī's feet. As per Hayagrīva, we learn from the tenth-century *Kālikāpurāṇa* (78: 76–8) that he was a demon killed by Viṣṇu, who eventually took his form. Viṣṇu-Hayagrīva is by all means considered an *avatāra* of Viṣṇu, and is celebrated for the slaying of Jvarāsura, the Fever Demon.[41] This has led Bhattasali (1929: 60), and others after him (e.g. Mishra 1999: 107; Shaw 2006: 196; Mukharji 2013: 270), to equate Hayagrīva and Jvarāsura. In fact, the only textual source mentioning both deities together is KāP. Although Viṣṇu-Hayagrīva is infected by Jvarāsura, a blemish that is countered with a purifying bath in a lake on the Maṇikūṭa hill (Assam), they are distinct characters. I thus suspect that Bhattasali's judgement might have been affected by his familiarity with ŚMKs, where Jvarāsura is the demonic attendant, or marshal, of Śītalā (also present in the steles). In fact, Hayagrīva is never mentioned in ŚMKs, nor are horse-headed renderings of Jvarāsura found in *maṅgal* songs or material culture associated with the Fever Demon of the ŚMKs.

What is interesting in the Dhaka steles is Śītalā's physiognomy. The goddess is an emaciated (old?) woman with loose hairs and pendulous breasts. Such rendering is highly evocative of tantric goddesses such as Cāmuṇḍā. Purāṇic literature confirms this. Cāmuṇḍā and some *yoginī*s (though they are not skeletal) have been represented riding an ass, or holding brooms and winnowers (see below p. 68).[42] It seems thus reasonable that tantric elements might have infiltrated legends of Śītalā in the east (hence the *maṅgal*-Śītala), just like goddesses associated with low classes (cf. *Puraścaryārṇava* 12: 80) have penetrated eastern Tantrism.[43]

Though there is sufficient evidence to say that, from at least the ninth century, Śītalā has been consistently represented, and visualized, as a naked ass-rider, this has changed considerably. The pale *digambara* goddess is not easily found in modern and contemporary Indian material culture. An example of this process is found in the Kalighat School of nineteenth-century Calcutta.[44] Thought standard tools are retained, Śītala is no longer naked, possibly in response to the taste and morality of customers (Bengali *bhadralok* and the British). She wears what look like bridal garments, i.e. a red silk sari, and red glass bangles (B. *cuṛi*). Her complexion is yellow, and the palms of her hands are red with henna (B. *mehedi*). The goddess is heavily bejewelled with necklaces, earrings, nose-ring, wrist- and ankle-bracelets. Though in some paintings Śītalā still has a *śūrpa* positioned on her head, she is most likely to sport a big crown pitted with gems, and her head is surrounded by a halo, a visual reminder of her divine status. This rendition, whether an original creation of Kālīghāṭ painters or a modification of current trends, would be destined to affirm itself as the standard iconography of the goddess. Contemporary non-religious art bears witness to it.

One such case is an oil canvas from the *Icons and Illusions* series of the Bengali artist Shuvaprasanna (b. 1947).[45] In his 'Goddess Shitala', the Cold Lady is three-eyed and has four arms. She does not hold any of her trademark tools. The goddess seems to fall down from height, or to float in empty space. A dark-red kameez covers the

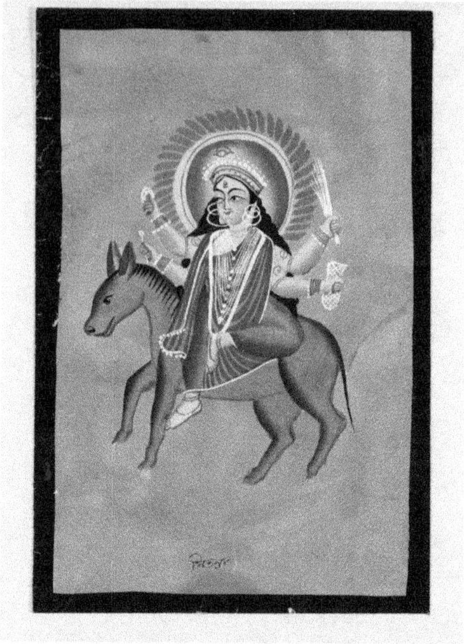

FIGURE 2.15 *Śītalā, Kālīghāṭ painting, opaque watercolour on paper, Calcutta, c.ca 1885, Victoria and Albert Museum, IS.607-1950 (Courtesy of Victoria and Albert Museum, London).*

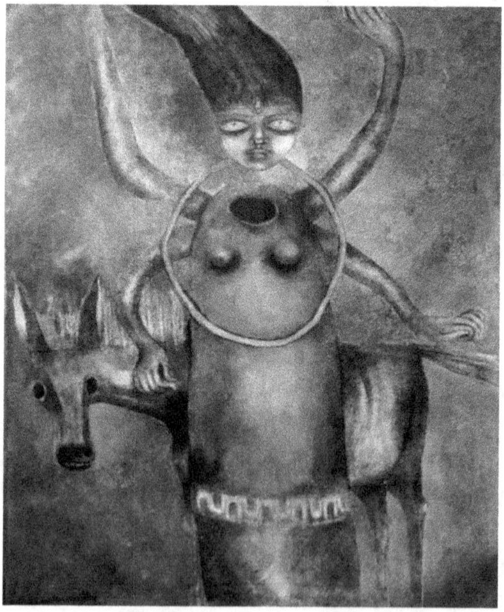

FIGURE 2.16 *Goddess Shitala,* Icons and Illusions, *oil on canvas, by Shuvaprasanna (courtesy of Shuvaprasanna Bhattacharjee).*

pale body of the goddess, whose cylinder-like form is featured by tiny breasts. Her head, as is the case for most goddesses in the *Icons and Illusions* series, is severed from the body, an artistic rendering of her necklace, but also a symbol of her detachment. Shuvaprasanna, who confirmed to me that his intention was to recreate the impassibility and calmness (*śītalā*) of the goddess who 'saves us from epidemics and disasters',[46] used a chromatic texture of choice to give Śītalā an aura of serene disengagement, a feature that is reflected in the lack of facial expression and in her eyes looking upward. In the background, there is a big grey donkey with hollow black eyes. This particular is the only one permitting identification of the goddess as Śītalā. This is not novelty. The ass has served as an indicator of the identity of the goddess not just for art historians, but for devotees of Śītalā too. A question, perhaps a naïve one, naturally emerges: Why the ass? Why should Śītalā – a goddess who heals and protects from scary diseases – mount an allegedly stupid animal? What is the meaning of the 'ass' in Indian culture? Answering such questions, I argue, could help to understand the nature of Śītalā as a natural healer, and a protector.

The ass *vāhana*[47]

A ubiquitous and consolidated presence in the standard iconography of Śītalā, the ass[48] is a marginal character in ritual and mythological literature. The ass is systematically mentioned in opening invocations (*cālīsā*, *ārti*, etc.), and its five names are invoked as auspicious in ŚAS 83–85. A *gardabha dhyānamantra* is given in PiT as propaedeutic to *pañcopacāra* (ŚPP 318; see below p. 187) and the praxis of feeding donkeys continues to be complementary to the observance of women's fasts (see above p. 12; cf. Forbes 1856: 327; Minsky 2009: 168–9),[49] even though the narrative elements (*kathā*) of *vrata*s do not confirm it. Notwithstanding its ubiquity, scholarly literature has virtually ignored it.[50]

Indian texts bear witness to the presence of the ass, an animal non-indigenous to South Asia, as early as Vedic times. Asses are described as strong and fast mounts that carry Agni (TS 5.1: 5; VS 11: 13) and the Aśvins, the physicians of the gods (RV 1.34: 9; 8.74: 7). At the same time, they are impure and ominous beasts. Indra is summoned to destroy the inauspicious ass (RV 1.29: 5) while the she-ass (jenny) is associated with witchcraft, and compelled to leave by means of powerful spells (AVŚ 10.1: 14). In both Vedic and post-Vedic literature, inauspicious goddesses ride (or are associated with) the ass:

1. Nirṛti ('Injustice', 'Disorder'): the Vedic goddess of death, decay and corruption. Early and late Vedic literature refers to her as a goddess to be kept away (RV 5.41: 17; 6.74: 2; 10.59: 1–10). There is little evidence suggesting Nirṛti was represented on an ass, although she has been later identified with ass-riding goddesses such as Jyeṣṭhā and Alakṣmī (Kinsley 1997: 178). According to Manu (second century BCE), to placate Nirṛti one is supposed to

sacrifice a one-eyed ass at a crossroad at night (Manu 11.119). In *Parāskara Gṛhyasūtra* (3.12: 1–11): 'a Vedic student who has violated his vow of chastity should sacrifice an ass to Nirṛti. He has to dress himself in the skin of the ass and eat a piece of the sacrificial victim cut out of its penis.'[51]

2 Jyeṣṭhā ('First [Wife]'): a goddess causing misfortune and disease. She usually has no mount, and is represented as an old dark woman with flaccid skin, pendulous breasts, loose belly and an ugly face. Traditionally, Jyeṣṭhā's vehicle and symbol is the crow. Yet, as Leslie informs us (1991: 118; cf. White 2003: 51), she rides an ass (*khararūḍhā*) in *Suprabhedāgama* 45: 3, and in the Sanskrit encyclopedic dictionary *Śabdakalpadruma* (1.1 p. 120), she is called *gardhabharūḍha*.[52]

3 Kālarātrī ('Black Night'): a tantric goddess identified with the fearsome aspect of Kālī,[53] or Bhairavī. Kālarātrī is worshipped as the seventh Śakti of Durgā and, as a goddess of destruction, is associated with everything leading to death, including disease. She is often worshipped along with Śītalā, and her images are found in many *śākta* temples. The goddess rides astride an ass, is black or dark-blue complexioned with long dishevelled curly black hair (see Fig. 2.23 below; cf. the goddess's *dhyānamantra* in ŚVK 4 and 12, where Kālarātrī is *kharasthitā*). In *Pratiṣṭhālakṣaṇasārasamuccaya*, an eleventh- to twelfth-century tantric text, she wears a garland of *javā* flowers (or, alternatively, skulls) and, naked, rides an ass (Bühneman 2003: 40).

4 Cāmuṇḍā (or Caṇḍamārī): the slayer of the demons Caṇḍa and Muṇḍa, described in *Vāmanapurāṇa* 29: 70, 73 and 87 in a way very similar to Śītalā, i.e. naked (*digvāsa*) and riding an ass. Cāmuṇḍā, among her many names, is also called Kālīkā. In this form, she is naked, rides an ass, holds a skull and is garlanded with red flowers (MaP 261: 37–8).

5 The *yoginī*s: a class of tantric semi-divine half-human female half-animal beings often represented in circles of 64. Reputed to be sorceresses or witches, the *yoginī*s in tantric culture are powerful and accomplished female ritual practitioners. Some *yoginī*s are represented as either standing on a donkey or as ass-faced females (e.g. Gandhārī and Vaināyakī in the Hirapur temple). Others have the ass as a vehicle. These are Hārārāvā (Hemādri's *Caturvarga Cintāmaṇi*, *Vratakhaṇḍa*, 1; *Pratiṣṭhālakṣaṇasārasamuccaya* 7: 327–400), Tālajanghā (*Matottaratantra* 20) and Piśītāśā (*Pratiṣṭhālakṣaṇasārasamuccaya* ibid.) (Dehejia 1986: 205–7).

6 Mātaṅgī ('the Intoxicated One'): one of the ten *mahāvidyā*s, she is represented as a richly adorned young woman, with firm breasts, long black hair, three eyes, green (or blue) skin. She sits on a corpse and her companion is traditionally the green parrot. She is known as the outcaste goddess and is associated with pollution and leftovers (stale food). In the fifteenth century *Caṇḍīpurāṇa* of Saralādāsa, Mātaṅgī has the donkey as her *vāhana* (Dehejia 1986: 200; Siṃha 1990: 150).

7 Raktāvatī ('Bloody'): Śītalā's servant or companion (see above, p. 26).

The ass, but also the mule (the offspring of a male donkey and a mare), is present in a number of South Asian narratives in relation to unruly demons, ferocious gods and diseases:

1 Kali ('Discord'): the demon of the Dark Age. In the *Kalkipurāṇa*, Kali confronts Kalki, the tenth *avatāra* of Viṣṇu, and tries to destroy the world. He rides an ass (21: 2) while his divine opponent – as many other solar deities – has a white stallion.

2 Dhenuka: a ferocious man-eating ass-demon living in Tālavana (Skt. 'grove of Palmyra tree'), near Vṛndāvana. Dhenuka, along with other ass-demons, was killed at the hand of Balarāma, Kṛṣṇa's brother (HV 57, BhP 10: 15; cf. *Viṣṇupurāṇa* 5: 8).

3 Rāvaṇa: the ten-headed lord of the *rākṣasas*. In a number of vernacular versions of the *Rāmāyaṇa*, and in related material culture,[54] Rāvaṇa is given the head of an ass above other heads to remind him of humility. Also, the demon king rides a chariot of asses (Rām 5.27: 24–5) and is brother/cousin to Khara, the Ass-Demon.

4 Khara ('Ass'): a ferocious and man-eating *rakṣasa* chief, brother (or cousin) to Rāvaṇa. Khara is described in his attempt to vindicate his sister Śūrpaṇakhā ('Fingernails like winnowers') whose nose was cut off by Rāma's brother Lakṣmaṇa. Eventually he is killed by Rāma (Rām 3: 30).

5 Gardabha ('Ass'): a child-devouring/snatching *yakṣa* living in Mathurā. He was converted by the Buddha (*Mūlasarvāstivādavinaya, bhaiṣajyavastu*, 2: 40–2).

6 Śani ('Saturn'): known as *graharāja* (Skt. 'King of graspers'), he has an inauspicious character. Śani is believed to be the source of several diseases, bad luck, negative possession and madness. As his younger brother Yama (the Lord of the Dead), Śani judges one's deeds in life and takes decisions in matters of punishment and reward.[55] Although no text I am aware of confirms that the ass is Śani's *vāhana*, there is an abundance of iconographic evidence from north-eastern India (circa tenth century) and, successively, in Madhya Pradesh and western regions (Mevissen 1997: 1274). In West Bengal and Odisha, Śani is regularly found alongside Śītalā and Jvarāsura.

7 Saṃvara/Heruka (Tib. Khrag 'Thung): a fierce and powerful god of tantric Buddhism, identified as a dangerous *piśaca* or, in KāP, a 'divinity of a

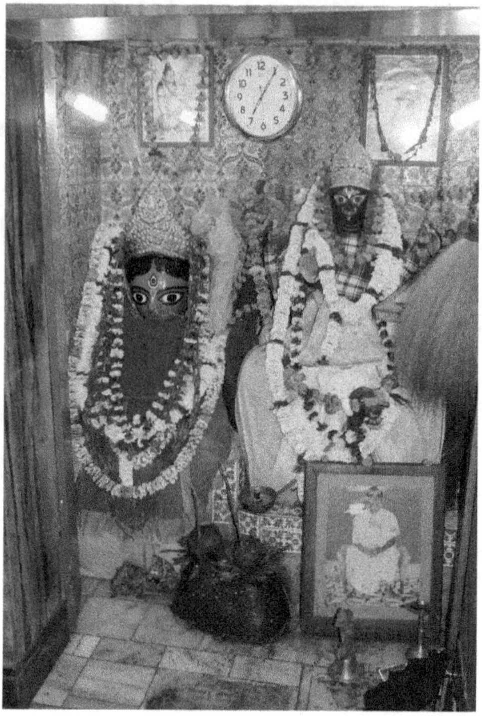

FIGURE 2.17 *Śītala (left), Śani (right) and Caṇḍī (aniconic), Bandhaghat, Salkia (photo by author).*

cremation ground' (Davidson 2002: 213). He assumes the form of a donkey in the *Yoginīsaṁcāratantra* (16: 14).

8 The Tibetan guardian goddess dPal-ldan Lha-mo (Skt. Śrī Devī): portrayed as riding a huge reddish mule (Jest and Rowis-Giorfani 1985: 15–16), possibly a kiang mule,[56] on whose back are two heavy bags made of ulcerated human skin full of the germs of virulent diseases (smallpox, cholera, leprosy, plagues, etc.).

South Asian narratives portray the ass following three trends. First, the animal is believed to be demonic, impure and a disease carrier (Rau 2012: 997). *Piśāca*s are believed to be asses (Filippi 2002: 105), just like *rakṣasas* (VS 24.40). The word *khara* ('ass') indicates any *asura*, particularly the *daitya*s (Bhattacharyya 2000: 110; cf. MBh 2: 275). The equid is associated with dogs, crows, *śūdra*s and 'untouchables' (BŚS 27.8, 28.10). Issues of purity have contributed to enhancing the reputation of the ass as an inauspicious (Manu 10.51) or demonic animal (Visuvalingam 1989: 170). The *Rāmāyaṇa* confirms this: 'If in a dream, a person sees a man going in a chariot, yoked with donkeys, the smoke of a funeral pyre will soon be seen ascending him' (2.69: 18). Similarly, in *Anaṅgaraṅga*, an erotic manual composed between the fifteenth and sixteenth centuries by Kalyāṇamalla:

> The Kharasatva-stri, [the woman] who preserves the characteristics of the ass, is unclean in her person, and avoids bathing, washing, and pure raiment: she cannot give a direct answer, and she speaks awkwardly and without reason, because her mind is crooked. Therefore she pleases no one. (*Anaṅgaraṅga* 4)

Parpola has found a number of references related to the impurity and inauspiciousness of the ass:

> The sounds of dogs, asses, jackals, vultures and crows forebode evil (Atharvaveda-Pariśiṣṭa 61,1,8), and Vedic recitation is to be suspended when dogs are barking, asses (*gardabha-*) are braying or jackals are howling (cf. Āpastamba-Dharmasūtra 1,10,19; Gautama-Dharmasūtra 16,8). Dreaming of camels, pigs, asses etc. forebodes evil (cf. Mānava-Gṛhyasūtra 2,14,11). In Rāmāyaṇa 2,63,14–16, Bharata's dream of a man driving an ass-chariot is explicitly stated to portend death. In spite of its fecundating power, the ass is an animal connected with Nirṛti, the goddess of Destruction, the guardian deity of the inauspicious direction of southwest. It is to her, Nirṛti, or to Yama (the god of death) that the ass is to be sacrificed in breaches of chastity and this in the wilderness (*araṇye*) (cf. Vasiṣṭha-Dharmasūtra 23,1; Baudhāyana-Dharmasūtra 2,1,30–5). The main reason for the ass's connection with destruction and death is, I suspect, the habitat of the wild ass, the lifeless salt desert. Indeed, in the Dhenukavadha myth [...], the wild ass is compared to the god of death (Antaka). (Parpola and Janhunen 2011: 71)

Thurston, writing at the beginning of the twentieth century, informs us that: 'Ashes from the burial ground on which an ass has been rolling on a Saturday or Sunday, if thrown into the house of an enemy, are said to produce severe illness, if the house is not vacated' (1912: 242). In contemporary India, stories of asses used to parade women accused of witchcraft or adultery are fairly common, and are widely reported in national and international media.[57]

Second, in Indic folklore the ass is known for its sexual voraciousness, a feature that goes along with its traditional stupidity and stubbornness (*Pañcatantra* 112–13, 152–4; *Hitopadeśa* 140–142). Sexual appetites are unambiguously associated with illicit behaviour (Manu 8: 370):

> A student of the Veda who has broken his vow of chastity should offer an ass (gardabha-) (cf. Āpastamba-Dharmasūtra 1,26,8; Gautama-Dharmasūtra 23,17; Vasiṣṭha-Dharmasūtra 23,1) and in this sacrifice the cut-off portion to be eaten by the sacrificer should be taken from the penis of the ass (cf. Kātyāyana-Śrautasūtra 1,1,13 and 17; Baudhāyana-Dharmasūtra 2,1,30–5). The Manu-Smṛti (11,122–3) instead prescribes that the guilty student should for one year wear the skin of the ass and proclaim his lapse while begging for his food. (Parpola and Janhunen 2011: 70)

In general, the ass is a symbol of transgressive, and excessive, fertility. In AVŚ (6.72: 3) a spell to make one's penis grow like that of the ass is reported. In the *Maitrāyaṇīsaṃhitā* (3.1.6: 7, 16) 'the ass is the most virile animal of all' (Parpola 2004–5: 34), a perception possibly derived from its well-known sexual voracity (cf. ŚB 6.3.1: 23; also *Pañcatantra* above). This exuberance is confirmed by the observation that 'whilst being one, double impregnates' (i.e. the mare and the jenny) (ŚB 6.3.1: 22-23; cf. AB 4.9). In that, the ass represents the two lowest *varṇas*, namely *vaiśya* and *śūdra* (ŚB 6.4.4: 12).[58]

Third, the ass is a strong beast of burden and *de facto*, a disease carrier. This is emphatically rendered in Bengali theatrical *maṅgalpālās*, where the equid serves only to carry the goddess and her heavy load of poisoned pulses. Alternatively, when Śītalā attacks with virulent diseases, she: 1) sits on an ass while other beasts of burden (oxen) carry the poxes (KD.ŚMK. 252); 2) sits on an ass and marches toward her enemies followed by a horde of diseases in form of horrid ghouls or demons (MG. ŚMK. 3); and 3) holds herself the load of poxes in the crook of her arm (ibid.) before unleashing the pestilence (MG.ŚMK. 5: 72–74; J.ŚMK. 1).

It has been suggested that Śītalā rides a donkey, actually a jenny, for the animal produces the milk that in 'folk medicine' was used to placate the burning heat of smallpox patients (cf. Bang 1973: 86; Mukhopadhyay 1994: 25; Bhaṭṭācārya 1997: 155; Nalin 2004: 1741).[59] Historical records, however, are extraordinarily vague. Svami Nirmalānanda reports a passage from the *Bhaiṣajya Ratnāvalī* of Govindadāsa, a popular Bengali medical compendium, in which the burning pain of *sphoṭa* is countered by drinking the milk of a jenny (*gardabhīr dugdhapān*), as well as its urine (*mutra*) (1413BS: 80). Bhaṭṭācārya (1997: 155) even suggests this medicine is prescribed in a number of āyurvedic sources (none provided). In fact, descriptions of this practice are wanting in Indian literature. Vāgbhaṭa informs us that: 'The milk of single hoofed animals (like horse, donkey, etc.) [*ekaśapha kṣīra*] is very hot (in potency), cures vāta disorders localised in the śākhās, (blood and other tissues), is slightly sour and salt and causes lassitude (lazyness) [sic]' (AHS.Sū. 5: 26).[60] Why should a cold goddess be associated with such a hot substance? Why should Śītalā treat a hot disease (*visphoṭa*) with a hot remedy when the traditional approach is to lower body temperature? I argue that the ass-*vāhana* is symbolic of heat, unpredictability, excess, disorder and inauspiciousness. This is balanced, actually countered, by Śītalā, a goddess associated with cool waters and the refreshing seasonal rains.[61]

The original habitat and the behaviour of the ass are both revealing. We learn from Parpola that *gardabha* is a loan from Proto-Dravidian **kaẓutay*, a word whose meaning is 'kicker of the salt desert' (from **kaẓ(i)*, 'saline soil', and **utay*, 'to kick') (Parpola and Janhunen 2011: 74). Indian literature confirms this. The animal is associated with desert landscapes and is called a voracious drinker (RV 1.16: 5; 8.74: 7; HV 57, 16). Alternatively, the equid is known as *ciramehin*, the one that long urinates. This depends on the urinary system of the ass and its capacity to drink enormous quantities of water (even salty water) in a very short time (up to one hundred litres in less than ten minutes) (Parpola and Janhunen 2011: 84). The only animal with similar features is the Indian Wild Ass (*Equus hemionus khur*) or khur, an Anglicized form of the Sanskrit *khara* (a sub-species of the hemione). The animal, unlike the donkey (*Equus asinus*, a sub-species of *Equus africanus*), is a large equid[62] from the salty deserts of north-western India (Rajasthan and Gujarat), and it has not been domesticated.

These and other features of the ass must have impressed Indians. In Sanskrit, the ass is given names that qualify it for its loud and unpleasant bray (*rāsabha, upakroṣṭr̥, rūkṣasvara, khara*[63]), long ears (*karṇin, lambakarṇa*),[64] dusty reddish colour (*dhūsara, reṇurūṣita*), strong hooves (*nighr̥ṣva*), strength in carrying loads (*bhāraha, bhāravāhana*), sexual appetite (*ramaṇa, smarasmarya*), similarity to horses (*grāmya aśva*), or its mischievous and unpredictable temper (*daśeraka*). In north Indian languages, the equid is called by forms derived from Sanskrit *khara, rāsabha* and, more often, *gardabha* (e.g. B., H. and Bhp. *gādhā*; G. *gadhēḍō*). This seems to point to the loud nature of the ass (Skt. *gard*, 'to roar'; but cf. above). In fact, *gardabha* is also used to indicate a (non-specified) skin disease. This is attested as *gardabhaka* in, for instance, *Agnipurāṇa* 31: 36 (*doṣā jvālāgardabhakādayaḥ*), and indicates a failure/blemish (*doṣā*) caused by small worms or insects whose larvae are found in dung.[65] These 'small asses' are the cause of various skin conditions such as *jvālāgardabha* (the [blemish of the] burning ass) found in magic texts like the pre-eleventh century *Kriyākālaguṇottaratantra* (28) or the *Gardabhadvādaśanāma*.[66]

Conditions known as 'blazing ass' are found in early āyurvedic compendia, where they are treated as (minor) ulcerative skin diseases. Suśruta calls *jālagardabha* a skin ailment (*-gardabha*) involving muscular, vascular, ligamentous and bony tissue (*jāla*). This affliction is listed with, among others, *gardabhī* and *visphoṭaka* (eruptions) (SuS. Cik. 20: 6–7).[67] In particular, *gardabhī* is an affliction of the windy (*vāta*) and bilious (*pitta*) humours causing a 'circular, wide, raised, slightly reddish patch studded with small eruptions'[68] (AHS.Utt. 31: 10b), whereas *jāla gardabha* is described as a 'śopha (swelling) caused by all the doṣas with the predominance of pitta, spreading from place to place slowly, not undergoing pāka (suppuration/ulceration), coppery in colour and producing fever [...]'[69] (ibid.: 13b–14a).

It seems that the same name has been used to indicate the ass and a series of ulcerative conditions of the skin, including *visphoṭaka*. Significantly, *gardabha(ka)* signals sarcoids, tumours involving epithelial, muscular and connective tissue which frequently appear on donkeys. Sarcoids can reach considerable dimensions; they often ulcerate and bleed, like big smallpox pustules. Verrucous sarcoids, the most common on donkeys, often occur on the head, chest, shoulder and under-leg and, lacking hair, they are easy to spot. Although no specific cause has been identified, their growth mostly appears in spring (*vasanta*) and early summer, when smallpox used to break out in South Asia, and in concomitance with changes in diet, humidity, solar radiations, surface temperature, routine and the presence of insects and parasites. The much-feared 'spring fever' (*vasanta rog*) was, with all probability, a loose label for all kinds of seasonal ailments affecting humans and animals (e.g. pox viruses and herpes viruses). Such ailments were believed to be caused by the sun's rays and their most evident symptoms were skin ulcerations and high body temperature. In fact, most non-orthopox viral diseases are transmitted by insects such as hematophagous flies or worms. The latter, first attested in *Atharvaveda* as *kṛmi* (Zysk 1993: 63–9), are known as voracious beings whose activity is more noticeable in the spring season, before the monsoon. (It is worth noting that, in Apte's Sanskrit dictionary, the ass is called *kṛmi*.)[70]

In conclusion, the ass is known for its hot temper, strength, insatiable thirst, exaggerated sexual appetite and fondness of precious medicinal plants (e.g. *dūrva*; hence the name Dūrvākandanikṛntana). This is combined with its propensity to contract diseases whose symptoms cause visible ulcerations and/or deformation of the epidermis. It may thus be that the hot, ominous and disease-carrier ass was identified with some of the most dreaded ailments that only a cold goddess is capable of healing. With time, the scary *gardabha* has become, like in many other cultures, a stupid beast of burden and, when associated with Śītalā, an animal to feed, for it carries the welcome Cool Lady (but cf. ŚMKs, where it continues to carry poxes). As the following ethnographic vignette shows, Śītalā is always a controller (*adhiṣṭhātrī*). By riding – i.e. controlling – the ass, she shows her cooling power over dreadful occurrences (droughts, infertility, fevers and skin diseases) popularly interpreted as unnatural states of hotness.

Ethnographic vignette 4: Śrī Dakṣiṇī Ādi Śītalā (Buṛhiyā Māī) Mandir, Banaras (Uttar Pradesh)

The central temple of the goddess Śītalā in Banaras is located on Śītalā Ghāṭ, contiguous to one of the city's most important and busy *ghāṭs*, Dāsāśvamedha Ghāṭ.[71] Śītalā Ghāṭ was developed in the first half of the eighteenth century, at the same time as the Dāsāśvamedha Ghāṭ is said to have been made *pakkā* (H. 'cooked,' i.e. made of bricks). The temple is presumably of the same period (Śaṅkar 1996: 78, 208). Visited on a daily basis by local devotees (chiefly Hindi-, Bhojpuri- and Bengali-speakers) from all *jātis*, the temple is included in the *pancakrośīyātrā*, thus attracting thousands of pilgrims from all across India and beyond.[72] The current *mahant* of the temple, Śrī Śiv Prasād Paṇḍey is assisted in his role by his son and a series of aides hired in various capacities. The Paṇḍeys belong to a powerful *gotra* (family) and are practitioners of the *śākta* tantric Śrīvidyā tradition.

The Dakṣiṇī Śītalā Mandir hosts various *mūrtis* of the goddess. The main one is centrally located, and faces the river Ganges. The *pratimā*, facing east, is a small golden head richly adorned with heavy garlands, *nīm* leaves and red drapes. The goddess sports a crown, and has large eyes. Her forehead is dotted with a large red *ṭīkā* and her lips are smeared with *sindūr*. In front of the main altar, on the bottom left corner, there is a small black stone tablet with Śītalā in bas-relief. (The image is very difficult to notice. It is regularly covered with flowers and one must lean onto

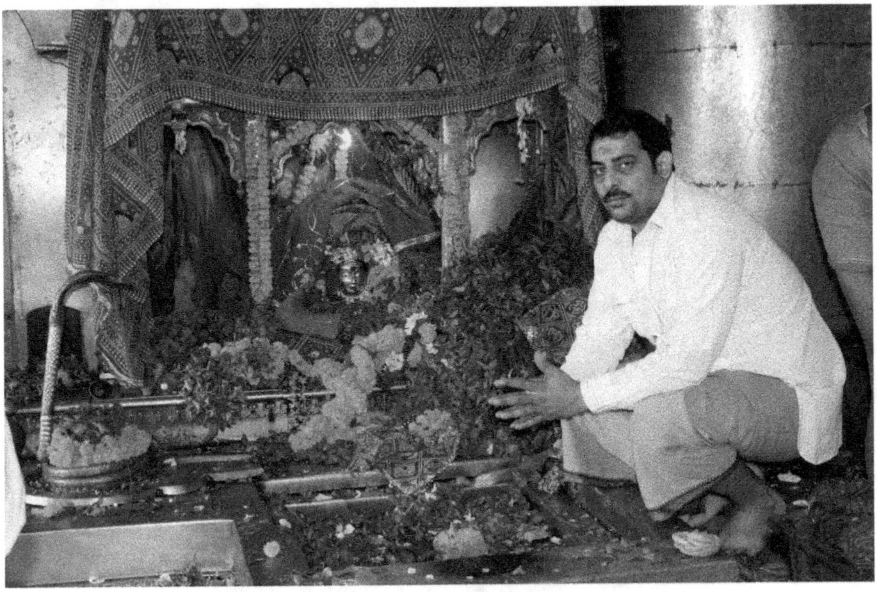

FIGURE 2.18 *Śrī Avināś Paṇḍey at Śrī Dakṣiṇī Ādi Śītalā Mandir, Banaras (photo by author).*

the goddess's sanctum to appreciate it.) This *pratimā* adheres to standard iconography. Śītalā is naked, rides a donkey, is crowned with a tiara and has four arms, each holding a different tool: *kalsā* (lower left), *jhāṛū* (upper right), *śūrpa* (upper left) and what seems to be a lotus flower (lower right). At the back of the temple there are other images. One is external to the main structure and enclosed in a small cage. Through the bars, one can admire a very small but vivid representation of the goddess riding her *vāhana*. Śītalā is naked and four-armed. This particular stone tablet is noteworthy for the goddess has bulging eyes, bright red lips and lolling tongue – a feature traditionally ascribed to Kālī. The lower left arm holds, instead of a lotus, what looks like a dagger. The last Śītalā *mūrti* is found in relief on a (recent) rectangular golden panel to the rear of the temple. The goddess sits on an ass, is richly dressed and has protruding eyes. Her neck is garlanded and she wears a big crown. At her feet, on the left, one can admire a series of very small black stone tablets from a pre-existing structure. Two are figurines of Śītalā. In both instances, the four-armed goddesses – whose facial traits have been completely eroded – are riding an ass, are naked and plump, and sport the same tools as in the above images.

One more *pratimā* is kept in the temple complex. This is worshipped in the *guphā* (H. 'cave', 'grotto') below the *mandir*, and faces south. In order to access the hidden chamber of Śrī Dakṣiṇī Ādi Śītalā, devotees (*upāsak*) are requested to enter through a small door in front of the Ganges. *Guphā darśana* is given every other Tuesday, or on

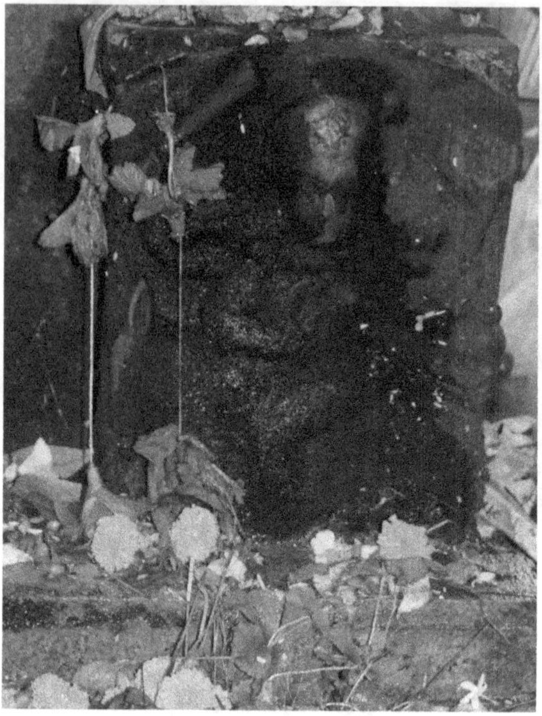

FIGURE 2.19 *Particular, Śrī Dakṣiṇī Ādi Śītalā Mandir, Banaras (photo by author).*

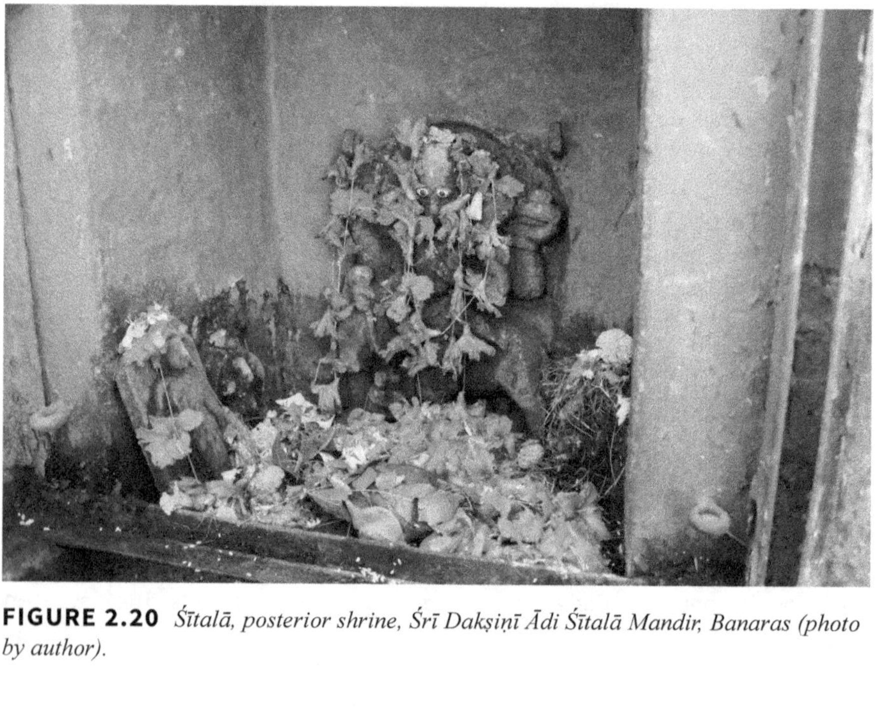

FIGURE 2.20 *Śītalā, posterior shrine, Śrī Dakṣiṇī Ādi Śītalā Mandir, Banaras (photo by author).*

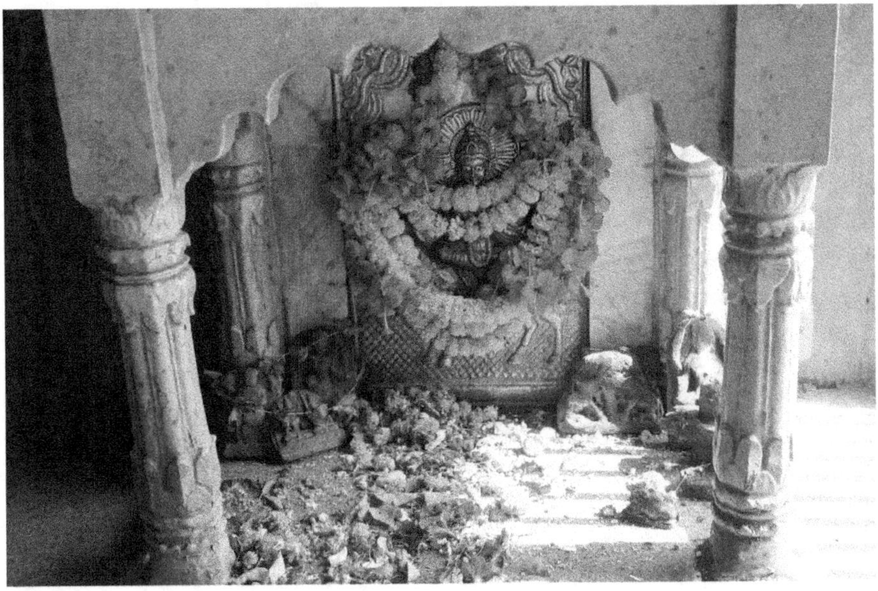

FIGURE 2.21 *Śītalā, posterior shrine, Śrī Dakṣiṇī Ādi Śītalā Mandir, Banaras (photo by author).*

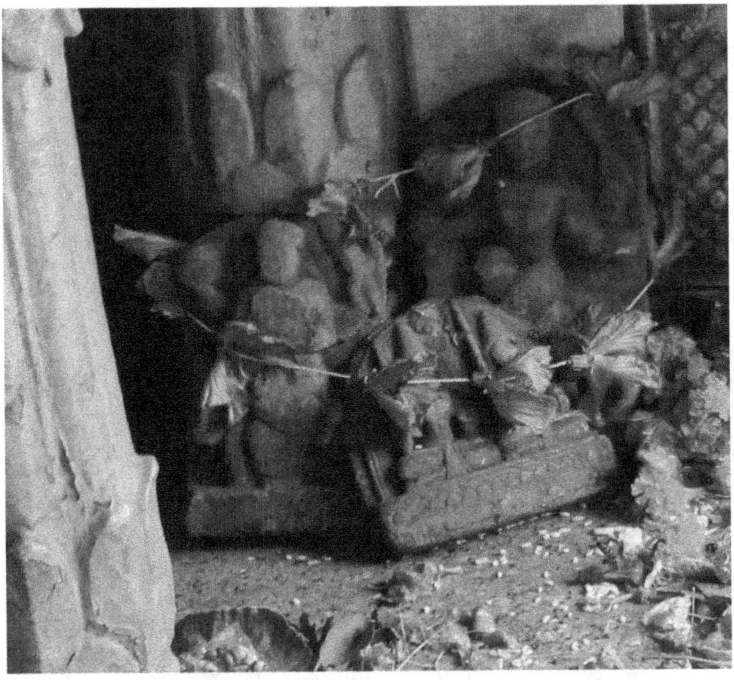

FIGURE 2.22 *Śītalā* pratimās, *particular, posterior shrine, Śrī Dakṣiṇī Ādi Śītalā Mandir, Banaras (photo by author).*

auspicious days (the celebration of *aṣṭamī* and *navarātrī*), from 6:00 to 11:00 and from 16:00 to 21:30.

The *guphā* is advertised as a sacred shrine where many *sādhus*, *svāmis* and *mahātmas* endured austerities (*tapasyā*) and meditated with firm mind (*sādhana*). On entering, the names of the *mahants* of the temple are listed on the right wall. The chain begins with Svāmī Avimakteśvarānand – the first of the *gotra* – and is followed by Svāmi Śrī Bhīm Rām Paṇḍey, who was given the title of Līṅgīyā[73] by Dārā Śikoh (1615–59), son of Mughal Emperor Śāh Jahān (1592–1666).[74] The Liṅgīyā title has then been transmitted to all the following *mahants*: Ātmārām, Dayārām,[75] Prabhunāth, Kanhaiyā, Parameśvar Prasād, Sūraj Prasād, Mahādev Prasād, Bhavānī Śaṅkar, the current *mahant* Śrī Śiv Prasād Paṇḍey and his elder son, Śrī Avināś Paṇḍey. A large wooden board presents the *guphā* as the site of the meditations of influential and charismatic figures such as Śrī Lāhiṛī Bābā (1828–95),[76] Tailaṅg Svāmī (d. 1887),[77] Svāmi Karpātrī (1905–80),[78] Svāmī Svarūpānanda Sarasvatī (b. 1924),[79] Bābā Kīnārām (b. 1601),[80] Avadhūt Bhagavān Rām (1937–92)[81] and others.

The grotto evokes tantric imagery. On the yellow-painted outer doors and on the white marble internal walls are painted in bright red *bījamantras*, e.g. *hrīṃ*, *hlīṃ*, *kriṃ*, *baṃ*, *śrīṃ*, etc. Upon entrance, a devotee pays homage to a large image of Ādi Kāla Bhairava Nātha. The *mūrti* is covered with a red cloth and surrounded by many *rudrākṣa mālas*. Only the face is discernible. The three-eyed moustached Bhairõ – as he is called in the local parlance – wears a richly decorated crown and two large earrings. Both his crown and eyes are pitted with gems. At the feet of the god is his loyal black dog. The animal is large and stands on an ochre-painted stone pedestal, on the edge of which is a pair of wooden-soled sandals. At the centre of the pedestal there is a triangular-shaped cavity hosting a human skull. To the left of Bhairõ, there is a small *mūrti* of Kālī.

Proceeding to the right, there is an icon of Maṅgal Gaurī standing on a niche hosting a *liṅga*. She is surrounded by *bījamantras*, and a huge human skull is painted on the wall. Finally, following the increasingly narrow tunnel, the devotee reaches the chamber of Śītalā. There is an anthropomorphic brass image of the goddess sitting on a white marble throne whose legs are lion paws. The back of the seat is richly decorated; on its top there is a huge *śrīyantra*. Śītalā is in full regalia. She wears precious jewellery, garlands and richly decorated clothes. The goddess holds a broom in her right hand, and a pitcher is positioned in the crook of her left arm. Her feet hang suspended at a short distance from the back of a miniature donkey. The syllables *auṃ* (right), *hrīṃ* (left) and *śrīṃ* (below) surround the goddess, along with the *mūrtis* of other deities, i.e. from left to right: Kālī, Kālaratrī, Rudraśaṅkara (Śiva), Kālī, Durgā and Hanumān (the latter stands above the names of Rāma and Sītā). Various brass *nāgas* (snakes) and marble tigers adorn the spot. On the left side of the chamber a series of steps lead down to the *rurdasarovar* (Rudra's pond, the ancient name of the *tīrtha* now known as Dāsāśvamedha Ghāṭ). The *sarovar* is symbolically rendered by means of a small square basin into which devotees throw water, milk, yogurt, ghee, rice,

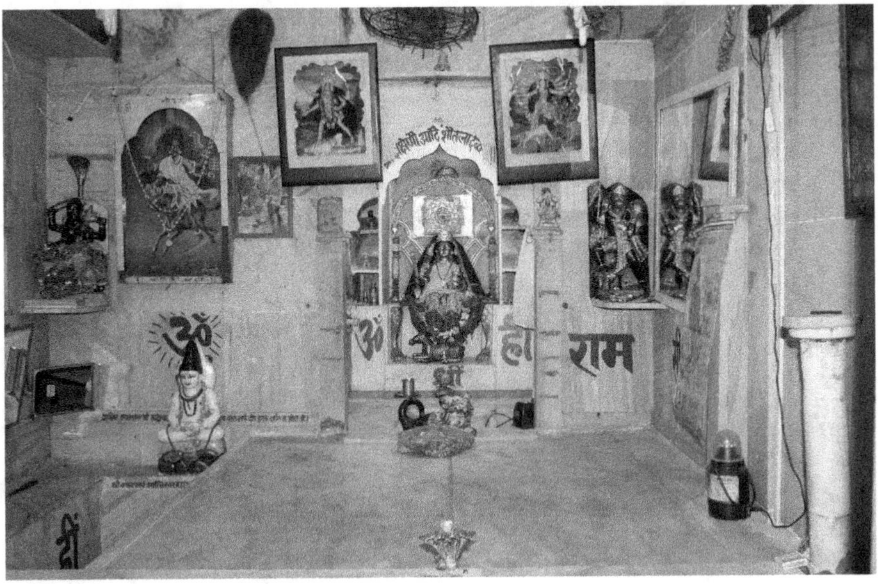

FIGURE 2.23 *Śrī Dakṣiṇī Ādi Śītalā, grotto, Śrī Dakṣiṇī Ādi Śītalā Mandir, Banaras (photo by author).*

clothes, money, fruits and various libations (*dhār*) in order to ask the goddess to fulfil their vows (*manautī*). The space is even more limited. It is impossible to stand and no more than two persons can stay. Śītalā is identified with Kālarātrī ('*bhagavatī śītalā hī kālarātrī haiñ*', ŚVK 4). This is confirmed by the *pūjā* performed with great pomp on the seventh day of *navaratrī* (i.e. the day of Kālarātrī), when Śītalā is meditated upon using the Kālarātrī *dhyānamantra*:

> She has one braid, china roses around the ears, she is naked, rides an ass, has big lips and ears and the body besmeared with sesame oil. On her left side, she sports a weapon made of iron thorns, [wears] a necklace [and holds] a head-chopper. O fearsome black Kālarātrī. (ŚVK 4)

The *kharasthitā* (ass-riding) Kālarātrī does not pass onto Śītalā her intimidating features. Rather, she magnifies the power to destroy chaos, disease and misfortune of the Cold Lady – a pattern that continues to be spectacularly rendered by means of controlling the unruly and scary ass. Ultimately, she conveys auspiciousness.

Besides women who meet on a daily basis to sing for the goddesses worshipped in the temple, the *mandir* is a popular venue for devotees of all ages, genders and backgrounds, particularly newlyweds. Śītalā is a remover of obstacles. The *Śrī Dakṣiṇī Ādi Śītalā (Buṛhiyā Māī) kā māhātmya* (ŚVK 3–5) says that the goddess protects from any illness, fever, nightmare, enemy, fear, bad encounters and ill fortune. Serving Śrī Śītalā or visualizing and meditating on the *śrīyantra* is mandatory to obtain joy (*sukha*), wealth (*sammpadā*), prosperity (*aiśvarya*), a long-living son (*putra dīrghāyu*), wellbeing (*ārogyatā*), health (*svāsthya*) and a safe environment (*paryāvaraṇ*). Devotees ask the goddess to cast her auspicious glance over their business, to grant fortune and glory and to give them *mokṣa*. The *māhātmya* indicates how to achieve all this. One should meditate on the *śrīyantra* and obtain *darśana* of the goddess. Ill persons should lie or sit in front of the image of Buṛhiyā Māī while the *pūjārī* will cut a lime (*nimbū*) and let its juice drop seven times in the small pool in the grotto. Alternatively, one can pour *gaṅgājal* seven times from a small pot (*loṭā*). The text repeatedly and unambiguously states that no *darśana*, *pūjā*, *vrata*, *yajña*, etc. is valid without the presence of the *guru*, the *mahant* or a *pūjārī*. The authority of Śītalā and her capacity to heal and to fulfil desires strictly depend on the presence of Brahman ritual specialists, and, naturally, on *dakṣiṇā*, the mandatory sacrificial fee. The first part of the *māhātmya* confirms this unequivocally. The goddess – the text explains – is actually called Dakṣiṇī Śītalā because in order to enjoy the fruit of one's offering or to be given *darśana*, the *dakṣiṇā* must be paid ('*ataḥ dakṣiṇī Śītalā kā darśan kar dakṣiṇā avaśya caṛhāvẽ*', ŚVK 3). The *māhātmya* further indicates that men are the right (*dakṣiṇa*) and women the left (*vāmā*). Once the left is victorious over the right, i.e. by worshipping in the proper way and paying the ritual fee, the goddess dispenses ultimate liberation (*mahāmokṣa*) in the form of Dakṣiṇī Śītalā. Eventually the goddess is the ultimate Śakti. Being equated to the ass-riding Kālarātrī does not transform Śītalā into an *ugra devī*. In fact, she is made part of an established order that expresses itself through sacred time (the celebration of *navarātrī*), sacred geography (the *pancakrośīyātrā*) and, ultimately, an epiphany of the sacred *per se* (Kālarātrī, the seventh Durgā).

Concluding remarks

The study of the iconography of Śītalā across north India confirms: a) her cold, auspicious, benign and protective nature; b) the lack of a disease-inflicting side; and c) her multiform and simultaneous presence. She is a welcomed goddess who, ultimately, grants liberation. In her most distinguishable aspect, she is the controller of disorder, a performance visually rendered by the action of riding the ass, a wild, unpredictable, thirsty animal associated with inauspiciousness, impurity, excess as well as dangerous and scarring ailments. But Śītalā is not just a controller. She is a destroyer and a remover of impurities, a task she completes with her broom, and a healer, who cools down the heat of her children with cold water and her winnowing fan. When Tiwari says that goddesses like Dhūmāvatī, Jyeṣṭhā, Kālarātri and Mahāmārī 'have collectively contributed to the formulation of Śītalā [...]' (Tiwari 1996: 455–6), he is eventually right. But, I argue, this 'formulation' is one dependent on narratives that have little in common with Śītalā *bhakti*. Textual investigation, study of material culture and extensive fieldwork show how Śītalā has been worshipped by her devotees: a form of control over injustice, unevenness and decay.

Notes

1 Temples hosting Śītalā in the form of *śilā* are ubiquitous in India. I am thankful to the *pūjārī*s and devotees of the small eighteenth-century Śītalā Mātā Mandir in Barkat Nagar, Tonk Phatak (Jaipur, Rajasthan), who, back in 1999, introduced me to this iconography.

2 This pattern is in no way specific of Śītalā. A number of male and female deities present virtually the same features. I observed this in West Bengal, where gods like Śiva (in his various manifestations, e.g. Pañcānan, Buṛa Ṭhākur, Nīleśvara, Kṣetrapāla, etc.), Dharmarāj, Śanibābā, etc. and goddesses like Caṇḍī, Manasā, Ṣaṣṭhī, Olā Bibi, Kālī, Ban Bibi, etc. are worshipped in this form.

3 This is also mentioned in Auboyer and De Mallmann 1950: 226. Minsky (2009: 167) reports the same names and signals Bhatti (2000: 134) as her source. Bhatti's list is identical to Crooke's, but it seems to be attributed to Rose (1919).

4 In several seven sister shrines, the actual number of stones or pitchers varies from a few units to more than a dozen. The seven sisters are more a collective name rather than an arithmetical concept. Further, it is not unusual to learn of *pūjārī*s who add stones as a sign of greater power of the shrine (Gold 2008: 167).

5 During my fieldwork I realized that informants often do not know, or do not remember, the names of all the seven goddesses. The icons may be collectively called Śītalā, or are addressed as manifestations of more popular goddesses (Caṇḍī, Kālī, Durgā, etc.). A similar case is discussed in Babb 1975: 129. Also cf. Freed and Freed (1988: 124): 'No single villager gave us a complete list of the Seven Sisters of disease. Usually, an informant would name three or four, sometimes identifying a specific disease with the wrong mother goddess, for example, Kanti Mata (typhoid) might be confused with Shitala (smallpox).'

6 On the seven sisters in West Bengal, see Basu 1405 BS: 93–5. Śītalā is not mentioned.

7 The worship of Śītalā as one of the seven sisters is found among Hindus outside Asia. For instance, in Suriname, Śītalā is listed along with 'Chuṭkī or Khelnī Kūdnī, Phūlmatī, Dhamsā, Ākāsgāminī or Jogjatī, Masānī and Koṛhiniyā' (Arya 1968: 25).

8 In the nineteenth and early twentieth centuries, when smallpox ravaged across north India, the temple was regularly scrutinized by the vaccinators of the IMS (see the report of Dr A. Ross, dated 4 April 1850, in RSC cixxii–cixxvii).

9 The site is also popular among businessmen who travel from all destinations to take advantages of Gurgaon markets, outlets and business facilities. A group of Gujarati entrepreneurs told me they regularly visit the temple in advance of business transactions to ask the goddess for good fortune (H. *kalyāṇ*; conversation in Hindi).

10 Ritual specialists in the temple are male Brahmans. However, on different occasions, I saw a Brahman woman coordinating *pūjā*.

11 This is different from the formal *cuḍākaraṇa*, the first head-shave, a compulsory rite of passage (*saṃskāra*) performed – often with great pomp – on the third year of the infant by a Brahman ritualist.

12 A huge board outside the *muṇḍan khānā* confirms this. It reads: *tathā baccõ kī lambī āyu ke lie muṇḍan karvāye jātẽ hai.*

13 Asterisks indicate a word has been used in English by informants.

14 Lalitā, also known as Ṣodāśī or Tripurasundarī, is traditionally one of the *dāsamahāvidya*. The list includes: Kālī, Tārā, Ṣodāśī, Bhuvaneśvarī, Bhairavī, Chinnamastā, Dhūmāvatī, Bagalāmukhī, Mātaṅgī and Kamalā.

15 The original temple founded by Siṅgh (alt. spell. Siṃha) is believed to be a small shrine near the Aravalli Biodiversity Park, 9 kilometres east of Masani Village. In some local narratives, Masānī is the main goddess and Śītalā her little sister/helper.

16 This story has been reconstructed from three similar oral narratives. I am not aware of any text reporting it. The names of the two kings are not mentioned by my informants. All of them, however, refer to Najīb Khān (i.e. Najīb ad-Dawlah) as the antagonist. This detail permitted the identification of the *rājkumār* (prince) and the *mahārāj* (the king) with, respectively, Javāhar Siṃha and Surāj Māl. It is worth noting that in this narrative the disease element is lacking.

17 A passing reference to this myth in found only in Rose 1916: 350.

18 Crooke informs us that in the village of Raiwala, south of Rishikesh (Dehra Dhun district, UP), Śītalā is identified, and worshipped, as Gāndhārī, the wife of Dṛtarāṣṭra – father of the Kauravas: 'When Dhritarâshtra, through the force of his divine absorption, was consumend with fire at Sapta-srota, near Hardwâr, Gândhâri also jumped into the fire and became Satî with her husband. Then, in recognition of her piety, the gods blessed her with a boon that in the Iron Age [presumably *kaliyuga*] she should become the guardian deity of children and the goddess of small-pox in particular' (Crooke 1978: 127, I).

19 A big banner in the courtyard of the temple says: *mātā śītalā devī ke pavitr tālāb kī miṭṭī nikālne se mānokāmanāe pūrṇa ho jātī hae* (H. 'By digging the sand of the sacred pond of Mother Goddess Śītalā, [all] desires are fulfilled').

20 Bhatti's report seems to have been taken almost verbatim from the description of Mātaṅgī/Masānī Devī found in Rose (1919: 354).

21 One of the largest temples I visited in Punjab is the Prācīn Śītalā Mātā Mandir (Śrī Durgayāṇā Tīrtha) of Amritsar. The temple, erected on a shrine dating back to roughly the fourteenth century, is a large building hosting the *mūrti*s of many pan-Hindu deities. In its present form, it bears witness to the worship of Śiva-Śakti. The *mūrti* of Śītalā, an anthropomorphic non-equestrian icon, diverges greatly with Bhatti's report.

22 The *śūrpa* is occasionally substituted with a *camar* (a flywhisk obtained from bovine tails), a ritual implement used widely across India to fan *mūrti*s. Hāphij (1978: 94) reports from Bangladesh that in rural areas married women used to dance in front of it to encourage the protective power of the goddess over their children.

23 White, as per the *dhyānamantra* of PiT (see below p. 186), is extremely rare. Surprisingly, colours traditionally associated with heat (various tones of red) are used for *pratimā*s. They are indicative of power – rather than rage (Beck 1969: 554).

24 Michael Meister, email communication, 31/12/2013.

25 The panel is regularly covered with *sindūr*, flowers, *nīm* leaves, *mauli*s and marigold garlands, thus making an examination difficult.

26 I first attended the pilgrimage in February 2012 and again the following year. The data gathered here is obtained from both visits.

27 Shri Chatterjee is an advocate and runs a marriage registration office in the room on the left of the shrine. He is helped in the administration of the temple by his wife and son.

28 In their 1986 documentary film on the rites in Salkia ('Sitala in Spring'), Elder and Sarkar mention 22 Śītalās.

29 Temple address: 23, Shri Aurobindo Road, Salkia, Howrah.

30 The *mandir* is a community temple located at 21, Bairagi Para Lane, Salkia, Howrah.

31 Temple address: 64, Shambhu Haldar Lane, Salkia, Howrah.

32 A similar arrangement is found at the Śrī Śrī Śani Mandir, a small shrine run by *sevāit*s from Odisha located near Banda Ghat where a ferry service to Ahiritola Launch Ghat in Kolkata stops. Here the cephalomorphic icon of Śītalā is positioned to the right of Śani. This *mūrti* is not paraded during the pageant (see Figure 2.17).

33 A log of wood fixed to a pivot, the husking pedal is a working tool used by women to crush the outer shell of paddy, pulses and grain. In Bengali folk culture, it appears in legends of Dharmarāj – a local sun god – where it is the vehicle of sage Nārada. The *ḍheñkimaṅgal* is a fertility motif sung by women (today very rarely). A version of the *ḍheñkimaṅgal* is found in Rāmāi Paṇḍit's *Śūnyapurāṇa* (78: 4), a Bengali text celebrating Dharmarāj. For fertility rituals and dances (*ḍheñkipūjā*), see my notes in Ferrari 2010a: 92–3. The husking pedal is also mentioned as Nārada's mount in MG.ŚMK. 9: 169–72.

34 Devotees traditionally ask for offspring, health, good crops, healthy cattle, timely rains and, more generally, wealth. This culture is still popular, and it is not unusual for younger generations to offer clay animals for achievements related to social advancement or economic gain (e.g. job interviews, university exams, new business ventures, etc.).

35 I observed snakes, owls, frogs, tortoises and geese in Bengali *grāmyer thanas* disseminated across the Rāṛh region.

36 In Mahesana district, precisely in Bhatta Paldi, there is a large Śītalā Mātā Mandir dated circa 1150. The temple, decorated with panels representing various gods and goddesses, does not host any icon of Śītalā but confirms her worship was not a phenomenon solely associated with village culture.

37 Cf. Abhayatilakagaṇi's commentary to Hemacandra's *Dvyāśrayakāvya* (7: 43) and the note in *Prabandhacintāmaṇi* (20) of Merutuṅga Ācārya.

38 Small statuettes are also found in the Archaeological Museum of Amer (Jaipur, Rajasthan), datable from the eleventh and twelfth centuries, and in the Musée Guimet, Paris (France), circa late twelfth century (Auboyer and De Mallmann 1950). Tiwari mentions statues of Śītalā from Tamil Nadu (1996: 457–9). I did not find evidence of this information.

39 The worship of Śītalā in the Pāla epoch is confirmed by a twelfth-century inscription of King Yakṣa Pāla who indicates a large Śītalā Mandir in Gaya. This, however, has not been confirmed archaeologically.

40 The label 'Śavara' is used across Indian texts as a cumulative term for *anārya* (non-Ārya) clans, or to specifically indicate the Saoras, a Munda-speaking large *ādivāsī* group of eastern India.

41 Hayagrīva is still associated with fevers and is worshipped in tantric Buddhism as a protector.

42 Jinah Kim has convincingly examined analogies between Śītalā and 'the tenth century images of yoginīs, especially those from Kancipuram in Tamil Nadu' (Kim 2013: 12). She further notes that '[…] one yoginī image from the Kanci set now in the Freer Gallery, Washington D.C., holds a broom and a winnower basket, the distinctive domestic tools associated with Śītalā's controlling power over smallpox as she sweeps and sifts the lentil-like smallpox. Another yoginī now in the Minneapolis Museum holds a dispenser and what seems to be a medicine jar. The full-bodied figure of the winnow and broom-bearing yoginī seems much distanced from the gaunt appearance of Śītalā, but in the same set of yoginīs we also find a similarly gaunt image with pendulant breast and haggard neck. The loose spraying hairdo in the yoginī image from Guimet [Museum, in Paris] is also comparable to the hair of the Bengali Śītalā image.' (ibid: 12–13)

43 I am thankful to Jinah Kim for sharing her thoughts on structural similarities between Cāmuṇḍā and the ass-riding Śītalās on the Dhaka Parṇaśavarī steles (also cf. Kim 2013: 7–14).

44 Kālīghāṭ painters initially recreated in a unique blend of Bengali and Western style episodes from the *purāṇas* and *maṅgalkāvyas*. Impressions of gods and goddesses were initially bought as souvenirs. With the consolidation of the market, artists obtained success among the British too. They portrayed various vignettes, including stories of saints, scenes of ordinary life, renditions of news from the local press and portrayals of animals, plants as well as customers (Jain 1999).

45 Shuvaprasanna Bhattacharya (b. 1947) is a Bengali artist initially associated to the 'Calcutta Painters'. His works have been exhibited all across the world. The series *Icons and Illusions* has been particularly successful for its originality and distinctive lyricism.

46 Shuvaprasanna, email communication, 20/07/2013.

47 An earlier version of this section has been published in Ferrari 2013.

48 The words 'ass' and 'donkey' are nowadays used interchangeably. However they were not synonyms. The term 'donkey' was originally a slang word to indicate a domesticated 'ass'.

49 See also the devotional movie *Śītalā Mātā*, when food offerings and blessing *ṭīkā* are given by women to a donkey (and a dog). The sequence can be found at the end of the movie, during the song *Suno suno jī* (H. 'Listen, listen!').

50 The only exceptions are works not immediately available to Western readers, i.e. Agrvāl (1958) and Paṇḍey Ārya (2037 VS) in Hindi, and Svami Nirmalānanda (1413 BS) in Bengali. Jinah Kim has recently presented a paper that, so far, is the most insightful problematization of the ass *vāhana* in the iconography of Śītalā. I am thankful to her for many informative conversations.

51 Translated by Parpola (2004–5: 33).

52 In contemporary Hinduism, Jyeṣṭhā overlaps with other inauspicious goddesses, such as Alakṣmī (see below) and Dhumāvatī ('Smokey'), the widow goddess. See also Mūtēvī ('Elder Goddess'), a Southern variant of Jyeṣṭhā. She represents ill fortune, discord and disease and is worshipped along with her younger sister Śrīdevī (fortune and prosperity). The goddess rides an ass, is dark-complexioned and holds a banner with the image of a crow (Sonnerat 1782: 160; Shulman 1989: 51).

53 Mahākālī is a protector, but in times of adversity she is a destroyer associated with ill-fortune and pestilence (*mahāmārīsvarūpa*) (DM 12: 38–41).

54 I am thankful to Joyce Flueckiger for informing that in Chhattisgarhi plains there are many such images (and for sharing some). Joyce Flueckiger, email communication, 16/05/2013.

55 *Śanimāhātmya, pradhanakarma*, in Svoboda 1997: 87–8.

56 The kiang (*Equus Kiang*, formerly known as *Equus hemionus kiang*), or Tibetan Wild Ass, is indigenous of the Tibetan Plateau, but is also found in Ladakh, Jammu and Kashmir and Nepal.

57 See the reports in *Times of India* 2009 and *Thaindian News* 2009.

58 Excessive fertility has possibly informed the practice of celebrating donkey marriages to call for rain in times of drought (Kattimani 2011; BBC 2003).

59 The business of donkey's milk in the subcontinent is still thriving, as this ingredient continues to be used as a remedy for skin eruptions and fevers. In 2001, the Department of Chemistry at the University of Lucknow was working on a project sponsored by the Uttar Pradesh Council of Science and Technology on the immuno-stimulant properties of donkey's milk. Clinical trials have been carried out in association with the Sanjay Gandhi Postgraduate Institute of Medical Science and the Central Drug Research Institute (ToI 2001).

60 Translated by K. R. Shrikantha Murthy.

61 This is paralleled in Vedic culture, where the Aśvin twins, the divine physicians, ride (control) asses. Unlike the Aśvins and Śītalā, all other ass-riding goddesses have a distinguished dangerous side and disease-inflicting nature.

62 In MG.ŚMK, Śītalā is seated on an ass, 'whose gait is like that of the Greatest among Elephants' (Nicholas 2003: 150).

63 *Khara* is in all probability an onomatopoeic noun.

64 Rau notes that: '*Equus hemionus* does possess shorter ears than *Equus asinus*' (2012: 991), the latter – donkey – being known as *karṇa* ('ear').

65 Cf. Monier-Williams's translation of *gardabhaka* as 'a cutaneous disease' (eruption of round, red, and painful spots) (1997: 349). On such basis I would attempt an alternative etymology: *garda-* 'crying' but also 'voracious' + OIA animal name suffix *-bha* and the diminutive suffix *-ka*, that is 'tiny hungry animals'.

66 The *Kriyākālaguṇottaratantra* has a chapter on treating the skin disease (*jvālāgardabha*) and it names twelve *gardabhas*: Kapila, Gaura, Mṛtyukāla, Piṅgala, Vijaya, Kalahapriya, Kumbhakarṇa, Vibhīṣaṇa, Candravaktra, Śveta, Kharadūṣaṇa, and Hiḍimba. This text, however, does not mention Śītalā. Conversely, the goddess is invoked as a protector in *Gardabhadvādaśanāma*, a single folio manuscript from the Nepal–German Manuscript Preservation Project (NGMPP H 334/24), where the names of the ass are given as per ŚAS 83–5. The manuscript bears no date, but it is likely to be no older than two hundred years. I am thankful to Michael Slouber for passing this material (Slouber, email communication, 05/06/2013).

67 A description of *jālagardabha* is given in SuS.Ni. 13: 13–17. Another pustular affliction of the *gardabha* type is *pāṣāṇagardabha*, a hard swelling (Skt. *pāṣāṇa*, 'stone') on the jaw which may suppurate. This too is considered *kṣudraroga* (cf. SuS.Ni. 13: 12 and SUS.Cik. 20: 5). Suśruta calls *kīṭagardabhaka* a class of dangerous insects that may cause serious illness (SuS.Ka. 8: 11).

68 Translated by K. R. Shrikantha Murthy.

69 Translated by K. R. Shrikantha Murthy.

70 Asses, employed for heavy work in the heat of the sun, are one of the main victims not just of 'worms' but of *Trypanosoma evansi*, a blood infection known as surra and transmitted via hematophagous flies. The symptoms of surra are high fever, fatigue, respiratory deficiency, anaemia, emaciation and lethargy. If untreated, case fatality rate in equines is near 100 per cent. Other symptoms of surra are very similar to *gardabha(ka)*. They include petechial haemorrhages, hydrothorax, ascites and enlarged lymph nodes (OIE 2009).

71 Shrines of Śītalā are disseminated in Banaras (Giri et al. n.d.: 75; Zeiler 2008: 162–8), and it is not unusual to see new *pratimā*s installed in temples (Keul 2012: 394 on Śītalā in Ātmavīreśvara Mandir).

72 The temple is the site where the righteous King Divodāsa installed the Daśāśvamedheśvara Liṅga (KKh 43–64).

73 Accomplished *yogin* who dedicated his life to learning and teaching *yoga*.

74 *Guphā kā prācīn itihās*, ŚVK 6–7.

75 Paṇḍit Dayārām Paṇḍey was conferred the title of *caudharī* (custodian) by the *pūjārī*s of all the temples of Kāśī (ŚVK 6).

76 Popularly known as Kāśī Bābā, he was a householder *yogin* originally from Krishnanagar (Nadia district, WB). He is associated with the practice of *krya yoga* to which initiated men and women from all social classes and religious backgrounds. He is known in the West for he is mentioned in Paramahansa Yogananda's *Autobiography of a Yogi.*

77 Originally from Andhra Pradesh, Tailaṅg (or Trailaṅg) Svāmī sojourned in Varanasi between 1737 and 1887. He was well known for his *siddhi* and longevity. A member of the Daśanāmi monastic *saṃpradāya*, he is remembered as the 'walking Śiva of Varanasi'.

78 The founder of the traditionalist Akhil Bhāratīya Rām Rājya Pariṣad (lit. 'All India Council of Rama's Kingdom').

79 A fighter for independence involved in the 'Quit India' movement, Svāmī Svarūpānanda Sarasvatī is the *mahant* of the Paścimāmnāya Maṭha in the Dwarka Pīṭha (Gujarat), one of the four monasteries founded by Ādi Śaṅkarācārya (eighth century CE). He became president of the Akhil Bhāratīya Rām Rājya Pariṣad and in 1982 he was officialized as the Śaṅkarācārya of Dwarka.

80 The founder of the Aghori tantric order. Aghorācārya Bābā Kīnārām, who is supposed to have lived for around 150 years, is believed to have been an incarnation of Śiva.

81 An Aghori saint and a social reformer.

3

Hosting Mā, feeding Mā. Controversies around *Śītalāpūjā*

Representations of Śītalā in Indian literature and material culture show that the goddess has been consistently worshipped as a protector and a healer. With the exception of the ŚMKs, where Śītalā is aggressive and disease-inflicting, the goddess is confirmed as a motherly figure who heals children, destroys disease (and the fear thereof) and assists women (particularly mothers) in their altruistic struggle to care for families. Her worship is functional to spread basic hygienic norms, but in purāṇic and purāṇic-derived texts, her power stretches to spiritual cleansing. The goddess is invoked to have sins (Skt. *pāpa*)[1] removed and to obtain *mokṣa*.

Textual sources are limited. The *Śītalāṣṭakastotra*, allegedly extrapolated from SkP, is found variously edited in *Bhāvaprakāśa*, *Picchilātantra* and a number of late-modern and contemporary texts across genres and territories. The *Picchilātantra*, though a minor text, is important in that it sets ritual *vidhi* (rules) in Bengal. Here we find unambiguous information about mandatory animal sacrifice (Skt. *balidāna*; B. *balidān*).[2] In fact, notwithstanding its popularity, especially in *śākta* contexts, *balidān* is a matter of social dispute. A growing number of Indians are unhappy about the slaughter of innocent beings on the occasion of religious festivals, and vociferously question the ethics of such manifestations of devotion. Animal sacrifice, however, is not the only contested practice. The worship of Śītalā includes a series of services (*sevā*) that increasingly meet the resistance, or dislike, of many, both in India and abroad.

In the following pages, I discuss animal sacrifice (*balidān*, or *paśubali*),[3] devotional possession and austerities. In particular, I examine objections to such practices as dependent upon class conflict. The goddess continues to enjoy enormous popularity among the peasantry and various working class sectors. But Śītalā is also an established presence among the educated and wealthy middle and upper-middle classes. Far from being a recent phenomenon, the divide between these social groups continues to impact heavily on ritual and devotional culture. Class-bound criticism will be discussed moving from three ethnographic sketches. The first two (animal sacrifice and possession) belong to the same event, the Choṭa Mā Yātrā in Salkia (Howrah District, WB). The third vignette surveys dramatic acts of mortification of the flesh on occasion of festivals of the goddess in Jammu (Jammu and Kashmir), Chandigarh and Patiala (Punjab) and Ahmedabad (Gujarat).

Ethnographic vignette 5: Animal sacrifice: feeding and thanking the goddess

The day after the Snān Yātrā of Salkia, the pageant of Choṭa Mā,[4] is dedicated to Baṛo Mā. This form of Śītalā, though worshipped as a benevolent mother, is known as *ugra* (powerful).[5] The goddess is naturally calm (*śānt*), kind (*śītal*), auspicious (*maṅgal*) and benign (*kalyāṇī*), but she may attack those who transgress social order by breaching norms of conduct (*dharma*). In order to feed her protective power, devotees offer her once a year a thanksgiving ceremony whose apex is the sacrifice and consumption of animal victims (goats). The ritual has contributed to the ambiguous reputation of Baṛo Mā and her votaries.

The practice of *balidān* ideologically divides the middle class from the working class, the social sector of most of Baṛo Mā's devotees. It so appears that divergent views in the matter of ritual and devotional service contribute to social blaming. Though Choṭa Mā is the *ṭhākur* of the *āñcal* and the queen of the pageant, Baṛo Mā is an extremely popular goddess, and her temple is the biggest in Salkia. Yet precisely because of *balidān,* a ritual performance growing obsolete in many Bengali temples, votaries of Baṛo Mā are negatively regarded. The *pūjārī*s (alt. spell. *pūjak*) in charge of the Śrī Śrī Baṛo Śītalā Māyer Mandir are accused of being backward, uneducated and violent.[6] Not only does this confirm the importance of social stratification in the study of myth and ritual, it also bears witness to the fact that – at least in this context – Śītalā is not one goddess but a fragmented persona shaped by the encounter with diverse communities, traditions, public policies and ethical discourses.

Coming back to the ritual killing of animals, the distinctive feature of the *vātsarik/vārṣik pūjā* (annual worship) of Baṛo Mā, this aims at pleasing, feeding and thanking the goddess for her protection. *Sevāits*, *pūjārī*s and devotees agree in considering *balidān* an obligatory (*nitya*) offering. Further it is a duty commanded in the *tantras.*[7] Yet notwithstanding its centrality, *balidān* – in Salkia as elsewhere – is increasingly objected to. Intellectuals, teachers, students, the upper and middle classes and the media are generally adverse to ritual performances involving violence. Sacrifice is currently dismissed and ridiculed (often aggressively) as a backward practice and a form of superstition. This has resulted in two opposing trends. On the one hand, a burgeoning number of devotees are deliberately editing (or renouncing) ancestral rituals, possibly in response to, or in imitation of, the concerns of the upper classes. On the other, I was able to detect diffidence toward what is interpreted as a biased *bhadralok* (bourgeois) and *videśi* (foreign) critique. Let us now examine the practice in Salkia.

The *balidān* is performed the day after the Snān Yātrā in the courtyard of the Baṛo Śītalā Mandir. The temple, a large three-storeyed building, is located on Shri Aurobindo Road, one of the busiest roads of the city. On the main altar, the *mūrti* of the goddess – who faces south – is enshrined along with Śani, Pañcānan and Manasā. The ceremony begins at around 16:00. Devotees, however, gather long before to secure the best spots to enjoy the show (*tāmāśā*). Despite the dramatic nature of the sacrifice and the high expectations of devotees, the atmosphere is festive. In the words of local informants, the whole spectacle is a display of devotion and aims at renewing the bond between the goddess and her children.

The sacrifice is performed by male Brahmans, who are responsible for all ritual arrangements. Assistants are also present. Their duty is to facilitate *balidān* by directing devotees offering goats (*vratadhār,* also called *bandak* or *bhaktya*), and making sure the crowd does not interfere with ritual action. The *sevāit*s are bare-chested and wear only their *poitā* (cotton thread), a *dhuti* (loincloth) and a *gāmchā* (lower garment) tied to the hips. There are practical reasons: the arena will soon be very warm and dirty with the blood of animals. Assistants – whose work is also considered a devotional service – sport a yellow *kamīj* (shirt) and a *dhuti*. They need to be easily identifiable.

The celebration is attended by men and women alike, although only male *vratadhārs* can bring animals to the altar and hand them to the *pūjārī*s or their assistants. Traditional rules of purity are temporarily suspended, as there are no class- or gender-based barriers.[8] In February 2012, I counted 40 male *vratadhār*s, including an 11-year-old child.[9] One of them was a *hijṛā*,[10] and the devotee presenting on behalf of her[11] community the biggest goat. Sacrificial animals are always male and black (only two were mixed colours), and they are expected to be unblemished.

The ceremony begins. Śītalā is invited with invocations (*nāmḍāk*), loud conch blasts and drum rolls. The chief *pūjak* – from inside the *garbhagṛha* – confirms the goddess is awake (*jāgrata*). Devotees now have only few minutes to rush into the temple and secure the best spots before the gates are barred with long bamboo poles. Havoc ensues, and often there are fights. The space is limited to the sides of the temple only, as nobody but the *pūjārī*s and their assistants can stand between the sacrificial area – emphatically marked by the Y-shaped stake (*hāḍikāṭh*) – and the sight of Baṛo Mā. When the space in the courtyard has been fully occupied, the gates are barred. Devotees and passers-by can only squat or stand to have a peep at the show. The crowd is impressive, and it causes several traffic problems on Shri Aurobindo Road.

The *balidān* is divided into ten stages. I was made aware that no ritual manual is in use. This is simply the way the *sevāit*s learnt the job from their fathers and grandfathers.

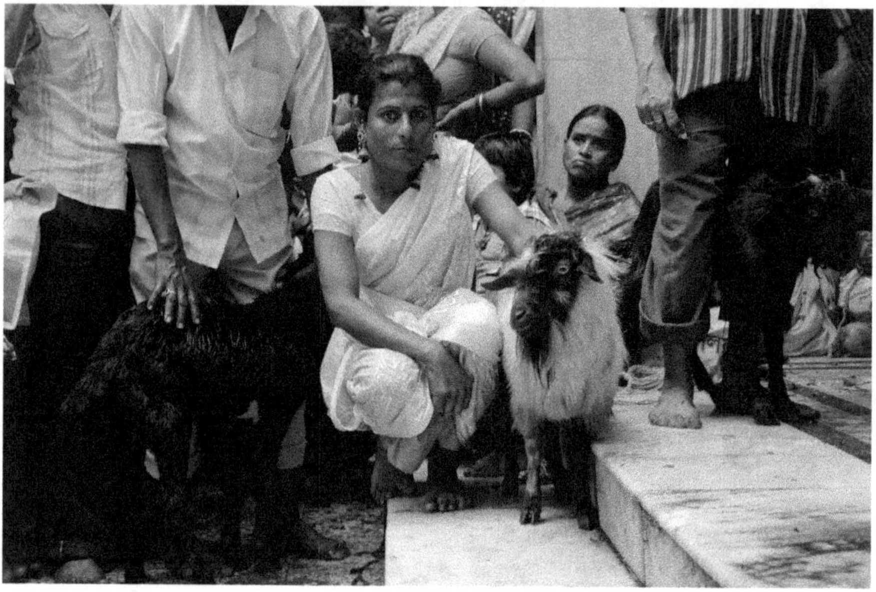

FIGURE 3.1 Hijṛa *devotee waiting for* chāg utsarga, *Śrī Śrī Baṛo Śītalā Māyer Mandir, Salkia (photo by Jayanta Roy).*

1 Presentation and dedication of the goats (*chāg utsarga*): the *vratadhār*s line up on the right side of the sanctuary. One by one, they are called by the chief *pūjārī* to present their gift (*bali*). Goats are brought in front of Baṛo Mā for they have to give consent to the killing. Animals are sprinkled with *gaṅgājal* and instinctively react by shaking their head. This is indicative of acceptance.[12] Animals are then cleansed and garlanded with fresh hibiscus flowers (*javā*). The various parties involved in the ritual, i.e. the recipient (Śītalā), the petitioner (the *vratadhār* and his family, or community), the medium (the *pūjārī*) and the gift (the goat), are now bonded together. After the presentation, the votaries go back to their original position and tend to their goat while waiting for the ritual to begin.[13]

2 Preparation of the *thālā* (clay platters): ritual assistants prepare rows of platters in front of the sacrificial stake. There are as many *thālā*s as goats. Each plate is placed on half a plantain leaf (*mājh pātā*) and contains a banana, a teaspoon of ghee, some curd and flowers. After each killing, the blood oozing from the headless body of the goat is poured on the plate assigned to it. At the end of the *balidān*, the plates are brought to the goddess as an offering and a sign of devotion. The carcasses of the goats go to the respective *vratadhār*s, whereas the heads stay with the *pūjārī*s as part of their *dakṣiṇā* (ritual fee).

3 Worship of the Y-shaped stake (*hāḍikāṭh pūjā*): painted in bright red, this sacrificial implement is cleansed and offered vegetarian edibles before being used for the killing of animal victims. The *pūjak*, after offering *praṇām* (obeisance) to the goddess and calling her name loudly, summons his fellow *pūjārī*s. They bring a small palanquin with a series of vegetarian presentations: cucumbers, a pineapple, pomegranates, oranges, papaya, guavas, grapes, *ḍāb* (green coconut), watermelon, hibiscus flowers and china roses. The offerings are then made available to Śītalā, who is supposed to guard the stake. This is then embellished with heavy garlands of hibiscus and jasmine, and perfumed with essences.

4 Calling the name (*nāmḍāk*): when the goddess is ready to receive the sacrifice, drummers and musicians are given a signal by ritual assistants. Loud drumming commences. This is followed by the blasts of conches (*śaṅkh bājāna*) and the festive melodies of the trumpet and *śānāi* players. This sonic exploit is followed by the invocations of the crowd who, directed by ritual assistants, repeatedly shout 'Jay Jay Baṛo Śītalā Mā!', while some women make the characteristic *ulu-ulu* auspicious sound (*uludhvani*) with their tongues.

5 Presentation of the blades (*khaḍga utsarga*): after music, drumming and invocations, there is a solemn moment of silence. The *pūjak* in charge of ritual killing presents a set of blades to the goddess and says: '*Auṃ khāḍgāya namaḥ. Auṃ asirviśāsanaḥ khaḍga stīkṣṇadhārodurāsadaḥ*.'[14] He approaches the director of the ceremony and is given four strings of white and yellow jasmine flowers, one for every blade. These are worn in a way to form a cross on his chest and, after presentation, are given back to the goddess.

6 Sacrifice (*paśubali*): when all ritual paraphernalia are in place, the first *vratadhār* is invited to pass his goat to ritual assistants. One by one all 40 goats are placed on the stake and beheaded with a single blow.[15] After the stroke falls on the animal and the head is detached, the crowd is incited by ritual assistants to call Śītalā's name loudly. One of the *pūjārī*s is given the head of the animal. This is presented to the crowd (sometime accompanied by merry dances to celebrate the auspiciousness of the moment) and then put in front of the *mūrti* of Baṛo Mā. Meanwhile, another *pūjārī* takes the headless body of the goat and quickly pours blood on one of the earthen plates. The corpse is then abandoned on the right of the altar.

7 Sacrifice of the pumpkin (*kumṛā bali*): after all the animals have been beheaded, one more offering must be presented. The pumpkins and cucumbers previously presented during *hāḍikāṭh pūjā* are ritually slain in a concluding ceremony.

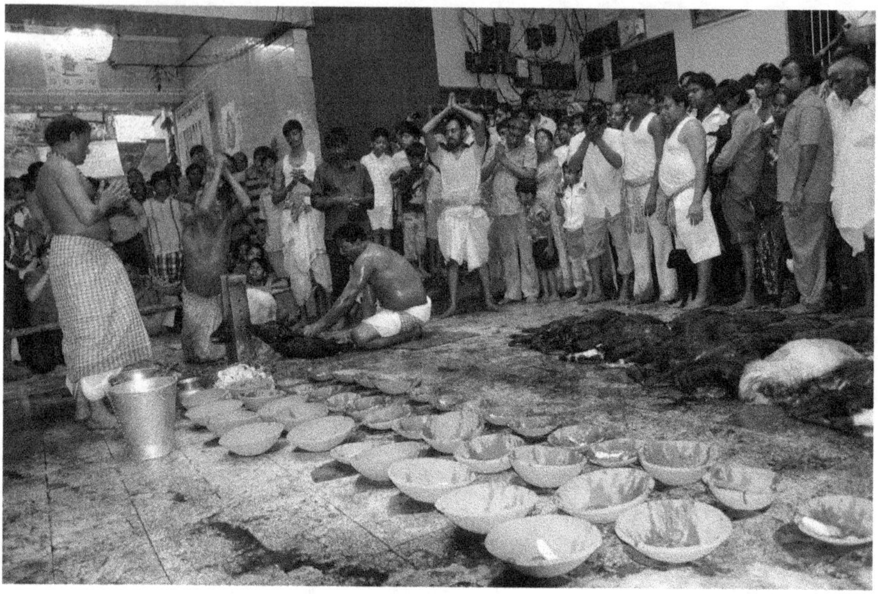

FIGURE 3.2 Balidān, *Śrī Śrī Baṛo Śītalā Māyer Mandir, Salkia (photo by Jayanta Roy).*

8 Salutation (*namaskār*) and release (*visarjan*): the *sevāit*s bow to the goddess, chant formulae of praises – seemingly the *dhyānamantra* from PiT (see below p. 186) – and let the goddess go.

9 Distribution of the food (*prasād*): pieces of pumpkin are given to devotees, who are now allowed inside the temple and rush toward the sacrificial spot. There is competition for the water that the *sevāit* pours into devotees' cups, pots and plastic bottles. A few drops of blood may be added too, on request, to enhance the power of the water. Meanwhile the headless bodies of the animals are sprinkled with water, offered incense and then given back to the *vratadhār*s and their families. They will decide whether to consume the meat with family, or to distribute part of it to the community, as a form of alms-giving. The heads stay with *pūjārī*s and ritual assistants, who will consume them.

10 Cleansing and purification: the chief *pūjārī*, with the help of attendants, starts cleansing the sacrificial area from blood and other organic material. The area must be purified as soon as possible as the presence of blood, flesh, hair, bone splinters, marrow and traces of the animals' excretions may attract the unwanted attention of competing deities or evil spirits (*bhūt*).[16]

Animal sacrifice is an important *sevā* for the devotees of Baṛo Mā. Though in the past it was celebrated on various occasions, it now takes place only once a year. This does not just depend upon the emergence of ethical debates. Funding is a major issue too.

A goat may cost ₹ 7,000 (£70) or above[17] but expenses are not limited to buying an animal. The majority of participants are on a low income and taking part in the *yātrā* often implies at least two days of leave from work. Travel and food expenses and, in some cases, overnight accommodation are a heavy burden to many. It should not be forgotten that celebrations like the Snān Yātrā (inclusive of *balidān*) are social events. Large family groups meet in Salkia, and money is spent on, for instance, new clothes, fees to the *sevāits*, offerings to the goddess (flowers, fruits, scents, incense, sweets), alms to *sādhus* and/or beggars, and gifts for children.

Notwithstanding public criticism and the expenses incurred, sacrifice continues to have an important meaning. While all agree that *balidān* is a way to feed and please the goddess, the reasons to offer the meat and blood of an animal are manifold. To some it is a matter of tradition, i.e. they are doing what their forefathers did.[18] The annual *balidān* is a treasured moment of commonality, and a way to confirm a tradition that for many is indissolubly associated with the notion of ancestral abode (*nivās*) and a powerful family-deity (*kuladevatā*). Alternatively, votaries offer a goat as part of a vow (*mānasik/mānat*),[19] a practice outspokenly associated with various material gains, such as improving one's personal (generally, financial) situation, or being able to take better care of the family. The offering is thus a way to attract the benevolent glance of the goddess on a new business venture, relocation or migration to another area, the prospect of a new job, or even in respect of university exams or pass tests. Protection is a key issue. Almost all my informants communicated to me the need to be blessed and protected. Some, however, were more insistent on this aspect than others. Members of the *hijṛā* community, for instance, are very emotionally involved in the ritual. Every year a representative of the community – who in the ritual setting is considered by her gender of birth (i.e. male) – offers Baṛo Mā a large goat. Every *hijṛā* contributes to the purchase of the animal, which is usually the biggest and finest specimen in the temple. Though they are a welcome presence, *hijṛās* experience a variable degree of social and economic pressure on a daily basis. This ranges from occasional stigma to major episodes of violence and discrimination. The sacrifice is not just a moment to seek the blessing and protection of a deity to whom they feel akin. (Śītalā– like *hijṛās* – is a virtual, i.e. non-functional, mother.) It is also a way to show their power in an authoritative arena. The link with Baṛo Mā, a powerful goddess worshipped for her power to grant fertility and to protect, confirms their place in society as mediums of the goddess.

Ethnographic vignette 6: Possession: bearing the visit of the goddess

There exists in South Asia the belief that some illnesses are dependent upon the influence of malevolent external entities (graspers, spirits),[20] wrathful gods, evil eye (caused by sorcerers, magicians, etc.) or the disembodied essence of powerful human beings (*yogis*, *pīrs*, etc.). Though the effects of such presences vary consistently, they are symptomatic of negative visitation.

As far as Śītalā is concerned, no textual source confirms possession phenomena as resulting from ritual or devotional practice. In fact, possession is an event succinctly documented in few ethnographic works only (Misra 1969; Ferrari 2007; Ferrari 2010b; Ghatak 2013).[21] A similar paucity of sources would suggest that Śītalā is not a goddess who possesses. Quite to the contrary, forms of possession resulting from manifestations of Śītalā are ordinary events (especially among women) on occasions such as festivals, pageants or other devotional public services. Alternatively, Śītalā may be invoked during exorcisms or other forms of ritual healing involving oracular or therapeutic possession (Misra 1969: 136; Hardiman 1987: 24–5),[22] though this is very rare. When this happens, the goddess is not the chief presence. She is mentioned along with a long list of deities (Gaṇeśa, Kālī, Viṣṇu, Śiva, Caṇḍī, Gheṇṭu, Śani, Hanumān, etc.) who are all equally beneficial to the healing process. In general, the presence of Śītalā is always auspicious (*maṅgala*), and her visitation is a performance resulting from devotion (*bhakti*), belief (*viśvāsa*) and suffering (*duḥkha*).

Visitations of the goddess are never malignant, and disease is not a form of possession, as argued by many (cf. Babb 1975: 130; Kolenda 1982: 235; Marglin 1990: 115; Oberoi 1992: 374; Arnold 1993: 123; Arnold 2004: 73; Pati 2002: 484; Samuel 2008: 248; Hauser 2012: 199).[23] This seems to be a quite widespread notion that needs rectification. The association of a deity with a pathology does not mean identity with it. Associating 'possession', or embodiment (as it is now more fashionable), with illness and suggesting that: a) fevers, poxes and measles are manifestations of Śītalā; and b) the patient is *de facto* Śītalā, are forms of disturbing cultural colonialism that do not correspond to beliefs and practices. Patients are not worshipped, and Śītalā is not a disease that possesses them. *Pūjā* is celebrated to summon the healing presence of the Cold Lady, and to ask her to stay.

In Salkia, as well as in the rest of Bengal, possession phenomena respond to a different logic. They are generally referred to as *bhar*, literally 'weight' or 'pressure'.[24] Hindi and Bhojpuri speakers, though they have assimilated the Bengali term *bhar*,[25] refer to Śītalā's visitation as *khelnā* (H. 'to play'; B. *khelā*). Both forms of presence are rendered as dramatic public performances that summarize the concerns of a devotee vis-à-vis complex social metaphors, implied meanings and codes of conduct. It can be thus argued that the rationale of devotional possession is to cause a reaction. Actors talk, collide, interject, quarrel, fight, agree, love, meet and depart. Śītalā is believed to respond to a call and to fill, *bharā*, or play, *khel(n)ā*, along with those who voluntarily 'empty' themselves by surrendering to the goddess in the context of a public devotional service (*sevā*). The pressure exerted by the goddess is the mark of a special relation.[26] This explains competition among devotees, and the ill reputation of those who are believed to fake *bhar*. Since possession is, among other things, a way to claim or challenge power in and across specific contexts (family, *jāti*, gender, etc.), it is not unusual for someone to be accused of cheating, or of being 'mad' (B. *pāgal*). Should this be confirmed, it has been explained to me in passionate conversations, Śītalā is likely to show her rage by heating up (*tāpāno*) and causing illness. Cheats must be discouraged.

Visitations of the goddess continue to be a powerful means of expression as well as a sign of the living presence of Śītalā. However, following the goddess's now-consolidated presence among the Indian middle class, *bhar* (and equivalent) has started to attract discordant opinions, incredulity or plain dislike. The fact that possession is chiefly a women's performance impacts heavily on such discourses. The reception of *bhar* during the annual Choṭa Mā Yātra in Salkia would serve to illustrate such dynamics.

During the walk that brings devotees to the various temples of the goddess, while many pilgrims are engaged in the practice of *daṇḍīkāṭā* (H. and Bh. *daṇḍavat*),[27] phenomena of individual possession are extremely common. The fact that a Bengali word is used to indicate 'possession', and that Bengali (or Bengalized Sanskrit) is the language of all ritual performances, is significant in that it confirms the ancestrality of Śītalā in the *āñcal*. A good number of pilgrims, however, are non-Bengalis, mainly Bihari migrants whose first language is either Hindi or Bhojpuri. These languages, as I had the chance to observe, are not used in public ritual settings but are spoken during possession. If a Hindi/Bhojpuri-speaker is visited by the goddess, then Śītalā expresses herself in these languages, and so communicates with other deities or human beings.

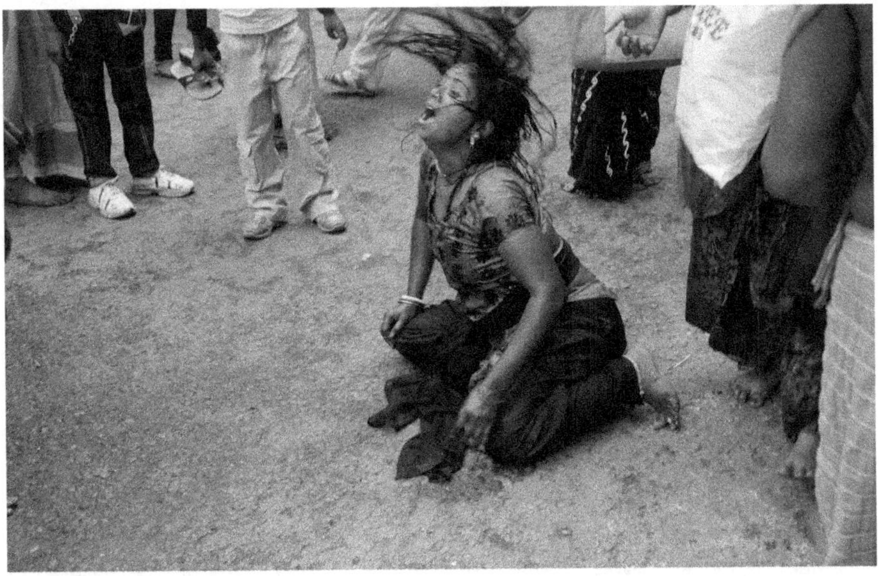

FIGURE 3.3 *Young woman during an episode of* bhar, *Choṭa Mā Yātrā, Salkia (photo by Jayanta Roy).*

The overwhelming majority of possessed persons are young women. During the time I spent in Salkia, I witnessed only four men giving signs of *bhar*. A limited yet important presence is that of *hijṛās*. Not only do *hijṛās* take an active part in important rituals, including those reserved for males (e.g. *balidān*, see above), they also share with the goddess her distinctive power to grant fertility. Their blessing is therefore much sought after. One of the most striking examples I observed took place during the communal bath at the end of the procession. A *hijṛā*, whom I will call Nandinī, apparently in a state of controlled *bhar*, was walking toward the *ghāṭ* surrounded by a considerable crowd making space for her. The immersion was eagerly followed by other pilgrims, who were waiting to touch her feet in a sign of respect. After the bath, the pilgrims' small water-filled *loṭās* were quickly poured on the head of Nandinī who, at that point, theatrically dishevelled her hair and let devotees collect the pouring water again in their small vessels as *prasād*.[28]

The relation between gender and possession is a tense one, especially during *bhar*, when women may express their objection to, and accusations against, male family members. The lack of a ritual agenda, and the exceptionality of an occasion in which gender and class boundaries are relaxed, permits forms of behaviour otherwise unacceptable, or discouraged. In open contrast to the altruism of *vrata* culture, the individualism and polemic approach of many *bhar* phenomena converge in forms of hedonism that contribute to generating contrasting interpretations, some of which are openly directed at casting stigma on the possessed one. Besides downgrading female devotees as *mad* or *hysteric*, sceptics suggest women are enacting a performance, or making a scene.

My informants reject the accusation of being cheaters but they do not seem to have any problem in admitting they know how to invite the goddess. As has been explained to me, this depends on the cultivated capacity of a devotee to concentrate on the feeling of sufferance, or its origin. Among my informants, two women in particular showed their willingness to discuss with me their experiences of *bhar*. Priyā and Mālinī (pseudonyms) are two cousins in their early twenties. Their families moved from Bihar at the end of the 1980s. Their first language is Bhojpuri but they are proficient in Hindi and have been educated in Bengali. (They both completed secondary education.) Priyā and Mālinī have been forced into marriage by their parents, and are now housewives. Their husbands, also from Bihar (recent migrants working in local factories), have the habit of drinking and minor episodes of domestic violence are regular. Both women confessed they do not find support from their families, and feel abandoned.[29] They fear that, should they conceive, the same destiny would affect their offspring, especially if female.

Women 'doing the *bhar*'[30] in Salkia, like Priyā and Mālinī, admit they know how to get possessed. Although the trigger may be different (some stories point to the frustration of being childless or unmarried, or the stigma that a particular condition attracts, e.g. vitiligo, poverty, or 'being ugly'), the manifestation is invariably aimed at denouncing a situation of relative injustice. What Priyā and Mālinī do on the occasion of the annual pageant of Choṭa Mā is not a matter of secrecy. In fact, for many women *bhar* is a way to find relief. The goddess gives them the power, and courage, to say publicly that they are not respected.[31] It thus appears that the practice of *bhar* can have serious social implications. Possessed devotees are neither 'health-seekers' nor sick persons. Rather they aim at reconciling a situation of imbalance that negatively affects their lives. Hence the dramatic outbursts of rage and aggression that features most *bhar* phenomena.

Violent or antisocial behaviour is typical of women. While men (and *hijṛās*) tend to undergo a trance-like state featured by immobility, speechlessness and gooseflesh (a set of symptoms often called *bhāva*, 'emotion'), women – to use the words of my (male) informants – go wild. *Bhar* is preceded by loud shrieks and cries of pain. This – as has been explained to me – is due to the physical pain of a person naturally resisting an unbearable external pressure. (Devotees complain of pressure on the chest, shoulders, neck and head.) Some women are then shaken by the incontrollable urge to get rid of the 'weight'. They twist their heads, roll on the ground and shout gibberish. Others seem to engage in an altercation. In this case the goddess, who by then has 'filled' their body, is recognizable by a different timbre, or accent. She indicates – or rather, accuses – those who contribute to the discomfort of her host. The dynamics of public blaming are particularly feared by male family members, who may be publicly accused of embarrassing secrets, i.e. domestic violence, cheating, homosexuality, impotence, incapacity to financially sustain the family, alcoholism,

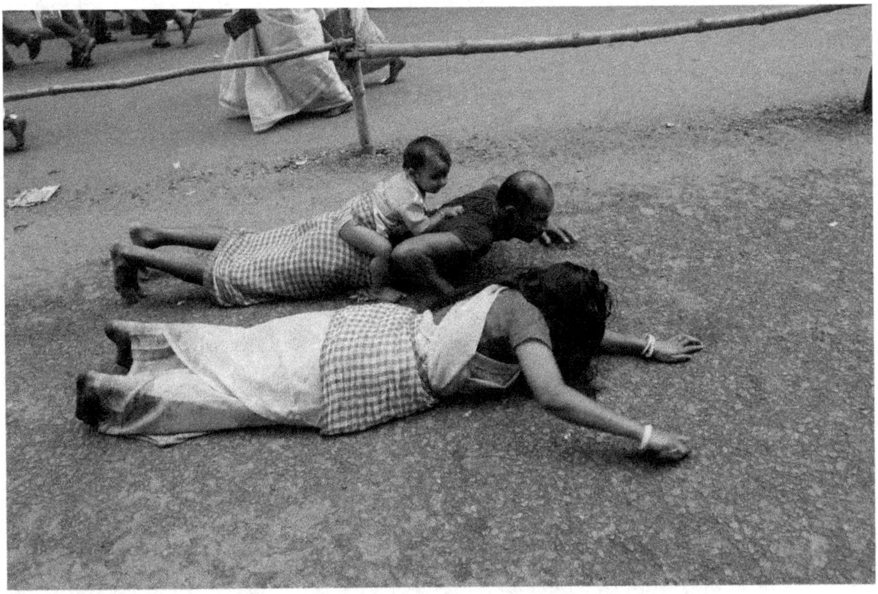

FIGURE 3.4 *Daṇḍīkāṭā, Choṭa Mā Yātrā, Salkia (photo by Jayanta Roy).*

etc. In short, what (human or divine) women say is dangerous. (It is fairly common for male family members to leave, or take part in the pilgrimage with other male relatives, if they sense the possibility of *bhar* among sisters, daughters, wives, etc.) Abusive language in the form of obscene sexual imagery directed toward men is not rare, neither are threatening behaviour, mocking fights and physical attacks against those who are indicted as guilty of causing sufferance. If the situation becomes dangerous, or unbearable from an emotional point of view, an older woman usually intervenes. Devotional possessions, unlike healing sessions, are unmediated events. Friends or family members, but also other pilgrims, make sure the possessed one does not injure herself or others. If that is the case, it is interrupted. The devotee is sprinkled with cold water and may be physically restrained. Mantras can be pronounced. If this does not work, an authoritative female intervenes and harshly orders the goddess to leave.[32]

Bhar is a way to find momentary relief, rather than an empowering performance whose effects are long-lasting. Since audiences are now mixed in terms of cultural and social background, a phenomenon depending on Śītalā's upward mobility, possession is liable to multiple, often contrasting, interpretations. Although *bhar* is far from uncommon, many question its legitimacy. It is posited that stories of possession do not figure in the 'texts of the goddess' (*meyeder vratakathā*s and *pālās* from *maṅgal* narratives). Furthermore, the practice of *bhar* is more common among the lower classes, migrants and (uneducated) women. This is an indicator of its lower (i.e. *laukik*, 'folk, popular') origin. *Bhar* is also discussed vis-à-vis the nobler *bhāva* (trance, ecstasy), *svapnādeś* (divine command in dream) or *svapnadarśana* (dream vision), two devotional events that do not depend upon public performance and do not negatively impact on the honour and dignity of the devotee (and her kin). Although doubts about the authenticity of trance and dreams may be raised, they are genuinely believed a safe way to experience the goddess and to respond to her call. Last but not least, it is worth noting that whereas *bhar* is an invitation provoked in a number of ways, dreams and trances are believed not to respond to such logic. It is the goddess who makes the call.

During conversations with Bengali middle class devotees in Salkia, I realized how *bhar* is often explained as a manifestation of fanaticism and superstition of the working class, or of non-Bengalis (mostly migrants from Bihar). Possession is at the centre of a class conflict. Educated social classes (mostly urban), new gentry and Westernized elites see themselves as different from 'the folks' precisely because of practices like *bhar* and *balidān*. These performances are exoticized, and are discussed as opposed to the 'modern' and the 'rational'. Some add a moral connotation to *bhar*, and judge those who 'do the *bhar*', especially women, as shameful, disgusting and laughable. Alternatively, the experience of possession is rationalized. Hosts of the goddess are labelled as cheats, who live off the credulity of the people, lunatic or attention-seekers. Women who are possessed are presented as victims of ignorance, backwardness and primitive beliefs. In light of this, *bhar* has become for many an embarrassing issue.

One more issue should be considered in relation to public manifestations of devotion such as *bhar*. The presence of young women acting wildly attracts predatory males only interested in the possibility of 'seeing something'.[33] Possibly because I was not supposed to understand Bengali, I overheard ungracious conversations and vulgar remarks coming from men of various ages attracted by young women rolling on the ground. The inappropriate comments of these spectators confirm the general idea that women doing *bhar* are not the goddess, but young females who make exhibitions of themselves and whose behaviour is likely to elicit unwanted attentions.

All these elements contribute to the increasing ill fame of devotional forms of possession like *bhar/khel(n)ā*. It is thus unsurprising that phenomena like the ones described in the above vignettes, though extremely popular, are more and more objected to. When possession takes place, it causes embarrassment among both relatives of the host and other devotees.[34] *Sevāit*s and *pūjārī*s often discourage, or show discomfort at, the presence of a habitual '*pāgli*' (mad woman). Though historical, economic and political factors have inevitably contributed to a general levelling of vernacular culture, the gentrification of many beliefs and practices is highlighting a gulf between social sectors. Many aspects of *āñcalik* culture are being eroded, or viewed as tourist attractions. Practices like *bhar* are being marginalized as something exotic or 'folkloristic'. While (female) devotees are chastised, Śītalā changes too. She is no longer the naked lady on the ass associated to Indian peasantry, but a richly decorated bourgeois young woman who acts as the bearer of the morality of twenty-first-century Indian middle class mothers.

Ethnographic vignette 7: Mortification of the flesh: Śītalā meets Māriyammaṉ

Ritual and devotional practices, and the beliefs that inform them, do not stay limited to small-scale *āñcalik* settings. Cultures are naturally fluid and open to innovation, irrespective of the resistance they may find. It is thus unsurprising that the migration of Indian labourers and peasants, their relocation in urban contexts and the response of indigenous communities have *de facto* contributed to shape alternative versions of Śītalā. The case of Bihari and Bengali working class devotees in Salkia is emblematic. It makes us reflect on the implications of the encountering of communities that express themselves in different languages in the same ritual/devotional context, and of the role played by uneven levels of education and wealth. Migratory waves, however, are not just limited to the movement of working class sectors across north India and their relocation, whether short-term, long-term or permanent. People from the rest of India too, from a variety of classes, are an established presence in several northern urban centres. Such is the case of Tamils, whose devotional culture, particularly the worship of the goddess Māriyammaṉ, has infiltrated local practices and rituals. My discussion is based on a general survey of the following festivals:

- Mātā Śītalā Devī Śobha Yātrā of Jammu (Jammu and Kashmir), celebrated for a week from the full moon of Āṣāḍha;
- Śītalā Mātā Utsav in Patiala (Punjab), on the *Śītalāṣṭamī* of Āṣāḍha;
- Śītalā Mātā Pūjā in Chandigarh (Punjab/Haryana), during the *amāvasyā* (new moon) of Śrāvaṇa;
- Śītalā Mātā Yātrā in Ahmedabad (Gujarat), on the Caitra *pūrṇimā* (full moon).[35]

The choice of Śītalā festivals is not casual. Māriyammaṉ and Śītalā share many features. Māriyammaṉ, like Śītalā, was known as the goddess of smallpox and epidemics, and continues to be worshipped to protect children from chickenpox, measles and fevers. Both goddesses are associated with cold and refreshing waters, and the rain. They enjoy much popularity among women, and are known as fertility goddesses. Though anthropomorphic renderings are not precisely akin – in her fierce form Māriyammaṉ has protruding fangs and weapons – such are the similarities that Śītalā is considered by Tamils the Māriyammaṉ of the north, and Māriyammaṉ is for locals the Śītalā of the south. Both communities, however, make it abundantly clear they are not the same goddess, thus contradicting an academic trope (e.g. Auboyer and De Mallmann 1950: 207; Tiwari 1996: 451; Craddock 2001: 150; cf. Harman 2012: 46 on this issue).

The Tamil goddess, unlike Śītalā who is intrinsically cold, oscillates between states of grace (T. *aruḷ*) and excess (T. *kōpam, ukkiram*) (Allocco 2009: 291).[36] Worshipping Māriyammaṉ, especially on occasion of her annual festival,[37] is a way to manage her excess power (*śakti*). Devotional austerities are supposed to incite the goddess, so that she might release her protective power. If, however, Māriyammaṉ is too excited, she may give voice to her fierce side, and cause harm (disease) (Harman 2004: 4; Allocco 2009: 294).

Māriyammaṉ is a transversal goddess. Like in Śītalā culture, her votaries are both Brahmans and non-Brahmans (Allocco 2009: 23). The Tamil goddess, however, is not stereotypically associated with low social classes, and her enculturation at all strata of the population is more persuasive. Śītalā , thought obsessively associated with myths of pan-Hindu powerful goddesses, like Durgā, Kālarātrī, Lakṣmī, Sarasvatī, Gaṅgā and Vaiṣṇo Devī, is known as one of the many *āñcalik devī*s (Bhaṭṭācārya 1997: 50).[38] Māriyammaṉ, conversely, does not need to be promoted among the top layers of society. Thought distinctively regional in character, her mythology is validated by authoritative Sanskrit and Tamil texts via the myth of Reṇukā (Biardeau 2004: 185–90).[39] Devotees from all regions and social backgrounds of south India (Tamil Nadu, Kerala, Andhra Pradesh, Karnataka, Maharashtra, but also Sri Lanka and many sites of the south Indian diaspora in Asia, Europe, Africa and North America) take part in her festivals. Such celebrations are featured by distinctive votive performances involving possession, oracular speaking (T. *aruḷvākku*), marching with firepots on the head, fire-walking (T. *tīmiti*) and austerities like *alaku*, a loose label indicating a series of devotional performances such as the piercing of the cheeks, tongue, bottom lip or back with spears, arrows and hooks.[40]

In the festivals celebrated in Jammu, Punjab and Gujarat, though ritual arenas are shared and there is the occasional overlap in terms of practice and performance (e.g. *pūjā*, *darśana*, *daṇḍavat*, etc.), each community stays loyal to the mythical and iconographic features of their goddess. This appears clearly in the liturgy, when regional languages are used, or on occasions of devotional forms of possession, mantric utterances, storytelling and songs.[41] The same is true for rituals. *Alaku* is performed by Tamil men and women only.

Austerities like *alaku* belong to a culture with its own texts, beliefs and practices. *Alaku* rites are so alien to local culture that there is not even a name to indicate them. They are generally called *tapasyā*, a term used for the asceticism of renouncers. Although I realized that not all are comfortable with such innovations, sharing festival arenas is normally not perceived as a problem. Tamils are encouraged by city councils – often in conversation with Tamil committees, cultural associations and the government of Tamil Nadu – to maintain and transmit community culture. By inscribing *alaku* in the annual festival of Śītalā, Tamils project their distinctive mode of worship, and affirm their ethos in a new *āñcal*. Indigenous communities seem to enjoy the festive mood of Tamil celebrations and their spectacular displays of bravery and endurance. Though ethnicity and culture inform different, and somehow divergent, dispositions in matters of ritual practice, Śītalā is not subsided by the presence of Māriyammaṉ. When *kōvil*s (T. temples) have been erected to worship Māriyammaṉ, the annual celebration of the two goddesses continues to be performed jointly. Notwithstanding the lack of community tension, three issues are discussed with increasing concern.

First, devotees (Tamil as well as northern Indian) are ambivalent about the growing presence of news operators and media coverage. Members of local temple committees and votaries are worried that the advertising of *alaku* and other spectacular devotional ordeals on a national and international level is likely to attract the bias of readers who are not familiar with the rationale of the celebration.[42] The lurid tone of media reports – invariably pointing at the eeriness and shocking nature of religious practices that involve self-harming – is generally not appreciated. Informants, including votaries who regularly take part in *alaku*, refuse to have their festival diminished to a circus performance, and tend to be defensive of their customs, especially when they are likely to be used to downgrade the nature of their *sevā*.

Second, participants in *alaku* are male and female of all ages, including minors. Women regularly take part in piercing rituals and, like male votaries, they actively seek possession, including *aruḷvākku*. Female devotees with tongues and cheeks pierced by arrows or spears (T. *vēl*) proceed in a state of trance along with men to the venue of the festival, usually a temple of the goddess and the core site of the *utsav*, where they receive *darśana* in exchange for their votive service. It has been explained to me that female ritualists are all 'Madrasis'; this was confirmed on more than one occasion as an important element in the discussion. Locals admire the bravery of Tamils and do not have adverse feelings toward those who take part in *alaku* rituals. If Tamil women wish, and are allowed, to do so, then they are pragmatically welcomed in the procession. After all, this is a matter pertaining to the Tamil community. No local women, I have been informed, have ever participated in *alaku* or similar rituals. That would be inappropriate, I was informed. The only austerity women regularly perform is *daṇḍavat* and various forms of fasting. As per the presence of minors, this has caused outraged reactions from both sides. Reporting from Chandigarh, Singh informs us that:

> devotees let their children [...] participate in orthodox rituals including piercing of skin, tongue, cheeks and what not. The entire proces [sic] is done without use of any ansthesia [sic], without any medical supervision and with self deviced [sic] surgical methods using instruments without any sterilisation. The administration fully aware of this happening year on year on the Amavasya of Shravanamasam, still no police, government officials seem to be interested to intervene in rituals like this, that to in a city like Chandigarh, boasting of having one of the highest levels of literacy in the country. (Singh 2009)

The Tamil and non-Tamil devotees I interviewed are unambiguously adverse to the inclusion of children in the practice of *alaku*, as well as other austerities. Though my informants are limited in number and more fieldwork is needed to assess the consistency of such a custom, there seems to be genuine concern, and incredulity. (None of my informants ever witnessed children with their cheeks pierced, as the one photographed in Singh's report, or other media sources.)[43] In this case too, there is a shared anxiety about the possibility of being negatively judged for the actions of few, an issue that points to the self-awareness of *alaku* as the source of ethical controversies among different audiences.

Third, the legitimacy of austerities in a devotional context, as posited by local *paṇḍit*s in Ahmedabad (Gujarat), is questioned. *Alaku* is interpreted as a form of *tapasyā* (austerity) that should be limited to *bābā*s only, i.e. ascetics like *sannyāsī*s or *sādhu*s. The rationale of such practices is to accumulate *tapas* (heat) and gain *siddhi* (power). Austerities are not about *bhakti*, and should not be performed by householders or, even worse, teenagers, children and women. This clearly contradicts Tamil views (as well as common praxis among many Hindu communities across the subcontinent).[44] *Alaku*, however, does not explicitly emulate the austerities of *sādhu*s. Even though similarities suggest the penetration, or imitation, of patterns from the ascetic tradition, Tamils consider their service a form of vow (T. *viratam*; Skt. *vrata*). By taking part in votive performances aimed at thanking the goddess or promising her devotional service in exchange for grace (e.g. healing, the gift of a son, protection and wellbeing), Tamils speak the same idiom of local votaries. Devotees going through such dramatic, and potentially harmful, rituals wish to prove in a public arena that the goddess is with them. Also, *alaku* is an offering, and a demonstration of love and faith. The ideology at the core of this performance, though different in practice, is conceptually similar to the various *mānat* dedicated to Śītalā in north India. The service is a sort of compensation for the goddess's many gifts and her enduring protection. The *kāmana* or *sakāma* (Skt. 'with desires' [attached]) nature of such votive acts is evident. Men and women perform *alaku* and other austerities in exchange for specific requests, such as marriage, career advancement or employment, offspring and, more generally, wealth and health. Devotees of both Śītalā and Māriyamman̲ are not uncomfortable with the allegation of seeking material gain from their service, an accusation famously coming from those who object to these forms of devotion. The goddess is a mother; as her children they have the right to ask her for practical goods.

Though controversies have been observed, the distinctive performances of Tamil devotees caused, perhaps unsurprisingly, positive backlashes (cf. Harman 2012: 53–4 and *passim*). Mass celebrations like *yātrā*s, *utsava*s, *annakūṭa*s, etc. featuring piercing austerities are seen by insiders as spectacles of devotion, and are contributing to the globalization of Śītalā, whose festivals now regularly feature in national newspapers and TV channels. The consequence of such attention is a spectacular growth in terms of participation. This has had beneficial implications for the economy at both local and national level, a fact interpreted as the protective presence of Śītalā and Māriyamman̲. Medium and small business ventures have grown, and the consolidation of annual festivals has resulted in burgeoning entrepreneurial activities such as *pūjā* kiosks, restaurants, pilgrim hostels as well as hotels and guest houses, sites for family entertainment, shops, malls and the development of the arts (musicians, storytellers, singers, etc. are hired on such occasions). Temple committees and *pūjārī*s have also benefited from joint and larger celebrations of Śītalā. Finally, roads and communication services have improved, and following requests from Tamil communities, there are plans to increase flight connections between Chennai and various northern sites.

Concluding remarks

Practices like animal sacrifice, possession and devotional austerities are at the centre of heated debates and community controversies. Educated upper and middle class devotees and outsiders perceive them as irreconcilable with the gentle nature of Śītalā or, broadly speaking, with modern India. Besides ethical debates, crucial to my discourse is the place of tradition with respect to: a) the social status of its adherents; b) its texts (or the lack thereof); c) the political responses it elicits; and d) its purported rationale vis-à-vis modernity.

Phenomena like *bhar*, *paśubali* and *alaku* (or equivalent) attract public contempt, for they allegedly diverge from conventional representations of Hinduism, or expectations about what Hinduism should be. This, however, is not novel. Since the late Vedic period, the place of animal sacrifice has been the object of debate and criticism from both within and outside.[45] This has culminated in the birth of dissenting (*nāstika*) traditions, notably Jainism and Buddhism, which rejected sacrificial practice and spectacular physical austerities. With the consolidation of *bhakti* ideologies, especially those informed by *vaiṣṇava* schools, we witness uncompromising objection to animal sacrifice (e.g. MaP 143: 13; BhP 4.27: 193). Prohibitions[46] and increasing pressure from NGOs,[47] anti-*bali* lobbies or animal rights campaigners have all variously contributed to consolidate the ill fame not just of animal sacrifice, but of those traditions – Tantrism, Śāktism and *ādivāsī* religions – that continue the practice. McDermott, who investigated the *balidān* controversy in West Bengal in relation to the worship of Durgā, Kālī and Jagaddhātri (2011: 197–223), has highlighted how various sectarian traditions (*vaiṣṇavas*, *bāuls*, the Brāhmos, monks from the Ramakrishna Mission), influential and charismatic intellectuals (notably, Rabindranath Tagore) and political parties (e.g. the Socialist Party)[48] have actively fought against the practice of *paśubali* (ibid.: 214–15). Yet especially in north-eastern India,[49] where there is a strong tradition of non-vegetarianism[50] along with a tantric (*śākta*) background, sacrifice persists. This has contributed to the exacerbation of tension. Many interviewees fear the raids of animal rights campaigners. Also, they expressed concerns about the tone of the debate, and the slander inevitably resulting from it.[51] Possession too, though a transcultural practice attested since Vedic times, has fascinated, and horrified, for centuries. Indian texts, colonial archives and media reports are replete with tales of possession and glosses commenting on its ethics, legitimacy and problematic position in Indian ritual and devotional culture. This is lucidly discussed in Kalpana Ram's recent analysis of women's possession in South India (Ram 2013), in which the author – who reports on the practice of possession and its perception as 'female disorder' – has identified in the public nature of these performances one of the key issues (ibid.: 53). I agree with Ram. The visibility of such practices and their performance in a public space are both the reason behind the criticism vociferously expressed by both insiders and outsiders, and the source of their self-invigorating power. The non-secretive, public and loud nature of services such as animal sacrifice, devotional forms of possession and austerities (from *daṇḍīkāṭā*/*daṇḍavat* to *alaku*) is an essential feature of the worship of Śītalā. The festivals of the goddess are charged arenas where power is openly critiqued, negotiated, affirmed and demonstrated. The fact that there is a critical response from the outside has in fact contributed to its empowerment. But just like in the ethical and epistemological criticism emerging in post-Vedic Indian texts, the long tradition of spectacularization, marginalization and blaming of alternative culture proper of much colonial, medical and missionary literature[52] has impacted heavily on the current perceptions, and the aesthetics, of these services. This is now continuing in contemporary India, where controversial practices are at the centre of heated social, doctrinal, political and epistemological debates.

Sacrifice, possession and devotional austerities, solidly rooted in local, regional and pan-Hindu traditions, are now presented as a marker of ignorance and backwardness. Such features are in contradiction with Śītalā's consolidated presence in the culture of educated, affluent Indian social strata. The goddess no longer has to threaten and scream '*pratiṣṭhā din*!' (B. 'establish me [in a temple]', i.e. worship me), as *maṅgal* poets told us. Upward mobility has determined a significant restyling of Śītalā's iconographical and ritual features. Inconvenient practices, i.e. rituals hard to accommodate in the new context, have been relegated to the realm of folklore – a label that in the popular parlance is associated with incoherent, lower forms of culture. Due to the gulf dividing class-borne practices, *paśubali* and *bhar* (or equivalent) have been surrounded by an aura of suspicion, and are perceived as quintessentially *tāmasik*,[53] thus fostering a rich imagery of impure, ferocious, blood-lusting and irate goddesses.

Unlike goddesses like Durgā and Kālī, who have a strong and healthy ritual and mythological textual tradition, Śītalā's devotees and ritual specialists cannot 'throw scriptures' to defend their practice. Śītalā is primarily associated with *Skandapurāṇa*, and *Picchilātantra* prescribes *balidān* as a duty. But these texts are eventually uninfluential. The *Śītalāṣṭakastotra* does not deal with either of the two practices discussed here. (In fact, the *stotra* is evocative of *vrata* culture.) As per *Picchilātantra*, it is not acknowledged as an authoritative manual. Eventually *pūjārī*s and *purohit*as revert to, and imitate, contemporary ritual compendia explicitly associated with the 'great goddess tradition', a culture increasingly informed by middle class values and outspokenly intolerant of the devotional practices of migrant labourers, the peasantry and the working class. In so doing, they contribute to the gentrification of Śītalā. Lacking social cohesion as well as economic and symbolic capital, subaltern sectors enact mimicry, edit controversial practices and actively contribute to the reshaping of the goddess.

Various political agendas have equally impacted on the restyling, and debasing, of controversial mythical, iconographical and ritual conventions. The rise of Indian folkloristics as a (political) response to British gazetteers has contributed to the editing of practices and beliefs irreconcilable with the ideals promoted by nationalist leaders (Korom 2006: 21–31; Mukharji 2013: 275). The trend continued after independence, when various political formations began to target folk beliefs. Socialist and communist militants, Hindu nationalists and Islamists operating in India as well as in Pakistan and Bangladesh are all expressions of the pressure exerted on a rich and diversified belief system. To this scenario, one should add the impact of the Indian entertainment industry, chiefly Bollywood. The presence of ritual practices in Bollywood movies, especially in *bhakti* movies, is either stereotyped in its representation of regional differences, or annihilated. Rituals whose focus is the promotion of widely acceptable ideals are presented as mainstream (e.g. *ārti*, *karvāchaut*, etc.), thus causing a process of imitation from below. Conversely, where a belief or custom may give rise to controversy, this is simply removed from the landscape.

Finally, the pathologization of devotional behaviour (trance, ecstasy, possession and austerities involving self-harming) along with the pharmacologization of Indian medicine have resulted in a progressive inhibition of the tradition informing the practices described above. As I learnt from Salkia residents, the number of *bhar*s used to be dramatically higher during pageants performed only ten years ago. Many are now ashamed of having relatives 'doing the *bhar*', and women are increasingly labelled as psychiatric patients. A similar discourse applies to sacrifice too (cf. Dr Suneelam's statement cited in McDermott, see p. 111 n. 48). When not aggressively challenged, devotees are lectured by animal rights campaigners that if the rationale of *paśubali* is health, the professional advice of physicians should be sought. Since Śītalā is generally invoked as a protector from childhood illnesses (exanthemata), infertility and mental illness (*graharoga*), there are now various opportunities to take advantage of affordable medical services and efficacious treatment. Animal sacrifice is discussed by activists as a cruel and contaminating custom which, eventually, may favour infections (due to bloodshed) and further disease. An ideological gulf dramatically emerges. Devotees do not look at *balidān* as a healing ritual but as a thanksgiving service that, incidentally, does not exclude medical treatment.

The moralization of tradition and the inculcation of rationalism have eventually proved crucial in the containment of Śītalā culture. Yet irrespective of the pressure exerted, the rituals and beliefs discussed in this chapter continue to be for large sectors of Indian society a culturally acceptable solution to, and an escape from, the immanent drama of an unfair history. Possession, mortification and sacrifice emphatically signal injustice and the willingness of the votary to overcome it. They are not rupture. They give voice to a long tradition that sees in the power of the goddess the capacity to acknowledge, manage and overcome the crisis.

Notes

1 On *pāpa* in relation to disease and contagion, see Das 2000: 58–9.

2 Animal sacrifice to Śītalā is relatively widespread in West Bengal, eastern Jharkhand, northern Odisha and western districts of Bangladesh. I am not aware of such practice in the western states I surveyed (Gujarat, Punjab, Rajasthan, Haryana and Uttar Pradesh). I heard discordant opinions as per the actual existence of animal sacrifice in honour of Śītalā in Bihar.

3 From Sanskrit *bali* (offering; gift) and *dāna* (presentation). The term *paśubali* specifically indicates the offering (*bali*) of a domestic animal (*paśu*). Animal sacrifice is colloquially called *bali*. The goddess Śītalā is primarily offered goats (B. *chāg*, *chāgal*), but I heard of sacrifices of buffaloes, pigeons and chickens. On a few occasions, I observed the offering of fish heads. Writing in the last years of the nineteenth century, Risley (1981: 177–8) reports on swine sacrifice to Śītalā. As per my experience, Śītalā is never offered piglets. Swine are offered to gods like Dharmarāj, or other *grāmya devas*, who are occasionally worshipped as companions of Śītalā.

4 See above pp. 54–7.

5 There exist *pratimā*s of the goddess that are considered extremely powerful. Such is the case of the *mūrti* in the temple near the Agam Kuāṅ, in Patna (see above pp. 52–4). Another form of Śītalā known for her excess power (*ugra śakti*) is the Dakṣiṇāśītalā in a small shrine near Kāl Bhairo Mandir, in Banaras.

6 Allegations come from outsider devotees and votaries from other Salkia temples. This is not unusual. Competition, especially on occasions such as pageants or other public festivals, may be fierce and narratives of discredit are often disseminated to gain prestige and authority. As per the *pūjārī*s of Baṛo Mā, my personal experience says otherwise. I was welcomed with very short notice at the busiest moment of the year, and took advantage of the knowledge, help and support of both ritualists and members of their extended families.

7 Votaries incessantly invoke tantric ritual digests as authoritative sources. Animal sacrifice, exhorted in purāṇic (KāP 57) and tantric (*Muṇḍamālātantra* 4; *Phetkāriṇītantra* 11: 20; *Bṛhannīlatantra* 6: 337; 12: 69–75) texts, including *Picchilātantra*, is a practice associated with ancestrality and tradition.

8 Children of all ages are also present. In fact, their presence adds significantly to the celebration. Crackers are thrown from the balconies onto pilgrims and pranks of various natures take place. This inevitably causes angry reactions among ritual assistants.

9 The following year I counted 38 votaries, but in 2014 a local informant communicated that the ceremony included 43 sacrifices.

10 Members of a community of transgender, transsexuals and eunuchs, often known as the third gender. The *hijṛā*, though heavily discriminated, are a consolidated presence in South Asian history and culture dating back to post-Vedic times (Reddy 2005: 19–30). Although *hijṛā*s are popularly associated with prostitution and lurid stories of child kidnapping, traditionally they are entertainers, and are welcomed on occasions such as weddings or children's rites of initiation. *Hijṛā*s are usually found at busy crossroads, markets and train/bus stations selling their blessings, which they activate with their characteristic handclap. The presence of a *hijṛā* during the *balidān* is a routine event: in the eyes of the goddess, a *hijṛā* is male (see below on *bhar*, possession). During the service of Baṛo Mā, *hijṛā*s are reserved a special place on the upper balcony.

11 *Hijṛās* talk of themselves as females. I will respect this convention throughout this work.

12 Should the goat not shake the head, it is expected to be released. This is reputed inauspicious for the votary and his kin.

13 Votaries show respect and affection for their goats. The animals are caressed, offered food and some play with them. Following conversations with some devotees, I was made aware of a sense of gratitude for the animal's self-sacrifice.

14 'Auṃ. Obeisance to the sword. The sword causes death. It is very sharp and cannot be destroyed.'

15 The *pūjārī* secures the forelegs of the animal in an unnatural, and arguably painful, position above its back. He holds the front and back hooves and stretches longitudinally the animal, whose head is blocked in the tight *hāḍikāṭh*. It has been explained to me that this is done to permit the blow to strike as close as possible to the lowest cervical vertebrae, so as to secure more meat.

16 In the alleys around the temple, I noticed some women started a protective ritual called *jhulāi* (lit. 'swinging'). They beat big winnowing baskets to cast away the evil eye. This seems to be related to the presence of hungry spirits who may taste flesh and blood, and then prey on humans (particularly children). The ritual, which does not seem prevalent in West Bengal, is a powerful protecting exorcism, and can be performed whenever the occasion requires.

17 The price varies depending on the quality of the animal, age and gender. Animals sold at the market before festivals are generally more expensive. In response to the economic crisis culminating in the 2013 devaluation of the rupee and the consequent rise in prices, goats for sacrifice now cost from ₹ 10,000 up to 100,000. Many devotees have thus resorted to *kumṛā bali* exclusively. Unlike the great Durgā and Kālī *mandir*s, Śītalā is generally worshipped in small shrines or modest temples, and devotees often have limited financial means. When *balidān* continues to be practised, as in the case of Baṛo Mā, this is limited to *vātsarik pūjā*.

18 This is usually the purported rationale behind the presence of minors. They are expected to carry on a family tradition.

19 Some men take part in the ritual on behalf of a female family member (in this case the motivation is often related to fertility issues).

20 Planetary affliction (Skt. *graharoga*) is a term used to indicate the external and malignant agency of 'graspers' (*graha*s). They are often identified with planets and asterisms, and are believed to be loose (H. *alag*; B. *ālagā*) forces that penetrate the body restraining knowledge and obfuscating consciousness.

21 It has been argued that actors impersonating Śītalā at open theatre performances (*yātrā*) are possessed by the goddess. This does not seem to be the case, as suggested by Katyal (2001: 100), and as I myself could appreciate after a series of interviews with itinerant performers. This is unambiguously confirmed by Chapal Bhaduri, a renowned Śītalā impersonator of the Bengali open theatre. When presented *sindūr* by women as Mā, he argues: 'I'm a man dressed as a woman.' (See below pp. 121–2.)

22 Both Misra and Hardiman rely on secondary sources such as late nineteenth-century ethnographic reports. No fieldwork seems to have been conducted to back up such conclusions.

23 Oberoi, Arnold and Pati, and others after them, base their conclusions not on personal observation or systematic interviews of informants. In fact, they derive the notion that a patient is possessed, and henceforth worshipped as Śītalā, by early twentieth-century journalists, or reports written by British surgeons, servicemen and civil servants whose agenda and techniques of investigation are, at the very least, unclear. See also the rendering of Lal and Van Loom (2005: 81) of Śītalā in their *Introducing Hinduism*, a booklet accompanying text with cartoons: A young lady with a backpack (presumably a Western tourist) asks a physician whether people invoke Śītalā to get smallpox. The doctor makes a point that the disease has been eradicated in 1980. A quasi-naked turbaned 'Indian' intervenes: 'The victim of smallpox was viewed as being possessed by the goddess. Smallpox epidemics are manifestation of Sitala.' Above, perhaps with some irony, Śītalā asks herself: 'So why should people have a Goddess of Smallpox?'

24 Forms of possession are alternatively discussed as *āveś*, a loan from Sanskrit (*ā-√viś*) indicating a 'confounded state of mind' or simply 'madness'. In medical jargon, this term indicates neurological disorders or psychiatric pathologies. To my knowledge *āveś* is not used in devotional contexts.

25 Possession in Hindi, Urdu and Bhojpuri is known as *peśī* (< F. hearing; appearance [in a court]). This, however, is not used in the context of the Choṭa Mā Yātrā. *Peśī* is a negative event. Those suffering from *peśī* are victims of the malignant visitation of *bhūts*, *jinns*, *pīrs*, etc. Other forms of possession involving the presence of evil spirits are called *caḍhnā* ('to climb', 'to mount'), *grahaṇ* ('seizing', 'grasping'), *dr̥ṣṭi* ('glance'), *najar* ('sight') and *ṭuk(ur)* ('intently gazing'). In cases of evil eye or various forms of negative possession, Śītalā is never indicated as the origin of sufferance. In fact, she is functional to healing (cf. SkP 5.13: 5).

26 *Bhar* is seldom an occasional event. In fact, it tends to be cultivated and re-enacted on occasions of other devotional services.

27 This form of votive austerity requires devotees to measure up with their bodies the distance of the pilgrimage from the bathing *ghāṭ* to the temple, and back.

28 This water, called *maṅgaljal*, was of special value to women wishing to conceive. It derives its power from a combination of circumstances: the *yātrā*, the purity of the Ganges's water and Nandinī's closeness to the goddess.

29 Elder female family members stayed discreetly around during the conversation, and did not object to the interview. They agreed the two husbands had been unfair, but they claim this is in the past. Further, they always helped Mālinī and Priyā.

30 It is significant that many informants say *bhar karā* (B. 'to do the *bhar*') as opposed to devotees, particularly women, who say *bhar haoyā* (B. 'to be filled', 'to be possessed').

31 This finds confirmation in the ethnographies of many: cf. Boddy 1994; Carrin 1999; Filippi 2002; Ram 2012.

32 I was surprised by the brisk tone of some matrons in cutting off the performance. For instance, an elderly and spirited Bihari woman addressed so the goddess 'playing' with a local Bengali young lady (unrelated to her): *O mā, chor do! Nikal tu!* (H. 'Hey, Mother, stop it! Get out!'). She was then warmly thanked by the relatives of the possessed one, who were standing speechless and scared at the unexpected and unprecedented exploits of the girl.

33 It may happen that during *bhar*, when the devotee is not primarily concerned with issues of modesty, frenzied movements cause petticoats or blouses to reveal few centimetres of bare skin.

34 I personally observed mothers fleeing horrified, stating they won't let their children witness such *shows*.

35 The list does not pretend to be exhaustive. Gujarati and Punjabi interviewees informed me of smaller towns where, with less grandeur, Tamils (whom they call 'Madrasis') join devotees of Śītalā in the celebration of their goddess. I learnt about these festivals from Indian media coverage and took advantage of brief sojourns between 2008 and 2009 and again in 2011. Since intensive fieldwork has not been conducted as elsewhere, my conclusions are provisional. Although I have been able to interview a good number of participants in Jammu, Patiala, Chandigarh and Ahmedabad, two elements have negatively affected my small-scale research. First, interviews have been conducted in Hindi and English; neither is the mother language of my informants. Second, a more in-depth study of archive material and historical records on the presence of Tamil communities in the above-mentioned sites is needed. Regretfully, for reasons of time and space, I have limited my work to other aspects of the worship of Śītalā.

36 My knowledge of Māriyammaṉ is entirely dependent upon academic literature, e.g. Younger 1980; Egnor 1984; Elmore 1995; Nabokov 2000; Harman 2004; Allocco 2009, 2013.

37 This is usually, but not exclusively, celebrated after the beginning of the hot season, in the Āṭi season (Allocco 2009: 269–371; Brighenti 2012: 128).

38 Many scholars have discussed Śītalā as the product of village folklore vis-à-vis the Brahmanic and Sanskrit ritual, devotional and medical tradition. See Arnold 1993: 121–5; Nicholas 2006: 107 and *passim*. A recent example of this disturbing trend is Behera, who says: 'The primitive mind, being incapable of any reasoning or logical analysis, believed in invisible and malicious spirits. This may be considered as nothing else than the existential meaning of religion in the folk-mind. From the above discussion it has been revealed that the worship of Sitala, the primitive disease deity, through the lapse of time has been identified with Hindu, Muslim, Buddhist and Sikh faith' (Behera 2013: 190). Cf. Gopalan and his argument that *Śītalāvratas*, and *vratas* in general, are not just superstition, but 'scientific explanations and functions holding true in those days and some even today' (Gopalan 1978: 117). In response to that, see the critique of Pati (2002: 485) and Mukharji (2013: 263).

39 Māriyammaṉ is associated with the deification of Princess Reṇukā. In Mbh 3.116: 1–20, Reṇukā is the *kṣatriya* wife of the *muni* Jamadagni. Tempted by impure thoughts of a sexual nature, she causes the angry reaction of her ascetic Brahman husband, who orders his five sons to kill her. Upon the refusal of four sons, Jamadagni makes them collapse as dead. The last son, Paraśurāma (Rāma with an axe), beheads his mother. Pleased with his loyalty, Jamadagni grants his son a favour. Paraśurāma asks for the resurrection of Reṇukā and his brothers, which is accorded. (An alternative version is found in the *Reṇukāmāhātmya*, incorporated in the late *Sahyādrikhaṇḍa* of SkP. Cf. Gerson da Cunha 1877.) The Tamil version of the myth has a different finale. In the fury of his murderous act, Paraśurāma beheads a dark-skinned washerwoman along with his mother. In haste, he attaches the wrong head on each body. Jamadagni refuses to take back his impure wife. So Reṇukā becomes the goddess Māriyammaṉ and the low-class woman becomes Mātaṅgī.

40 Piercing rituals are performed by Tamils in other diasporic contexts (e.g. Collins 1997; Bauman 2006). I am not aware of devotional ordeals specifically dedicated to Śītalā. I heard devotees invoking Śītalā on occasion of the *caṛakapūjā* ('hook swinging') during the celebrations featuring the *gājan* in West Bengal (Ferrari 2010a). This, however, is a *śaiva* festival, and does not usually feature Śītalā (cf. Nalin 2004). Contrary to my previous conclusions, it seems Śītalā is currently included in some Bengali *gājan* traditions. A short documentary has been recently produced: *Śītalā Gājan* (2013). Devotees swing on fire, roll on thorny branches and have their tongues pierced. The short video has been shot in Pilkhan village, Khanakul police station (Hooghly District, WB). The rationale of the performance is healing and the protection of newborns.

41 Language barriers have contributed to keep the two goddesses apart. Devotees of Māriyammaṉ – though proficient in local languages (Hindi/Urdu, Punjabi and Gujarati) – continue to transmit the mythology of the goddess in Tamil, a language that is unintelligible to locals.

42 Informants mentioned piercing rituals in general and, particularly, the spectacular nature of austerities like the pulling of cars with ropes tied to hooks piercing the back of a devotee, a devotional performance associated with a strong bravado component.

43 Online versions of Indian newspapers, as well as web pages of amateur ethnographers or websites for the sharing of photographs, do not bear enough evidence to suggest this is a common practice.

44 Devotional ordeals are far from uncommon in India. See my study of the *gājan* festival in West Bengal (Ferrari 2010a). Also cf. Obeyesekere 1978; Oddie 1995; Collins, E. 1997; Ferrari 2005; Bauman 2006; Nicholas 2009; Brighenti 2012; Schröder 2012.

45 Vedic texts show concern with the inauspiciousness that may derive from bloodletting as a result of the beheading of animals at the sacrificial stake (*yūpa*). This practice – known as *paśubandha* – was slowly substituted by the tying of the animal and its suffocation, a ritual that avoided the spilling of blood (Schmidt 1973).

46 The Indian constitution objects to cruelty against all living beings, and the Animals and Birds Sacrifices Prohibition Act has been implemented from 1950 in some states of the union (Andhra Pradesh, Gujarat, Karnataka, Kerala, Pondicherry, Rajasthan and Tamil Nadu). Yet even when *balidān* is forbidden by law, there is no formal objection from the authorities. See, for instance, *Times of India* 2012 on *balidān* at the Agam Kuāṅ shrine in of Patna (Bihar).

47 Some of the most active in West Bengal are Compassionate Crusaders, People for Animals (Kolkata), the Indian chapter of Beauty Without Cruelty and Love N Care for Animals. PETA India has also members operating in West Bengal.

48 With reference to the ongoing ritual killing of hundreds of animals in the Kāmākhyā Temple in Assam, 'the Samajwadi Party national secretary, Dr Suneelam, retorted: "People who sacrifice animals are mentally disturbed. The party does not believe in it"' (cited in McDermott 2011: 215).

49 West Bengal, Odisha and the Seven Sister States (Arunachal Pradesh, Assam, Meghalaya, Manipur, Mizoram, Nagaland and Tripura).

50 Bengalis, including Bengali Brahmans, are stereotypically portrayed across India as avid consumers of *chāg* (goat), *māch* (fish) and *bhāt* (rice).

51 An erudite *paṇḍit* and *purohit* of an urban *śākta mandir* in Kolkata (who asked to remain anonymous) was vociferous about the way in which anti-*bali* campaigns are conducted. He noticed that the trend is to systematically downgrade and exclude ritualists, devotees and intellectuals (e.g. historians and other academics) from the debate. He showed me a series of articles and print-outs from web pages of Indian newspapers featuring random and incoherent voices from illiterate and semi-literate devotees suggesting that if the goddess (most papers referred to Kālī) is not given sacrifice, she will punish everybody. Such simplistic arguments are opposed to the objections of powerful, well-educated and visible leaders (e.g. Maneka Gandhi), Indian and Western NGOs, intellectuals, volunteers and even pupils from elite primary and secondary schools.

52 Sacrifice, austerities and possession have been systematically objected to – and in some cases outlawed (Oddie 1995) – in response to the moralizing campaigns of British authorities and Indian reformers. Further to that, one should consider the importance of the missionary element and the penetration of Protestant and Catholic churches in the subcontinent. From a Christian point of view, *bhar* and *khelnā* were equated to the diabolic possessions of the Bible and the Gospels, whereas sacrifice was a horrific practice associated with pagan cults not worth their space in a country governed by a Christian monarch.

53 According to a philosophical notion powerfully enculturated at all levels of Hindu culture, everything that exists is featured by one of the three qualities (*triguṇa*), or a combination of them. These are *sattva* (purity), *rajas* (dynamism) and *tamas* (obscurity, ignorance).

4

The smallpox myth and the creation of the goddess of smallpox

The gentrification of Śītalā, a phenomenon largely, but not exclusively, imputable to upward mobility, has resulted in various forms of critique of her culture. The spectacularization of the goddess should be included in the landscape. This phenomenon is one beginning as early as the seventeenth century in lower Bengal, when Śītalā was made the protagonist of *maṅgalkāvyas*. Presented by their authors as folk literature, these texts have portrayed Śītalā as aggressive, capricious and disease-inflicting. The myth of the smallpox goddess begins here. This was disseminated in three stages: 1) seventeenth to eighteenth centuries: the production of *maṅgal* poems and the circulation of selected sections (*pālās*) by means of the Bengali open theatre (*yātrā*). These are fictionalized stories designed to entertain, and therefore thought to meet the tastes of large audiences; 2) nineteenth to the first half of twentieth century: in the middle of the smallpox crisis in colonial Bengal, the British – eager to know more about indigenous medicine and prophylaxis – learn about Śītalā, possibly from *pālās* but most likely from public *pūjās*. It follows the uncritical, Orientalist construction of the 'goddess of smallpox of the Hindoos'. This view radicalizes with the introduction of Jennerian vaccination and the colonial struggle against smallpox. The process culminates in the banning of inoculation/variolation (B. *ṭikā*; see below p. 133), a practice that, with time, had been associated with Śītalā; 3) 1960–80: the myth of the smallpox goddess is advertised globally in the years of the WHO SEP (Smallpox Eradication Program) in India and Bangladesh, and particularly through reports and medical narratives of the 'smallpox warriors' as well as of other medical personnel. A trend largely dependent upon uncritical acceptance of the *maṅgal*-Śītalā has emerged in successive studies, thus transforming a literary character into the goddess herself. In the following pages, I will disengage Śītalā from her consolidated image as a smallpox/disease goddess, and explain how this rendition has penetrated global culture.

Ethnographic vignette 8: The Baṛī Śītalā Mandir of Adalpura (Uttar Pradesh)

One of the most popular sites of worship of Śītalā in Uttar Pradesh is the Śītalā Dhām, the 'abode of Śītalā'. Situated on a mound near the small market town of Adalpura (Mirzapur district), around 25 kilometres south of Banaras, the Baṛī Śītalā Mandir ('temple of the old Śītalā'), as it is officially known, is a rectangular construction whose extant structure dates back to the 1970s. In fact, the site is an ancient one. Singh and Rana have dated the walls of an earlier structure back to the beginning of the eighteenth century, but it seems it was used for worship already in the twelfth century (2006: 272). The population of Adalpura is divided into 15 or 16 *jāti*, but the Śītalā Dhām is administered exclusively by *mallāh*s, traditionally boatmen and fishermen. Informants in both Banaras and Adalpura suggest the site was originally a settlement of the Niṣādas, a coalition of various hill-dwellers mentioned several times in MBh (e.g. 6.10: 50) and in other texts.[1] This is unsurprising, since the *mallāh*s claim ancestry from the Niṣādas.

To enter the temple one must pass through a huge gate where a eulogy to the goddess – 'Jai Mā Śītalā' – is displayed in big bold red characters above a brass bell with two tigers by the sides.[2] Once past the portal, one enters the bazaar. Mostly dealing in *pūjā* articles (posters, bandanas, flags, stickers, small figurines for car dashboards, CDs, video-CDs, and activation codes to get *bhaktigān* ringtones), the market includes food, tea, *lassī* and juice stalls, toy kiosks, artisans' shops and repair businesses. The town, which is well connected to surrounding cities (Mirzapur, Allahabad, Banaras) via bus services, has a post office and one bank branch. Its population is limited (c.ca 2,500), but it rises considerably during every full moon, on the occasion of the monthly celebration of Śītalā. During the *navarātri* of Caitra (March–April) and Aśvina (September–October), when large *melā*s (festivals) are arranged, it may reach half a million (Singh and Rana 2006: 272).

In the premises of the Śītalā Dhām, the goddess is represented according to her consolidated iconography, i.e. a young woman richly dressed, holding a pitcher and a broom and riding a donkey (there is no sign of the winnower). Such images disappear once entering the temple. The Śītalā of Adalpura is a riverine goddess.[3] Local narratives and devotional songs in Hindi and Bhojpuri do not mention her mount – a means of transportation she does not actually need. According to local *āñcalik* culture, the goddess revealed herself to a poor *māṁjhī* (a boatman) some 400 years ago.[4] She gave indications through *svapnādeś* (command in a dream) about how to retrieve an ancient *pratimā* lying on the bottom of the river Ganges. The next morning the fisherman threw his net and caught a small stone slab. This was placed in a humble shrine on the banks of the Ganges and there it stayed until the goddess decided it was not a sufficiently decorous place. She appeared again in her devotee's dreams and ordered the building of a proper *mandir*. In exchange she promised protection, good health and fortune.

An alternative and lesser-known tale exists. According to such narrative, Mātā Devī (i.e. Śītalā) appeared to the Niṣāda boatman (*kevaṭ*) who helped Rāma, Lakṣmaṇa and Sītā to cross the river on their way to their 14-year exile in the wilderness.[5] The goddess was very pleased with the boatman's service, and decided to reward him. When the boatman asked who she was, the lady said that in the *kali yuga* her name is that of Śītalā (cf. SkP 7.1.135: 1–2). The goddess then granted him the exclusive right to administer her *pūjā*, and became the protector of his clan.

In the holiest place of the temple, one can only see the silver face of the goddess. Baṛī Mā is entirely surrounded by marigold garlands, *nīm* branches and red drapes. The actual *pratimā* is entirely hidden from the sight of devotees. Over the goddess hang two silver *chatra* (parasols) while in the background there is a huge silver panel with two columns on each side and carved floral motifs. Below the goddess, at the centre of the panel, is represented a small pitcher surmounted by a coconut and auspicious *harā pattā*s, while on each side there is the bas-relief of an ass. When I asked the reason for using an iconographical element, namely the *gadhā vāhan* (H. 'ass mount'), that does not find a confirmation in local culture, I was given contrasting answers. Several informants never considered such issue, and some let me clearly understand I was too much concerned with meaningless details, thus spoiling the devotion behind Śītalā worship. Some *mallāh* ritualists, however, explained that the

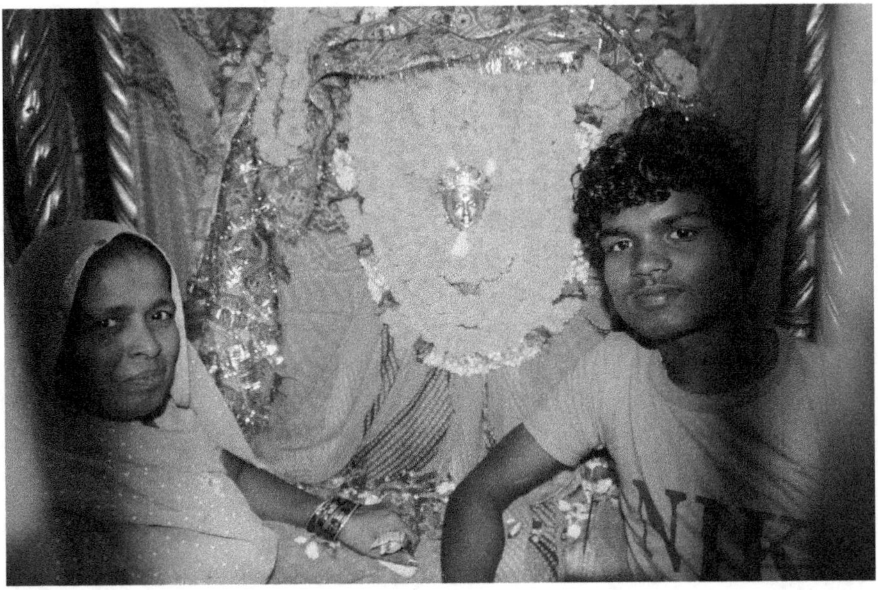

FIGURE 4.1 *Baṛī Śītalā surrounded by* mallah pūjārīs *(mother and son), Śītalā Dhām, Adalpura (UP) (photo by author).*

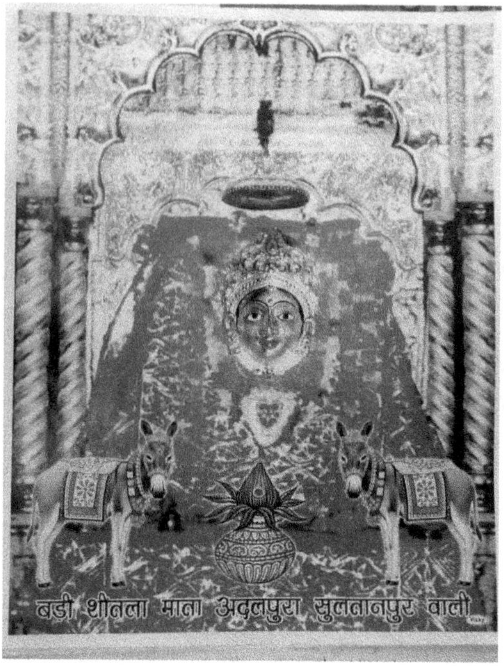

FIGURE 4.2 *Baṛī Śītalā, Adalpura, poster (author's collection).*

iconographic material reproduced and displayed in the temple and the surrounding bazaar is not a local product. It reflects a Hindustani custom. Adalpura Mahimā has no mount but, I was told: 'We know that this [indicating a postcard with the goddess on a donkey] is a very popular aspect of Śītalā. And we love it too.' Further, as I learnt from other informants, 'all good goddesses have a *vāhan!*'.

By reflecting on the conversations I had with local *pūjārī*s and *bhakta*s, I gained a profound awareness of, and appreciation for, the multiform ways in which the goddess Śītalā manifests and is represented. There is however a major hiatus between the general perception of Śītalā and the goddess worshipped as Adalpura Mahimā. The latter is not a deity chiefly related to illness. For the *mallāh*s of Adalpura and Banaras, Śītalā is an auspicious mother who grants fertility, good luck and prosperity. As the protector of their business, she is the goddess of the *mallāh*s, not the 'goddess of smallpox'. Baṛī Śītalā does not cause diseases, and healing is believed to result from her auspicious presence. The worshipping pattern is also different from the extremely ritualized one I observed elsewhere, for instance in nearby Banaras. *Mallāh pūjārī*s are neither Brahmans nor healers, and their intervention is minimally invasive. They are administrators and coordinators more than ritual specialists. The mass of devotees is controlled by assistants with bright orange T-shirts while red-clad temple *pūjārī*s pass their (vegetarian) offerings to the goddess, receive donations and give *prasād*. Śītalā is a gentle presence, a benevolent goddess who helps the *mallāh* community of the districts around Banaras in the turbulent waters of their often difficult lives.[6]

Notwithstanding the strong localism of the foundation myth of the Adalpura site and its enculturation in community life, the *maṅgal*-Śītalā has found a way to express herself. This depends on the diffusion through new media, chiefly the world wide web, of the smallpox myth. The following is an excerpt from the unofficial blog of the Adalpura Śītalā Dhām:

> In Hinduism, Goddess Shitala, or Sheetala Mata, is considered an aspect of Shakti. Popularly she is the Hindu goddess of small pox in North India and is known to spread the dreaded disease and cure it. In rural India, she is also considered as an incarnation of Goddess Parvati and Durga, which are two forms of Shakti. Goddess Shitala is popular as Mariamman in Tamil Nadu. She is undoubtedly one of the most popular rural deities and her origin can be traced to the days of Nature Worship. Legend has it that Goddess Shitala wears a red-colored dress and rides around the villages in North India on a donkey (ass) and inflicting people with the dreaded pox – small pox, chicken pox etc. Symbolically, she represents Nature's power of generating viruses causing disease and Nature's healing power and is of tribal origin. She is depicted having four hands. In her four hands she carries a silver broom, winnow fan, small bowl and a pitcher with Gangajal, holy water from River Ganga. Occasionally, she is depicted with two hands carrying a broom and pitcher. Symbolically, Goddess Sheetala idol also emphasizes the need for cleanliness. According to Puranas, Shitala, the cooling one, was created by Lord Brahma. She was promised by Brahma that she will be worshipped as a Goddess on earth but she should carry the seeds of lentils. In folktales in North India, the lentil is 'Urad dal'. She then asked for a companion and she was directed to Lord Shiva, who blessed her and created Jvara Asura (the fever demon). It is said that he was created from the sweat of Lord Shiva. Shitala and Jvara Asura remained in Devaloka along with other gods and goddess. They used a donkey to transport the lentils wherever they went. But the lentil seeds one day turned into smallpox germs and start to spread the disease among gods and goddesses. Finally, fed up with Goddess Shitala, gods asked her to go and settle in heaven where she will be worshipped. Shitala and Jvara Asura came down to earth and started hunting for a place to stay. They went to the court of King Birat, an ardent devotee of Shiva. He agreed to worship her and give a place in his kingdom but she will not get the respect given to Shiva. An angry Shitala demanded supremacy over all other gods and when King Birat did not budge, she spread different kinds of pox on the land and finally, the King had to agree to her wishes. Soon the disease and all its after effects were miraculously cured. The most important festival dedicated to her takes place in Chaitra month, the Ashtami day after Purnima (full moon) in the month is observed as Sheetala Ashtami. [. . .] (Sahani 2011)

The above myth is not the one of Adalpura. The story of Śītalā's birth and her exploits with Jvarāsura (a demon that only appears in Bengali narratives of Śītalā) in the kingdom of 'Birat' is loosely extrapolated from the *Virāṭapālā* of Nityānanda Cakravartī.[7] Sahani's log is indicative of the way in which aspects of Bengali *maṅgal* narratives have slowly but dramatically penetrated the goddess culture at the point that Śītalā's vernacular aspects have merged in the global *maṅgal* narrative of the goddess of smallpox. In this and similar websites or blogs, Śītalā is presented as Śakti, or a form of pan-Hindu goddesses. Her 'low' (i.e. rural, folk) origins are always mentioned. She inflicts poxes and is known in the south as Māriyammaṉ. The internet is replete with similar descriptions. For instance, the Wikipedia entry 'Shitala' – in all possibility the most accessed and accessible resource – provides readers worldwide with a description highly evocative of the Bengali *maṅgalkāvyas*:

> Shitala is accompanied by Jvarasura, the fever demon, Oladevi, the cholera goddess, Ghentu-debata, the god of skin diseases, Raktabati, the goddess of blood infections and the sixty-four epidemics. Shitala is represented as a young maiden crowned with a winnowing-fan, riding an ass, holding a short broom (either to spread or dust off germs) and a pot full of pulses (the viruses) or cold water (a healing tool). Among low-caste Hindus and tribal communities, she is represented with slab-stones or carved heads. Sometimes, she is said to be carrying a bunch of neem (Azadirachta indica) leaves, an ancient Ayurvedic medicinal herb that is believed by some to be an effective remedy to most skin diseases even today.
>
> Shitala is form of goddess katyayani (adi shakti). She gives coolness to the patients of fever. According to Devi Mahatyam when a demon named Jwarasura gave bacteria of fever to all the children, goddess katyayani took herself in the form of Shitala to purify children's blood and to destroy the bacteria of fever in blood. In sanskrit [sic] fever means Jwar and Shital means coolness. Shitala is also sometimes depicted with a shady woman called Raktavati (Possessor of Blood). She is often worshiped with Oladevi, another disease goddess.[8]

Similar problems affect academic reference works (and their online editions) whose often uncritical use has nurtured the diffusion of the myth of the goddess of smallpox (e.g. Lochtefeld 2001: 632; Jones and Ryan 2007: 405). Two among the most recent cases can be found in the *Encyclopedia of Hinduism* (Cush, Robinson and York 2008) and the *Brill's Encyclopedia of Hinduism* (Jacobsen, Basu, Malinar and Narayanan 2009). In the former instance, Cynthia Bradley informs us that Śītalā is 'also known as Olācandi [sic] and Olabibi' [sic] (2008: 798). We also learn that 'she is accompanied by Jvarasur [sic], the fever demon, and her serving woman, Rāktabāti [sic], 'the Bloody One'. The myth of origin of the goddess is then given, i.e. the story of the birth of Śītalā in Nityānanda Cakravartī's ŚMK. The message is that Nityānanda's 'smallpox goddess' is the South Asian Śītalā. Bradley then mentions Kolkata temples only, and concludes by saying that: 'At her urban temples, Śītalā is not seen as a fierce, disease-bringing goddess, but as a gentle, kind friend who gives general protection in the lives of her devotees' (ibid.) It seems thus implied that there exist two Śītalā: the gentle mother worshipped in urban centres and the scary disease-inflicting goddess of the rural folks. This is somehow confirmed in the second source. Half of the 'Śītalādevī' entry authored by Rebecca Manring (2012), a specialist in Bengali literature, relates to the goddess of the ŚMKs without acknowledging that these works are entertaining/ imaginative literature (Curley 2008: 4). Manring's contribution, like many other studies, bears witness to an overall dependence on studies of the goddess in Bengali literature and culture only. (Her sources include: Bhattacharyya 1955; Bang 1973; Dimock 1982; Mukhopadhyay 1994; Stewart 1995; Nicholas 2003.) An exception to this trend is the very short, but extremely accurate, 'Śītalā'-entry authored by Susan Wadley in an encyclopedia of South Asian folklore (2003: 561–2). Wadley, in a concise style, offers a general introduction to the worship of the goddess across north Indian regions and literary genres, and highlights the role of the goddess as a protector whose worship permits the transmission of hygienic norms.

The authoritative and influential nature of academic and medical resources has fostered the 'smallpox myth' in various facets of contemporary culture. It so appears that Śītalā:

- **a** is a folk/village/rural goddess;
- **b** continues to be the Indian goddess of smallpox, even though the Certification of Smallpox Eradication is dated 1979;[9]
- **c** is associated with deities and demons that appear only in (some) of the Bengali ŚMKs;
- **d** is a protective-cum-malign goddess who inflicts smallpox and other diseases if dissatisfied with the behaviour of human and divine beings.

The internet, as a global medium for the dissemination of knowledge, is contributing to a dramatic editing of the history of the goddess and her relation to health issues. This trend, as I will show in the next sections, began in late premodern Bengal and was favoured by the intensification of the struggle against smallpox in colonial and post-colonial India.

Disease and ambiguity: The construction of the 'other' in the Bengali *maṅgalkāvyas*

Śītalāmaṅgalkāvyas have been regarded as a minor – in both quantity and quality[10] – chapter of the *maṅgal* tradition of premodern Bengal. Studies conducted by Bhaṭṭācāryya (1998), Mukhopadhyay (1994), Nicholas (2003), Dimock (1982), Stewart

(1995) and more cursorily by Zbavitel (1976), Curley (2008) and Bhattacharya (2000), among others, have indulged in three, partially overlapping, issues: 1) the ambiguous nature of the goddess Śītalā; 2) the social history of Bengal; and 3) the production of this literature as a response to the smallpox emergency. It goes without saying that just as ŚMKs are not representative of Śītalā worship, they are equally not representative of the *maṅgal* genre in its entirety. Each chapter of *maṅgal* literature is informed by a variety of texts as part of an increasingly fashionable genre, and should be read with awareness of its own specificity and, where possible, uniqueness (Lotman 2005: 206). There are however some features – ideological and political – that have been neglected. So far, all studies on ŚMKs have insisted on their devotional and folkloric nature. I argue differently. Constructed on class-bound mythopoesis and a substantial revision (and reinterpretation) of Bengali folk culture for entertaining purposes, ŚMKs have shaped a new profile of the goddess that eventually impacted on renditions and understandings of Śītalā in colonial and post-colonial Bengal, in the rest of India and, eventually, abroad.

The Śītalā celebrated in the *maṅgalkāvyas* is not akin to the goddess worshipped in north Indian households, both in villages and urban centres. I use the verbs 'to celebrate' and 'to worship' purposely. Śītalā is a ritual goddess. Although there is evidence of at least two clusters of narratives (the auspicious lady of the *vratakathās* and the ambiguous smallpox goddess of ŚMKs), Śītalā is not a deity primarily dependent upon storytelling. Myths of the goddess are retold to transmit ritual praxis. Yet the narratives contained in ŚMKs are neither interested in ritual nor in practices conducive to healing. A significant gap thus separates the Bengali ŚMKs from other narrative elements of Śītalā culture. The former are *bona fide* fabrications inspired by the customs of Bengali peasant folklore. The latter are tales or hymns about ritual, or supporting ritual performance.

In *maṅgal* poems, Śītalā appears when humans refuse to worship her. In particular, the appearance of the goddess is triggered by the conscious and stubborn refusal of powerful people to acknowledge her divine status. ŚMKs, however, do not indicate ritual and remedial practice. They make a case for complete surrender. Only occasionally are the rituals of the folk mentioned. These, however, are not supported by detailed instruction. In fact, they point at the spectacularization of ritual while invigorating the underlying menace typical of the *maṅgal* genre:

> He [the tall collector] erected a winsome temple on the banks of the Gaṅgā River and had there installed the Queen of Smallpox, Śītalā, the Cool One. 59. He had her worship performed, offering the full gamut of appropriate sacral items. From that the wicked and base were frightened into good and honest people! 60. Goats and rams were sacrificed with satisfying production, and her worship was consummated with reverent concentration and attention. (*Madanadāsapālā*, KD.ŚMK)[11]

The goddess of the ŚMKs loudly demands to be acknowledged as a powerful and praise-worthy deity. But she does not say how. Worship depends upon absolute surrender. If her divine status is disregarded, Śītalā strikes gods and humans with poxes and other debilitating diseases. Only after destruction has been inflicted do survivors learn that Śītalā is a powerful *devī*. The happy ending depends on submission, and *bhakti* responds to fear.

Chapal Kumar Bhaduri, a celebrated Bengali female impersonator well known for interpreting Śītalā and an open-air theatre (*yātrā*) star,[12] speaks thus while playing the goddess in a *Śītalāpālā*:

> O King, thou art noble, thou art all powerful
> Render onto me thy fervent deference
> I know the Celestial medicine-men rule here –
> The Ashwinikumaras and Dhanwantary[13] –
> And the world accepts their medications
> No mortal dares question their judgment.
> But have they any cure for the vile pox (*vasanta*)
> To relieve mankind from this dreaded
> Summer affliction that curses so many?
> No! yet these established ones gain men's respect.
> But one who has no status in society,
> Thought she's ever so worthy, will always be ignored.
> That is the eternal law. Therefore O King,
> I demand you establish me (*pratiṣṭhā din*).
> I demand, O King, the recognition that is due to me!
> And the world shall hail your noble deed forever.
> (Chapal Bhaduri as Śītalā Mā, *Ārekṭi premer galpa*, 2010)

Ambiguity is unproblematic to Bengali devotees, for they are fully aware of the 'simultaneously contradictory iconography' (Katyal 2001: 104) that features the *pālā*s. Contemporary Bengali folk theatre reflects this trend. An interesting case is that of the New Loknath Opera (Katyal 2001). The mean of the message may well change, but the philosophy of the *maṅgalkāvya* tradition remains unaltered:

> Compelling drumbeats, loud music, pulsing lights, and the tale of the goddess is brought to life. Sweeping gestures and lofty lines. The hunger for recognition, for worship, the vengeful violence against nonbelievers, the protection of devotees who call her name. Repeatedly, the call for offerings, for worship, to earn the blessings of this awesome deity. Bowed heads and folded palms, coins held in work-worn hands, offered in appeasement, in devotion, in desire, in fear. (Kishore 2001: 115)

See also the implied threat in the following handbill distributed in advance of the representation of a *Śītalāpālā* by the New Loknath Opera:

> The Mother is coming! The Mother is coming! The Mother is coming! Bearing a basket of the deadly pox on her head, to village after village, comes the mother of all the poxes, Devi Sitala. That is why, in every village, there is the worship and puja of Devi Sitala. Along with the worship of the mother one must utter her sacred name, have devotional songs in her praise [...] (Handbill distributed by the New Loknath Opera theatre company, cited in Katyal and Kishore 2001: 96)

Given what is at stake, actors must be credible. They carefully reproduce the standard features of the goddess: white paste to recreate the pale complexion, a big third eye across the forehead, a bright red sari, heavy golden ornaments, a winnowing tray secured to their wig, a *jhāṛū* or a *camar* in their right hand and a metal or earthen pitcher in the crook of their left arm (cf. Kishore 2001: 114). The actor impersonating Śītalā is expected to bless the audience. Here we see how the popularization of selected *pālās* and their adaptation for public consumption have permitted assimilation into ritual practice, an essential feature of Śītalā culture.[14] Chapal Bhaduri himself expresses surprise at the practice of receiving offerings in exchange of *darśana*, i.e. his performance as Śītalā:

> This Shitala pala ... I still do it, it goes on, it starts in the Spring. As for this sindoor custom ... I once asked this young woman how come you put sindoor on me and let me put sindoor on you? That's a custom only women share. But I'm a man dressed as a woman, and your husband is sitting right here, doesn't he mind?[15] But she said: 'No, you're Ma Shitala. Say what you will, you're not Chapal da. You're Ma.' (Chapal Bhaduri, in *Performing the Goddess*, 1999)

The eulogies of ŚMKs are reframed in a novel set of physical and behavioural features of the goddess that spectacularly affirm themselves by means of an entertaining performance. Contradictions, however, emerge. See, for instance, how the opening invocation in Kavi Jagannāth's *maṅgalkāvya* combines purāṇic heritage with typical *maṅgal* ideology:

> The matted locks on Your head surpass the yak-tail fly-whisk. On Your forehead there is vermillion mark. [...] Your limbs are adorned with many ornaments. I salute You, Devī Śītalā, and worship Your feet. Wearing royal garments (*rāṭbastra*), yet You are space-clad (*digambarī*, i.e. nude). In Your right hand a broom [?], in the crook of Your left arm a water-pot [...]; You have with You pox-incense (*basanter dhup*). A golden broom in Your hand, a golden pot on Your left side. Come Ruler of Disease (*Roger Rājā*), accept the worship that is rightfully Yours, and offer salvation through Your unique quality. (Kavi Jagannāth, *Bardhamānapālā*)[16]

This is even more evident in Nityānanda Cakravartī's ŚMK, a text composed circa two decades later. Though maintaining traditional elements borrowed from ŚAS, Śītalā's miraculous birth among the gods is told:[17]

> Listen carefully, devotees, while I tell the story of Mother Śītalā's birth. King Nahuṣa was performing a sacrifice to obtain a son. Who could count all the sages and seers who came! They performed the sacrifice with the offerings, unimpeded, and the whole ceremony came off peacefully. At the end of the sacrifice, they put out the fire. In it they found a radiant young woman. She emerged with a winnowing tray on her head. When Brahmā caught sight of her, he politely asked, 'Who are you, lovely girl, whose wife? Why were you in the fire? Tell us the story!' 'A goddess! I was born in the fire pit. Where do I go now, what do I do? I'm bewildered.' Brahmā replied, 'You were born after the sacrificial fire had cooled, so your name is Śītalā, the "Cool One". I hereby send you straight to earth, where you will be worshipped in many ways. As Śītalā you will be proclaimed throughout the world. Take all these peas, lentils and chickpeas and go into the world of mortals for a great celebration.' (*Janmapālā*, NC.ŚMK)[18]

The ambiguities are not over. In ŚMKs, the goddess is worshipped as a charming young woman, crowned with a tiara, heavily bejewelled, with garlands of fragrant flowers and dressed in a red silk sari (e.g. J.ŚMK. 1). But she often wanders in disguise (e.g. J.ŚMK. 2; MG.ŚMK. 5: 73). She may appear to humans as a poor and old Brahman lady, a witch or a village madwoman, wearing ragged clothes and matted hair (as in Jagannāth's *Bardhamānapālā* above). Her traditional nudity offends and scares (NC. ŚMK-B.) and her dream visitations are ominous presages. Most *pālā*s emphasize her aggressiveness, vengefulness and murderous intents, this depending on her double (hot/cold) nature (H.ŚMK. 150). In fact, *maṅgal* poets seem to have constructed their Śītalā on lurid details of tantric goddesses, or *yoginī*s and *ḍākini*s (cf. NC.ŚMK-B. 61; H.ŚMK. 156–7) or spectacular and exotic renditions of the beliefs and customs of 'the folks'. This has resulted in the affirmation of Śītalā as Rogeśvarī, the fearful Lord of Diseases (e.g. NC.ŚMK-B. *Vivāhapālā* 45–6; *Indrapūjāpālā* 47, 50, 53, 56). In such guise, she is described at the head of armies of plagues, or followed by dangerous demonic assistants:

26 The *Cāmudal* (Skin Eruptions) went, with the sixty-four disease; the *Rakta-muṅga* (Bloody-mawed) pox got ready gaily.

27 The exceedingly terrible *Beṅgcya* (*baiñcā*, Jujube) pox, that jeopardizes life and has Death as an ally, prepared.

28 *Tilyākalyā* (Sesamum-cake), the *Kāṭhalya* (Jack-fruit) of terrible strength, and the *Musuryā* (Smallpox, lit. pox resembling *masur* pulse) and *Dhukuṛyā* (? Pox associated with a coarse sack) eruptions (*cāmudal*) got ready.

29 The Agni-*muṅgā* (Fiery-mawed) pox, most terrible, lined up; in its burning, life goes away, taken to the house of Death.

30. The *Biṣmuṅgā* (Poison-mouthed) poxes of various kinds got ready, as did the *Atika* (Bundle) pox, with the *Ḍumuryā* (Fig) for company.

31 *Garula* (*garal*, poison) and *Tẽtulyā* (Tamarind) – these principal poxes prepared themselves, and the rambunctious *Batryā* (?) and *Ṣiphuryā* (?).

32 The *Alkusyā* (Cowage) pox got ready in great glee; and the *Ṭiuryā* and the *Chapryā* (? Blotchy) readied themselves along with *the Biśālyā* (Huge).

33 The accoutred *Milāmilā* (Measles) went with the *Mataryā* (resembling *maṭar* pulse), which, one it seizes hold, does not let go while life remains.

34 The *Suci-muṅgā* (Needle-mouthed) pox got ready swiftly; and *Paṭalyā* (*paṭal*, a small cucumber-shaped vegetable) and *Pāniphalyā* (Water-chestnut), the intractable ones.

35 The *Luā-garā* (Iron-clad) pox accoutred itself in great style, [the one] that appears after a person dies, on the stiff corpse.

36 Many a *Dhān-śisā* (Rice-whisker) pox rushed forth, [as did] the *Mādāryā* (*Mādār*-fruit) and the *Nīl-badan* (Blue visage).

37 *Galagaṇḍa* (Goiter) got ready with a sinister passion, and all of the *Khos* (Scabies) prepared, together with the *Biṣphoṭak* (Poisonous boils).

38 In this way the various species of pox readied themselves; they came to the Goddess's feet and saluted.

39 Said Śītalā, 'I have a great desire to hear what power (*pratāp*) each one of you has, so tell me.'

(MG.ŚMK)[19]

The goddess of the ŚMKs is rough, violent, mysterious and passionate. Only when pleased (*santuṣṭī*) with human and divine recognition, she calms down and leaves. One could even wonder whether, according to such texts, Śītalā's presence is truly auspicious. As a matter of fact, the manifestation of the goddess is often symptomatic of her rage, and anticipates disease and destruction. The more Śītalā is distant, the more likely are humans and gods to avoid contagion. This is the reverse of ritual praxis, when Śītalā is invited to stay, as her awakening guarantees protection.

The oscillations of Śītalā's behaviour are a grotesque mockery of the *ugra-sāmya* paradigm featuring Śaktis like Kālī, Tārā and other fierce tantric goddesses.[20] Unlike Dimock (1982: 185–87), who associates the manifestation of the goddess with the Christian theological concept of *charisma* (Gr. 'grace') and suggests that *maṅgal* poems impart 'well-being, beneficence' by means of the *līlā* (Skt. 'play', 'game') of the goddess (i.e. epidemic and information), I see Śītalā's presence as a performance depending upon exaggeration, hyperbole and sharp dichotomies. It is so that along with stories of absolute devotion, we have intimidating tales of death, horror and blood:

> In Virāta, at the foot of a banyan tree, on an extensive piece of ground eight miles in length and breadth, Śītalā established a marketplace for ghouls. In heaven, the sun, the moon, Death, and the gods of the ten directions trembled when they observed her play. Demons sounded drums, a great uproar arose, and with arms uplifted the diseases danced. Having gathered all the corpses, male and female ghouls put them on abundant display in shops, and bought and sold. Getting the stench, crows and kites in hundreds of thousands came, and flies buzzed around. An old grandmother ghoul sold intestines of corpses, calling them jackfruit [...] and human heads as coconuts and rotting heads of elephants as ripe Palmyra fruits. The ears of corpses were sold in the market as *pān*, and the pupils of their eyes as rice. Female ghouls bought bags of brains of corpses as lime, and rotting melting corpses for perfume. Pairs of ears were sold as incense, finger and toe nails as husked rice, and the penises of boys as dates. Palates were sold as ripe cantaloupe, and human heads as vegetables. Vomited blood is the best loved drink of male and female ghouls; human blood is sugarcane juice for them. Demons bought and ate the breasts of dead women as if they were custard apples or pomegranates [...] and the female ghouls bought and wove garlands made of human heads and fingers and toes and hands and feet. Blue and yellow ghouls sold brains, having broken open skulls and emptied them. Heads of men and women were lined up, and heads of children, and elephant tusks were sold as radishes. Human ears were hibiscus flowers, flywhisks were made of skin with hair, and blood and pus were sold as sandalwood paste. (*Virāṭapālā*, NC.ŚMK)[21]

Not only does the fascination with dread pervade various sections of ŚMKs and their public representation, it also features opening invocations, whose function was, and still is, that of welcoming the auspicious presence of the goddess:

> I praise the Cool One, Śītalā, goddess of smallpox and dread diseases, perched on her donkey, and I make obeisance to her feverdemon, Jvara, and to Śītalā's blood-thirsty servant of dread diseases, Dāsī Raktāvatī. (Excerpt from Gayārāma Dāsa's *Madanamañjarīpālā*)[22]

ŚMKs have a devotional component. But this, I argue, is functional to their mundane scope, that is, to entertain. I had the chance to witness this aspect on several occasions. During a short sojourn in Vishnupur (Bankura District) in 2010, during the annual *pūjā* of the goddess, I observed a one-night theatrical representation of the myth of Śītalā loosely adapted from Nityānanda's *Virāṭapālā*. The story was well known to everybody, and the festive atmosphere contributed to making the event appealing and enjoyable. I noticed, however, that many amid the crowd, particularly youngsters and children, were eagerly waiting to see monsters and demons (*bhūt-piśāc*). Actors impersonating vengeful skeletons, horned and hairy demons and ferocious fanged ghosts were welcomed with a big cheer. Their performance was made even more convincing by the use of a language pitted with profanities and a series of animal-like tones (high-pitched screeches, guttural sounds, roars, incomprehensible blabbering and what I understood as voluntary syntax errors).[23] This was a much-anticipated aspect of the representation. Although one can appreciate extensive references to globalized horror culture (particularly the Hollywood zombie and vampire stereotype), the gory narrative elements of ŚMKs continue to be a common theme within *Śītalāpālās*.

This brings us to the didactic rationale. What sort of teaching do these poems convey? Like other *maṅgal* poems (Curley 2008: 10; cf. Kaviraj 2003: 516), ŚMKs recommend imitating human protagonists. In particular, they narrate about the refusal of *upajāti*s, or powerful people, to worship Śītalā, and their inevitable capitulation (advertised as *bhakti*) after tasting the wrath of the goddess. I thus oppose the idea that the *maṅgal* genre is just 'village poetry', as Dimock summarized in an early essay (1963: 6).Similarly, I do not see in the *bhakti* of ŚMKs a form of pedagogy, as Dimock does when he notes that: 'They enable us mortals, with limited vision and small intelligence, to learn from discrete experience, to fit that experience into larger divine scheme of things. We are kept aware of the presence of the goddess, and of her grace, and by devotion to her we are blessed' (Dimock 1982: 187). In fact, I argue that ŚMKs are folklore as professional (Brahman) literati wanted folk culture to be.

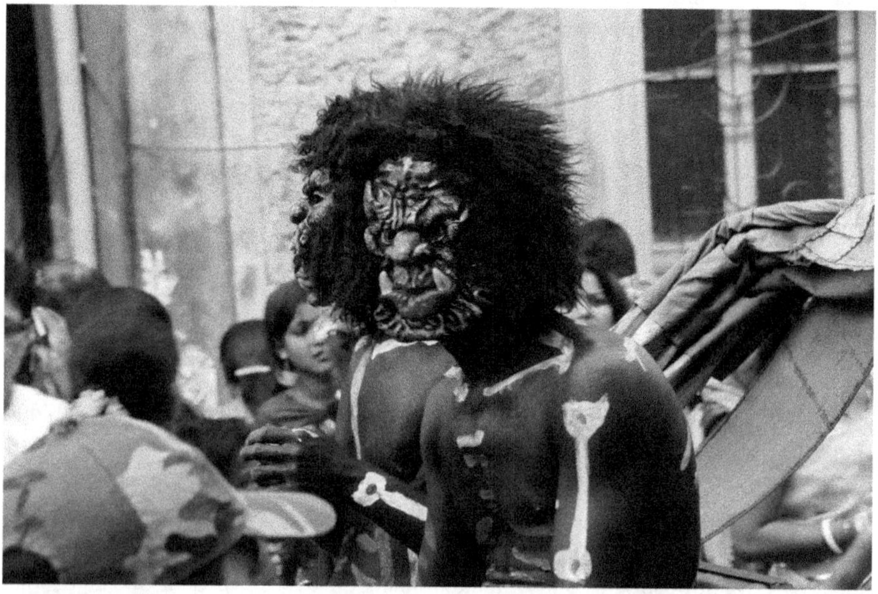

FIGURE 4.3 *Actors impersonating monsters, Salkia (photo by Jayanta Roy).*

The ŚMKs give voice, in a poetic and captivating fashion, to the (*bona fide*) prejudice of educated and wealthy elites toward the peasant classes and their religion, which they describe as a form of utilitarian *bhakti* informed by fear and ignorance. *Maṅgal* poets portray the people and their narratives as primitive, just like nineteenth- and early twentieth-century anthropologists did with the culture of extra-European non-Christian people. This ideology has been so persuasive that a long line of scholars have accepted ŚMKs as genuine expression of folk culture, and never questioned the possibility of an alternative reading. See, for instance, Āśutoṣ Bhaṭṭācārya on *maṅgal* texts in general:

> The lower society of the *maṅgal-kābyas* was unable, because of its narrow-minded limitations, to appreciate the ideal of merciful and benefactory deities conceived by the advanced Aryan society. Therefore the gods of the *maṅgalkābyas* are low, selfish, cruel, revengeful, ungrateful and deceitful. The devotees never bow to them in reverence and devotion voluntarily, nobody takes refuge with them, attracted by their greatness; people pronounce their names only out of fear, in order to protect themselves against their groundless persecution. (Bhaṭṭācārya in Zbavitel 1976: 160)

The ŚMKs are a grotesque portrayal of peasant culture. The auspicious narratives of the goddess Śītalā are constructed on the commodification of *bhakti*, and tell a story that confirms social boundaries and class-bound prejudice. Not only does this explain the spectacularization of folk culture,[24] it also provides an alternative way to understand social dynamics in relation to disease and its diverse – often contrastive – exegeses.

Finally, I find it revealing that health issues and healing practices are not mentioned in ŚMKs. For a literary genre celebrating a goddess associated with disease and widely worshipped as a protector, *maṅgal* poets, unlike the composers of purāṇic hymns, *dharmanibandhas*, *vratakathās*, tantric manuals or *pūjāpaddhatis*, are surprisingly reluctant to discuss medical knowledge and/or prophylactic/hygienic norms. This may well be a narrative device to highlight the necessity of submitting to the goddess as the only way out of misery – just like the anonymous author of ŚAS did. In fact, it says that village culture is a world deprived of knowledge, where the only remedy for disease (or chaos) is surrendering to a superior power, and respecting the rules. Or else.

In the words of Kaviraj: ‘the religious spirit animating the *maṅgalkavya* stories leans toward the magical, in contrast to the more intellectual and rationalized preoccupations of orthodox or developed *bhakti* doctrines’ (2003: 516). Unlike the *kathā* supporting the ‘ritual Śītalā’ in *vrata* culture, Bengali *maṅgalkāvyas*, as wisely noted by Curley (2008: 4), are ‘imaginative works of literature’ and should not be looked at as ‘reports or documents’.[25] They are not even religious texts. They are plays based on a non-original subject.[26] This is made abundantly clear by *maṅgal* poets themselves, who describe Śītalā as the protagonist (*nāyak*) of a drama (*pālā*), and invoke her to protect the performing party (*āsar*) and the poetical structure of the verses (*gānthani*) of the play (cf. Nicholas 2003: 149 on MG.ŚMK). Exaggeration responds to the necessity to entertain and captivate audiences.[27] See, for instance, Jvarāsura's advice to Śītalā:

> Jvarā said, 'Hear, Oh Mother Devī Śītalāi! All of these diseases will not get You worship. The Gods churned the ocean, and thereupon Dhanwantari (the heavenly physician) was born. If you go to him with these diseases, he has medicines for all of them. If people take medicine, the fever disappears and they become well, and they will not give You worship. If You are to receive worship at Bīrsiṃha's seat, then call those diseases for which there is no cure.'
>
> Having heard [the advice] of Jvarā, the Goddess [summoned] the poxes [by name]. Receiving the command of the Goddess [...] the poxes came. (*Bardhamānapālā*, J.ŚMK)[28]

The plot can be summarized as a tragic *do ut des* (NC.ŚMK-B. 42–3). If Śītalā's expectations are not met, she mercilessly kills everybody, including the innocent. In the text of Jagannātha, at the apex of her fury, the goddess infects and kills a child whose only guilt is to be the son of the King of Bardhamān. In turn, the king was responsible for not renouncing Viṣṇu for an old crone (i.e. Śītalā). Contagion, the goddess confesses, is the only way to be worshipped (J.ŚMK. 10). The king concedes that the sole condition for establishing the worship of Śītalā in Bardhamān is the resurrection of the young prince (J.ŚMK. 12; 14). Devotion is not a noble feeling in *maṅgal* narratives. It is motivated by fear only. The same logic is found in KD.ŚMK (*Madanadāsapālā* 52, 56), when a smallpox-stricken toll collector bargains health for the establishment of Śītalā's vessel (*ghaṭapratiṣṭhā or ghaṭasthāpana*).

Punishment is the rationale of *maṅgal* tales. This is emphatically actualized by means of spectacular murder. But Śītalā does not just react to injury, offence or neglect. The pain and death she inflicts is sometimes a mere caprice. In the *Lavakuśapālā* of his ŚMK, Mānikrām Gāṅgulī (1966: 285–93) tells the story of Śītalā who summons Jvarāsura and reveals her intention to kill with smallpox Lava and Kuśa, the sons of Rāma.[29] Even Jvarāsura shows some piety (2: 10–21). He mentions the troubles of Rāma and Sītā, their exile, the abduction of Sītā, the struggle with Hanumān against Rāvaṇa, the victory and the unfortunate banishment of Sītā. The two boys should be left in peace. Śītalā reacts with surprise. There is no other way to be worshipped (2: 22). After assembling a horde of demon-poxes (see above pp. 123–4, cf. NC.ŚMK-B. 62–3), the goddess marches toward Munipur and poisons the royal twins with her lentils. Then she orders Jvarāsura and the others to enter their bodies (6: 113; 8: 137), and to massacre the rest of the city. The happy ending (healing and recovery) depends upon Śītalā's satisfaction, i.e. the public acknowledgement of her glory.

The process mirrors the dynamics of power regulating exchanges between the working class and agricultural proletariat, on the one hand, and the power bloc (landowners, local *rājās*, wealthy merchants, physicians, tax collectors, etc.), on the other. Just like villagers present a tithe to the local *jamindār* or royal families and must show a respect regulated by strict rules in matters of purity, or more practically, economic power, every human present in the *āñcal* visited by Śītalā is expected to act in the same way. Gods are not spared. In fact, they are terrified by the presence of the goddess (see Dhanvantari's reaction on hearing of Śītalā torturing Lava and Kuśa from Hanumān in MG.ŚMK. 9: 192–4). A divide thus exists between the semi-fictional Śītalā of *maṅgal* poets and the ritual-bound goddess worshipped widely across north India. In the former case, the ontological affirmation of Śītalā and her justification depend on a hierarchy imposed by a capricious power. In the latter, worship – constructed on sacrifice and devotion – is a measure to invite and welcome the goddess as 'one of us', regardless of social norms and hierarchical constraints.

Stories of Śītalā have been composed from the perspective of *upajāti* professional poets, rather than that of the peasants whose culture they were supposed to represent. Their authors, though solidly rooted in the background they describe and certainly familiar with the language and culture of the Bengali peasants, are in no way 'organic intellectuals', as posited by Gramsci (2007, Q4 §49).[30] Their production does not aim at class-consciousness, nor does it suggest a conscious proposal to give voice to, or empower, marginal strata of the Bengali population. *Maṅgal* poets have *de facto* appropriated and manipulated vernacular folklore, though – I believe – not with malice.

With this in mind, I am not convinced that the construction of an alternative mythology in *maṅgal* literature should be simplistically discussed as 'hegemony', just as it is a gross misunderstanding to identify the 'popular' with the 'subaltern' (cf. Hauser 2012: 99). I am sceptical that *maṅgal* poets represent, or give voice to, a central apparatus of coercive power vis-à-vis the lack of a coherent effort in constructing consensus among local peasantry. *Maṅgal* poets might well have been sincere lovers of Bengali folklore who used their professional skills and artistic creativity to create a fashionable product for a variety of purposes, including material gain. I am thus more inclined to discuss the manipulation of Śītalā as the convergence of genuine fascination with local folklore and an unproblematic effort in classifying the goddess's devotees and their modes of life and expression. It thus appears that mythologizing, rather than myth, is an important aspect for understanding how Śītalā evolved in premodern and modern Bengali culture. This process inevitably ends up with the production of a materiality fitting the needs and agendas of authors and audiences.

The variants emerging within Śītalā's semiosphere, the continuum of the 'multivariant semiotic models situated at a range of hierarchical levels' (Lotman 2005: 206), mark economic and political changes in linear time (history), yet are empowered by their alleged mythical origin. As Barthes admonished us, 'the fundamental character of myth is to be appropriated' (2009: 143). If language and meaning are easy prey of the dynamics of power, then what empowers narrative is not just content, rather the way in which things are said (ibid.: 131), or not said. The myth of Śītalā in *maṅgalkāvyas* is shaped by an irregular balance between fixity – a 'paradoxical mode of representation' that 'connotes rigidity and an unchanging order as well as disorder, degeneracy and daemonic repetition' (Bhabha 2007: 94) – and mimicry, a discourse 'constructed around ambivalence' where there appears to be 'a desire for a reformed, recognizable Other, as a subject of a difference that is almost the same, but not quite' (ibid.: 12). The creation, replication and editing of selected micro-myths or behavioural features are indicative of conservatism, a feature that may or may not be intentional. Regardless of the actual *intentio auctoris*, ŚMKs inaugurate the 'smallpox myth', an ideology they construct on the sharp division between *laukik* (folk, popular) and *grāmya* culture on the one hand, and *mārgīya saṃskṛti* on the other.

Barthes's theorizing offers further help to evaluate such still ongoing praxis. Moving from the premise that myth is a tool to achieve the 'dream' of an elite (2009: 178) and is then enforced on otherized subjects, I have adapted Barthes's seven-point analysis (2009: 178–83) to the ŚMKs:

1. *The inoculation*: admitting accidental evil (smallpox epidemics) to conceal principal evil (the manipulation of the 'other').
2. *The privation of history*: history evaporates in front of convenient truths. This is enforced by the idea of the 'irresponsibility of man' vis-à-vis the power of the goddess.
3. *Identification*: the scandal that the other represents is epitomized by simplistic, stereotypical, renditions of the folks, including their deities. The 'other' cannot be really imagined and so 'any otherness is reduced to sameness'. The result is misrepresentation.
4. *Tautology*: in a world deprived of knowledge, the only way out of drama is magical thinking – that is the murder of reason and language.
5. *Neither-norism*: folk culture is examined from a 'prudently compensatory perspective' aiming at equilibrium between opposites: illness/health, hot/cold, protective/malign, high class/low class, man/woman, human/divine, etc.
6. *The quantification of quality*, or the commodification of *bhakti*.
7. *The statement of fact*: the refusal of any explanation and the affirmation of an unalterable hierarchy are once and for all legitimated. ŚMKs are the consecration of common sense.

ŚMKs, and possibly other *maṅgal* poems, have perpetuated a to-date unacknowledged patronizing reading of *āñcalik* culture. The convergence of new technologies[31] with the intensification of smallpox outbreaks, the collapse of indigenous political power, the presence of the British, the emergence of a (Anglicized) Hindu gentry, a powerful hyper-territorial medical machinery and the way in which ŚMKs have been represented, have contributed to the rise of the ambiguous 'goddess of smallpox', and a large-scale dispersion of *āñcalik* culture. On a positive note, the perspective of the

ŚMKs, regardless of its bias, is an open window on premodern Bengal's fascination with indigenous folk culture and their gods. These poems and their representations make us ponder on the way peasant culture was imaged and idealized in new arenas and audiences (royalty, landowners, urban *bhadralok* and Bengali nationalist intellectuals).

The consolidation of the smallpox myth: The struggle against smallpox

One of the most radical innovations of the *maṅgal*-Śītalā is her aura of danger and aggression. Bengali professional literati, in response to their understanding of folk *bhakti* or, possibly, to conform to fashion or external requests (patrons?), created a goddess who could fit the spectacular *ugra-sāmya* paradigm of tantric imagery. It is thus that Śītalā changed from a protective mother into a grotesque peasant Śakti, and the scary goddess of diseases (Rogeśvarī). The popularization of the Lord of the Pox (Vasanta Rāy), however, should not be imputed to *maṅgal* poets *tout court*. The *Śītalāpālā*s, theatrical *adaptations* of selected material from ŚMKs (chiefly, Nityānanda's), have profoundly impacted on public renditions of Śītalā as an irate goddess who punishes men and women with terrible diseases if not properly worshipped.

Bengalis, however, just like other Indians, are perfectly capable of distinguishing the modes of on-stage narratives from ritual praxis and the beliefs informing them. Although devotees continue to attend *pālā*s celebrating the goddess, especially on the occasion of large festivals, in their daily practice Śītalā remains the protective mother that Indian cultures celebrate by means of *pūjā*, *ārti*, *vrata*, *yātrā*, *balidān*, *gīti*, etc. The difference between fiction and praxis, however, was less obvious to other spectators, i.e. the British – whose presence in Bengal was established since 1600 – and the new urban gentry (*bhadralok*). Both have, in different ways, uncritically received and transmitted the myth of the goddess of smallpox.

Given the popularity of Śītalā, and the threat posed by the disease she was associated with, it is not surprising that British residents in Bengal learnt about the Cold Lady. The open theatre (*yātrā*), and its place in big festivals, must have been an important medium. In the eighteenth century, theatrical companies used to perform regularly in and around Calcutta. The *yātrā*, a genre informed, among others, by *maṅgal* myths, was an extremely popular form of expression that was included in annual *pūjās*, religious festivals and other auspicious occasions. Further, representations of *pālā*s were social events aiming, among other things, at the display of the wealth and prestige of the patron and his *gotra*. It seems safe therefore to assume that landowners, royalty and influential families must have welcomed the British.[32] Although it is not easy to prove a consistent British presence on occasions of *yātrā* representations – specifically, *Śītalāpālās* – we know that colonial authorities scrutinized attentively Bengali theatre, and were perfectly aware of the contents of folk performances like *vijaya*s and *yātrā*s. This is confirmed by the text of the Dramatic Performances Act (DPA), implemented in 1876 to prevent, and punish, the dissemination of anti-British sentiments.[33] Article 12 of the DPA tactically says that: 'Nothing in this Act applies to any jatras [sic] or performances of a like kind at religious festivals.'

A more convincing testimony of the British interest in Śītalā in the very same period is documented in the reports of physicians, sanitary commissioners, surgeons and magistrates. Such interest was not due to ethnographic or artistic curiosity. The control of contagious diseases, notably malaria, smallpox and cholera, among the indigenous population was central to policies in matters of public health and sanitation. Quarantine, for long the only method of containing epidemics, proved not viable in the case of smallpox.[34] It is thus that the Indian Medical Service (IMS) began to scrutinize indigenous medical literature (mostly Āyurveda), and sought advice among local *kavirāja*s (i.e. B. *vaidya*s, āyurvedic physicians). Paradoxically, the only remedy against smallpox was found outside the realm of official medical systems. The practice was known as *ṭikā* (B. 'mark') and is known in English as variolation or inoculation.[35]

The first report on the practice of variolation in India dates back to 1767, when John Holwell presented to the College of Physicians in London a detailed description of the practice (Dharmapal 2000: 151–7). Holwell mentions the 1725 *History of Physic from the Time of Galen to the Beginning of the 16th Century* of John Friend, in which the author reports of a 'Gootee ka Tagooran' (B. Guṭikā Ṭhākurāni, the Lady of the Pustules), whose worship is allegedly found in the 'Aughtorrah Bhade' (i.e. *Atharvaveda*) (ibid.: 153). Holwell does not mention Śītalā in his report. However he indicates that variolators – who are described as 'a particular tribe of Bramins' [sic] – were, at this stage, extraneous to ritual worship:

> [...] these instructions being given, and an injunction laid on the patients to make a thanks giving Poojah, or offering, to the goddess on their recovery, the Operator takes his fee, which from the poor is a *pund of cowries*, equal to about a penny sterling, and goes on to another door [...] (Holwell 1767: 19)

Inoculation was 'largely restricted to the Bengal Presidency, with isolated pockets of the practice also occurring in northern and western India' (Banthia and Dyson 1999: 659; cf. Arnold 2002: 72).[36] By 1865, approximately 85 per cent of Hindus were protected by inoculation (BSC 60). Due to its success,[37] inoculation, originally a non-ritual practice, was soon adopted by British residents (Arnold 2004: 72; cf. ICM 14–18).[38] Professional inoculators, mostly Brahmans (Ainslie 1829: 63), were known as *ṭikadār*s or *ṭikāits* ('markers'). Ainslie (ibid.) calls them '*Tikar Brahmens*'. The Reverend W. Ward refers to inoculators as a 'lower order' of Brahmans, and informs us that inoculation was performed at any time of the year, but preferably on the seventh, eighth and ninth days of the waxing moon (Ward 1822: 174). The business of inoculation in the Bengal Presidency was alternatively administered by low professional *jāti*s such as *mālin/mālākār* (flower sellers, garland makers) and *nāpit/nāī* (barbers). Muslims too acted as variolators.

Marking doctors inoculated infected dried pus previously extracted from smallpox victims' pustules for a variable fee (depending on age and gender).[39] The inoculation was meant to cause a milder form of smallpox followed by immunity. Here follows the description of variolation as reported on 10 February 1731 by Dr Oliver Coult:

> The operation of inoculation called by the natives *tikah* has been known in the kingdom of Bengal as near as I can learn, about 150 years and according to the Bhamanian records was first performed by one Dununtary [Dhanvantari], a physician of Champanager, a small town by the side of the Ganges about half way to Cossimbazar whose memory is now holden in great esteem as being thought the author of this operation, which secret, say they, he had immediately of God in a dream. Their method of performing this operation is by taking a little of the pus (when the smallpox are come to maturity and are of a good kind) and dipping these in the point of a pretty large sharp needle. Therewith make several punctures in the hollow under the deltoid muscle or sometimes in the forehead, after which they cover the part with a little paste made of boiled rice. When they want the operation of the inoculated matter to be quick they give the patient a small bolus made of a little of the pus, and boiled rice immediately after the operation which is repeated the two following days at noon. The place where the punctures were made commonly festures and comes to a small suppuration, and if not the operation has no effect and the person is still liable to have the smallpox but on the contrary if the punctures do suppurate and no fever or eruption ensues, then they are no longer subject to the infection. The punctures blacken and dry up with the other pustules. The fever ensues later or sooner, according to the age and strength of the person inoculated, but commonly the third or fourth days. They keep the patient under the coolest regimen they can think off before the fever comes on and frequently use cold bathing. If the eruption is suppressed they also use frequent cold bathing. At the same time they give warm medicine inwardly, but if they prove of the confluent kind, they use no cold bathing, but (keep) the patient very cool and give cooling medicine. I cannot say any thing of the success of this operation or of their method of cure in this disease, but I intend to inform myself perfectly when the time of this distemper returns which is in April and May. (Coult, cited in Dharmapal 2000: 149–50)

With Edward Jenner's publication of *An inquiry into the causes and effects of the Variolæ Vaccinæ* in 1798 and the success of vaccination, variolation became obsolete. Yet when vaccine reached India in 1802, practical difficulties in disseminating Jennerian vaccination dramatically emerged (see below p. 136). At a practical level, inoculation continued. Furthermore, in some areas, such as in the Dinajpur district of the Bengal Presidency, mantras to the goddess Śītalā began to be pronounced by inoculators treating children, thus suggesting the *ṭikā* has been included in elaborate *pūjā*s (Buchanan 1833: 70). At the same time, in many rural villages, *pūjā* and basic hygienic norms (transmitted via ritual praxis) were the main, if not the only, preventative measures (Ainslie 1829: 59; RSC xviii, xxiii, xliii, lxxxvi). Writing in the first decades of the nineteenth century, James Wise, civil surgeon in Dacca, reports on the service offered by *mālin*s in the Dacca District. There is no evidence whatsoever of the practice of inoculation. In fact, the *mālin* intervenes strictly as a ritual specialist, and only after the *kavirāja* acknowledges failure of medical science.[40] The ritual practice of the *mālin* aims at lowering the temperature of the patient and inviting the goddess with cold edibles and cool water that is copiously sprinkled on the patient and the *mūrtī* of the goddess with *nīm* branches. Remedies to counter fever and the itch of pustules are not specific of Śītalā culture, but belong to various folk traditions (e.g. turmeric, flour, shell-sawdust and milk). After such operation, the ritualist says various mantras (unspecified) and tells lengthy stories ('*kissa*', H. *kissā* < A. *qiṣṣa*).[41] We then learn that:

> When the pustules are mature, the Málī dips a thorn of karaundá (*Carissa*) in til oil, and punctures each one. The body is the anointed with oil, and cooling fruits given. When the scabs (dewli)[42] have peeled off, another ceremonial, called 'Godám,' [*godān*, the 'gift of a cow' to a Brahman][43] is gone through. All the offerings on the waterpot [rice, a coconut, sugar, plantains, a yellow cloth, flowers and *nīm* leaves] are rolled in a cloth and fastened round the waist of the patient. These offerings are the perquisite of the Málī, who also receives a fee. (Wise, cited in Risley 1998: 62, II)

In the meantime, in Calcutta and its vicinities, inoculation was far more popular, and was increasingly included in various forms of worship. The incorporation of the ritual element seems to be coincidental with the burgeoning animosity of the government toward *ṭikadār*s, a situation that was to escalate with the 1865 prohibition by the Bengal legislature to practise inoculation in Calcutta and its suburbs (BSC 60). At the beginning of the nineteenth century, the Superintendent General of Vaccine Inoculation, John Shoolbred wrote in his report to the Medical Board at Fort William: 'The small-pox has not prevailed, epidemically, in Calcutta and its neighbourhood, since the introduction of vaccine, owing, I have no doubt, to the judicious prohibition of variolous inoculation by the police, ever since that time' (Shoolbred 1805: 64). A few decades later, the then Superintendent General of Vaccination, Duncan Stewart notes how:

> The Seapoys [sic] even, and some of the more intelligent natives are so given to *superstition, idolatry* and *fatalism*, that our best endeavours to benefit them

> are often marred and defeated. Their blind reliance on fate can only be equalled by their firm faith and dependence on the protective power of Seetla Mata, the goddess of Small Pox. (Stewart 1844: 15)

Stewart finds confirmation of this in the words of a Baboo Russomoy Dutt:

> I cannot but think [...] there is hardly any medical treatment, the recovery is more relied on under the superstitious belief on the mercy of *Sieutula* (the presiding Goddess over Small Pox) than on any medical treatment. A passage in the prayer usually offered to Sieutula runs: 'No Charms or Medicines exist for the wicked disease.' [ŚAS 78] (cited in Stewart 1844: 49)

Robert Pringle confirms this pattern:

> Religion seems to have been so mixed up with the whole practice of inoculation, that it partook more of a religious ceremony than exhibition of medical skill; while the goddess of smallpox 'Seetla' by name, was propitiated by gifts to her priests and her shrines, and special hymns were sung in her honour. (Pringle 1885: 740)

In his study of indigenous responses to variolation and vaccination, Brimnes, who bases his findings on the report of Shoolbred (1885), notes how: 'The most significant measures taken after the operation were to pour cold water over the head of the inoculated person until the fever came on and to ensure that an offering was made to Śītalā, the goddess of smallpox in Bengal' (Brimnes 2004: 207). Previously unnoticed, all of a sudden Śītalā is consistently mentioned in reports on the smallpox crisis. Colonial sources associate the goddess with the practice of inoculators, or the reluctance of Indians (including professional variolators) to take the more efficacious cowpox vaccine. Medical historians have given a series of explanations.

Bhattacharya highlights the intrinsic protective nature of the goddess, and notes how not only (potential) victims of smallpox worshipped Śītalā. Those who were vaccinated also used to take an active part in celebrations, either because they did not trust vaccination or 'fortify' the effect of a non-indigenous remedy. 'This trend was sometimes also noticed among government servants, who were able to successfully separate their official and private lives [...]' (Bhattacharya 2006: 240; see also ibid.: 245). Bose has investigated Śītalā's relation with 'imminent social and religious dangers to the community' (2006: 39), thus suggesting the goddess is in fact a social defensive measure against (possibly threatening) change. Vaccination, thought to be dispensed free of charge by British authorities (BVA 6), was actively discouraged by inoculators who argued against its doubtful purity (cf. Wujastyk 1987: 153). The lymph for the vaccine was initially transferred arm-to-arm and the only vaccinifers available were often low-class people. When calf lymph vaccination was introduced, many Hindus expressed concern about violence inflicted on cows (Chacko 1980: 15; Arnold

1993: 142). Beside purity issues, many thought that 'the practice of taking down personal details of every vaccinated person was a prelude to either a captivation tax or transportation' (Brimnes 2004: 210). Others looked at vaccination as a threat to religion (Bhattacharya et al. 2005: 66–9), or even the prelude to the annihilation of the indigenous population (Bose 2006: 40).

An organized anti-colonial resistance toward vaccination is difficult to prove.[44] It seems more likely that practical implications of a social and economic nature might have impacted on the choice of most Indians, especially in rural areas. Peasants and labourers, who could not afford to miss work due to side-effects, continued to disregard any form of prophylaxis, not just vaccination (Bhattacharya 2001: 256). Another reason to explain the reluctance toward vaccine can be found in the likely loss of income for a predominantly agricultural population (Wujastyk 2001: 141). Mass vaccination campaigns were scheduled during the harvesting season – a crucial moment of the year for peasants. Further, cattle owners were reluctant to sell farming animals to extract calves' lymph. Separating cattle calves from their mother often resulted in the latter's infertility and incapacity to produce milk (Minsky 2009: 181). The impact on the population of the side-effects of vaccination (WHO 2009), which was given great and protracted attention (anon., cited in Bose 2006: 45–6), was another major issue. Finally, it emerges from the studies of Arnold (1993: 156) and Bhattacharya (1998: 50–1) that a two-tiered system of vaccination was in place in India from 1850. The urban vaccination scheme was informed by the latest technologies, whereas the vaccination programme in rural areas was less reliable. Humanized unattenuated lymph was used when the preserved calf lymph was damaged during transportation or by the hot climate. This naturally resulted in a long list of side-effects, and the aversion of the rural population to vaccination.

As per the fear to offend Śītalā, this seems tangential to the discourse on the resistance of inoculation, and should not be regarded as a dominant pattern (Stewart 1844: 221; Bhattacharya, Harrison and Worboys 2005: 222; Arnold 1993: 122–3). Arnold informs us that: 'Although worship of the goddess was not integral to the inoculators' craft, Śītalā's assistance was often tactfully invoked by variolators as they began their work' (Arnold 2004: 73; cf. Arnold 1988: 50). Marking doctors, fearing the quite likely possibility of losing income and prestige, began to disseminate the notion that inoculation was (part of) *pūjā*, a way to keep quiet the ambivalent 'goddess of smallpox' whose scary stories were by then endemic in Bengal. By the mid-nineteenth century, inoculation was inextricably associated with *Śītalāpūjā* (RSC 36).

Indigenous variolators, however, were not opposed to novel medical treatment *per se*. The argument proposed by Marglin that 'Resistance to vaccination in the name of Śītalā is a rejection of politically repressive dualistic conceptual structure' (2001: 124) is highly problematic.[45] 'English' medicines, if efficacious, were recommended. The main concern of 'marking doctors' and other indigenous healers was their downgrade and, quite understandably, loss of capital. I thus argue that the conflict was one between the authority and power of different classes of health specialists, not between opposite beliefs/technological systems. It is thus unsurprising that many variolators, as soon as they were offered alternative employment and realized the efficaciousness of vaccination, gave considerable help to the IMS (Stewart 1844: 135–6; cf. Minsky 2009: 174).

Historical records show that the opposition toward vaccination eventually contributed to cast ill-fame on Śītalā, by then widely known as the goddess of the marking doctors. In order to counter such a trend, we learn from the 1850 Report of the Smallpox Commissioner that the natives were invited to reveal names and addresses of those who continued to take advantage of variolators. A questionnaire was then developed to better understand the norms in the matter of variolation, and submitted to a committee of *paṇḍit*s in Calcutta:

> **1** Is there in the holy shasters [*śāstras*], any distinct commandment enjoining Smallpox Inoculation, as a religious duty, or recommending it as a commendable Act?
>
> **2** Is the omission to be inoculated considered a sin, or a disreputable act?
>
> **3** Is there any penalty in this world for this omission, or punishment in the next, and if so, how may it be atoned for?
>
> **4** What religious observances are enjoined on those who contract Smallpox naturally?
>
> **5** Supposing it to be proved that the Vaccine disease is really a modified form or variety of the Smallpox, should not all the religious ceremonies, observed in cases of Smallpox, be practised during Vaccination by good Hindoos?
>
> (RSC xiv)

Bengali *paṇḍit*s, in a series of letters from March to April 1850, confirm that inoculation is a practice extraneous to Manu, *purāṇas*, *itihāsa* and other Sanskrit sources. Nothing suggests that one should be punished for not being inoculated. By analogy, failure to be vaccinated (inoculation with cowpox) is not something that should be disciplined. Finally, the *paṇḍit*s observe that, according to *Skandapurāna*, *Bhāvaprakāśa*, *Kr̥tyatattva* (cf. p. 36n. 27) and *Śabdakalpadruma*, in case of smallpox infection the worship of Śītalā is a duty (RSC xiv–xxvi). This confirmed the suspicion of the British against inoculators, the goddess and her worship, a custom symptomatic of superstition and irrational resistance to scientific progress (Harrison 1994: 82). In 1844, the Superintendent General of Vaccination in Calcutta went so far as to report that 'smallpox was annually introduced into Calcutta by a series of inoculators' (ibid.: 83). Draconian measures followed:

> Variolation did come under increasing attack from British physicians. In 1831 Dr W. Cameron blamed tikadars in and around Calcutta for recurring epidemics of

> smallpox and for spreading 'falsehoods and ridiculous stories' about vaccination. The Smallpox Commission of 1850, in comparing variolation to sati and infanticide, declared that the time had come to suppress 'this murderous trade'. (Arnold 2004: 72–3)

Meanwhile, the worship of Śītalā as the practice of cooling down patients continued:

> The usual treatment followed by Natives is essentially 'cooling' and expectant. One of the *benignant* [emphasis added] Divinities of the Hindoo Pantheon, variously named Seetulah [Śītalā], Bowanny [Bhavānī], and c. is specially the *guardian* [emphasis added] of those affected by Small Pox, and at her shrine prayers are offered and vows made by relatives. I possess a curious ancient gold coin, of about half an inch square, which represents the Goddess in her usual attitude, viz. seated naked upon an ass bedecked with flowers and jewels; she holds in one hand a broom, representative of the duty of cleanliness; resting on the left hip, and supported by that arm is a large round jar indicative of the necessity of ablution and coolness. On her head she carries a winnowing sheaf or fan to be used as a ventilator. Medals of the same description of gold or silver are very commonly worn as amulets – but I fear that the primitive duties enjoined on the worshippers of Seetula are too much neglected for the more important ones of priestcraft, incantation ceremonies, and propitiatory offerings. (Stewart 1844: 48-9)[46]

Stewart – though generally showing a considerable familiarity with Indian culture – does not escape the contradiction of opposing science to religion, thus blaming Śītalā for the delay in enforcing vaccination:

> To the conciliatory firmness of Dr Shoolbred, to the evident disinterestedness of his proceedings, to their publicity, as well as to his very high character among all classes as a benevolent and skilful Surgeon, must be ascribed the great success of vaccination at that time in Calcutta, and the almost magic conversion of the bigotted [sic] worshippers of *Seetula* to a new faith. (Stewart 1844: 137)

Similar feelings are confirmed in the reports of Indian informants (RSC clxxxi) and physicians, such as that of Shamachurn Sircar, sub-assistant surgeon in Gaya. After a detailed description of the inoculation process, we learn that:

> No medicine is given to the children when they have a high degree of fever, and the eruptions become confluent and the life of the child is in hazard; the parents as well as the Inoculators leave them to the divine protection of *Situla* (Goddess of Smallpox) and at the same time allow them any kind of food they ask for. (Sircar, cited in RSC clv)

In a letter dated 18 March 1850, the Superintendent General of Vaccination in Calcutta requests 'to obtain specific information as to the actual *number* of *Ticcadars* at work' and 'to ascertain their proceedings during the past 12 or 18 months; and whether in any or many cases fatal results have followed from their operations' (RSC xxvii). A questionnaire was then prepared and distributed among informants (ibid.). The result of the investigation is a list of names of 'native inoculators'. The statements of *ṭikādār*s, the majority of whom are Brahmans, then follow. [47] We learn from these interviews that Śītalā is invariably mentioned as a protective goddess whose *pūjā* follows inoculation (ibid.: xxxi, xxxiii). Only one informant, Baboo Govind Persad Bose (who was not a *ṭikādār*), reports that:

> It behoves here also to notice a false prejudice under which some of the Hindoo families totally refrain from having recourse to any kind of protective whatsoever, on a tradition that in the days of yore their ancestors were visited by Smallpox without Inoculation, which they interpret *Itsha* or a favourable visitation of the *Goddess Situla*,[48] and have thence made it a family rule never to adopt any kind of protective by which they apprehend that the goddess will be incensed, and it is chiefly in these families that the malady first appears till it becomes general [...] (Bose, cited in RSC xliii)

Although by 1850 Bengali urban gentry were abandoning inoculation in favour of vaccination – as we learn from the words of Pundit Moodusooden Guptu, one of the inoculators interviewed by the Smallpox Commission (1850: xxxi–xxxii) – the majority of the rural population, immigrants and the poorest social sectors continued to consult the marking doctors (ibid.: xxxvii). In this climate, W. H. Elliott, Magistrate in the 24-Parganas, writes to Duncan Stewart, Superintendent General of Vaccination, that '[...] Inoculation is *the* evil to be contended with [...]' and that he is 'most anxious to see Inoculation altogether prohibited by Legislative enactment, and severe penalties prescribed' (ibid.: xxxviii). Elliot's wish was to be fulfilled three decades later. In 1880 it was promulgated the Bengal Vaccination Act and, on 9 July of the same year, the prohibition of inoculation was included in Section 6 of the Central Government Vaccination Act:

> In any local area to which the provisions of this Act apply, inoculation shall be prohibited; and Inoculated persons not to enter, without certificate, local area subject to Act. No person who has undergone inoculation shall enter such area before the lapse of forty days from the date of the operation, with out a certificate from a medical practitioner, of such class as the State Government may from time to time by written order authorize to grant such certificates, stating that such person is no longer likely to produce small-pox by contact or near approach. (James 1909: 32)

Despite prohibition, marking doctors were still in demand. In 1909 IMS Officer S. P. James publicly admitted that smallpox outbreaks could be traced to the business of variolators (Harrison 1994: 83). Historical records confirm the manipulation of Śītalā's personality in response to professional needs, class values and governmental policies. The picture offered by reports and narratives included in the documents of the IMS is however incomplete. There are virtually no records of the voices of local peasantry and the working class. Further, we know very little of vaccinifers and inoculators either.[49] 'Popular sources from the colonial era, including newspapers, journals, and pamphlets, represented well the ideas, activities, and demands of urban middle and upper-class healers, bureaucrats, professionals, merchants, moneylenders, and landowners, but not those of the lower classes' (Minsky 2006: 166). This pattern tends to continue in post-colonial medical literature. While historians have noted the various facets of Śītalā and her worship, and have examined literary and archaeological sources, often integrating them with valuable fieldwork, WHO medical personnel have not delved into the complexities and multifarious modes of expression of Śītalā culture. Rather, they have favoured narratives of a protective-cum-malign goddess. I do not want by any means to diminish the achievements of SEP and the 'smallpox warriors'; though sometimes there is ground to question the ethics of vaccination enforcement squads in India (e.g. Gelfand 1966; Brilliant and Brilliant 1978: 359), one should keep in mind both the context and the aim of the operation. The risk is otherwise to incur a dangerous exercise of cultural relativism, such as Marglin (2001: 122), who argues that 'the success of the smallpox campaign has been achieved at a high political and cultural cost and that smallpox could have been successfully controlled rather than eradicated had other approaches been followed'[50] (cf. Mitter 1996). While I appreciate that epidemiologists and physicians had a different – and praiseworthy – agenda, it is nevertheless significant that, in the long term, the Śītalā emerging from the narratives of most medical personnel operating in South Asia between the 1960s and 1970s is the dangerous 'goddess of smallpox'.

The first and foremost concern of the WHO Intensified SEP, launched on 1 January 1967 under the guidance of Dr Donald Henderson, was to define a strategy for mass vaccination. While inoculation had virtually disappeared, *Śītalāpūjā* and the hygienic norms associated with it continued unchanged. A substantial difference in the tactic of the WHO personnel was to take advantage of this custom. In their final report on the eradication of smallpox from India, Brilliant and Conrad inform us that 'the temples of Shitala Ma [...] became strategic observation posts for finding smallpox cases and offering vaccines' (2010: 77). This is corroborated in other sources:

> As in other countries, the discovery of suspected cases was usually accomplished by questioning village leaders, schoolteachers and their pupils, and people attending weekly markets. In Rajasthan and in many other parts of India, there were two additional methods, unique to India, by which cases could be detected. One consisted in questioning visitors to the Sītalā mata temples. Many villagers came to give thanks to the goddess for recovery from smallpox or to offer homage in the hope that they and their families would be spared visitation by the

> goddess. Cases could also be detected in villages when, as was customary in many areas, branches from the neem tree were hung over the front door of a house in which a patient lived. The leaves of the neem were considered to have special cooling properties when applied to the skin of the patient and other, less tangible, properties when hung above the doorway. (Fenner et al. 1988: 740)

On the basis of these and similar observations, the general understanding that Śītalā is smallpox, or that she is feared because she inflicts poxes, is fortified. This view, however, does not come from premodern Bengali poems or indigenous inoculators. The myth of the goddess of smallpox is disseminated by authoritative Western scientists and medical practitioners whose writings eventually influenced global audiences.

Śītalā is yet again advertised as unstable and vengeful, and naturally intolerant to vaccination. For Hindus, we are told, medical prophylaxis is an offence to the goddess, and her *pūjā* is not a performance aiming at inviting her, but remedial practice (Brilliant 1985: 1–5; Brilliant and White Conrad 2010: 76–7; Koplow 2003: 159, Fenner et al. 1988: 793; Chacko 1980: 15; Hopkins 1988: 1590). Davida Coady, an epidemiologist working for the SEP in India from 1974–5, remembers her time in India thus:

> One thing we noticed was [...] that the Indians, they wanted some conversation before they were vaccinated. They wanted an explanation and their views of the goddess and her role in all this varied really from village to village, and sometimes – in one village they wanted us to come back next Tuesday because that's what the goddess wanted us to do instead of vaccinating people then. I think we finally agreed to do that, it was just easier, but many times they would say, "No, the goddess doesn't want us vaccinated;" and we'd sit down and go through all the explanations and just at the point when we were convinced they were never going to let us vaccinate anyone, they'd say, okay now we understand that it's a disease and it's not a goddess and please vaccinate us." I remember one elderly man, he said, "No, I don't want to be vaccinated because I'm getting ready to go to God;" and my husband looked him right in the eye and said, "I really think God would like you better vaccinated;" and I was just thinking "Oh my!" And the man said "Oh, alright fine," and he said, "Please, please vaccinate me." So a lot of it was just listening and realizing that nothing worked fast in India. (Coady 2008)

With only few exceptions, there is an overall tendency to talk about Indians, their beliefs and practice as if a homogenous cultural group. Slogans such as the popular 'Worship the goddess, and also take a vaccination' (Brilliant 1985: 4) are indicators of this prevailing sentiment. Indians are portrayed as dependent upon their religion at the point of not seeing the advantages of medicine. Their religious beliefs are interpreted as a form of *do ut des* inspired by fear; just like in the ŚMKs. Śītalā is a capricious *dea irata*. There is, however, a major difference: the ŚMKs were designed to entertain, and so they were received by their target audiences. In medical memoirs and reports, Orientalist fascination prevails.[51]

When, on 23 April 1977, the WHA33.3 Resolution was issued – 'the world and its peoples have won freedom from smallpox' – a dreaded disease that was responsible for around two million fatalities every year (not to mention blinded, crippled and scarred survivors) was no more. What about Śītalā? The *British Medical Journal*, one of the world's oldest and most prestigious publications on general medicine, bears witness to the parable of public renderings of the protective goddess and her transformation into the capricious 'goddess of smallpox'. The following article appeared on 27 March 1880:

> An Indian paper reports that the following is said of Shitala, the goddess of small-pox, in Skandapurana. As small-pox invariably attends the goddess, it may be called the goddess herself, and the fever which accompanies it is called violent fever. There are seven kinds of small-pox. Fever is generally felt beforehand; then within a week the eruption comes out; in the second week it becomes mature; and in the third it dries. But, if the pustules break, the smoke of the dung of a wild cow should be taken. The branches of the nimb or neemb (Melia-azaderata) tree should be waved in order to drive out the flies. Cold water should be used, and the body should not be rubbed even at the time of fever. The man suffering from it should be placed in a clean (well-ventilated), cold, and lonely room. A dirty or unholy man should not touch him or go to him during that time. Almost all the physicians do not prescribe medicine at all, but a few only do so. The only treatment for it, as prescribed in the Shastras, is *japa* (prayers), *homa* (oblation), *dana* (donation), *sedastayana* (aversion of evil),[52] and the worship of Brahmin, cow, Shiva (the well-known god) and Gauri (the wife of Shiva), and a holy and faithful Brahmin should recite the praise of the goddess Shitala before the patient, and the eruption will be cured. Skanda (the son of Shiva) requested his father thus: "O great god of gods (Shiva) kindly recite fully before me the auspicious praise of the goddess Shitala, which, being uttered, cures the small-pox for ever." Shiva said: "I bow before the goddess Shitala, riding on an ass, having the points of the compass for her clothes (i.e., quite naked), holding a broom and jug with both hands, and her head is adorned with a winnowing basket. I pray the goddess Shitala, the destroyer of all diseases, and by whose grace no fear of small-pox exists any more. If a man suffering from burning sensation utter [sic] the word 'Shitala', 'Shitala', the fear of eruption will suddenly disappear from him. O goddess Shitala, if a man placing you within cold water, worship thereby, he and his descendants have not to fear the eruption any more. O goddess Shitala, you are the only medicine to men suffering awfully from inflammatory fever, having an ill smelling body and losing eyes for ever. O goddess Shitala, you are the infallible curer of all pains arising in the human body, and you shower the heavenly nectar over the man who suffers

> from eruption. No Mantra (incantation) nor medicine can effect [sic] any benefit to the man who is suffering from bad diseases but only you, and no other goddess is the curer of the same." (BMJ 1880: 490)

The goddess is clearly associated (equated?) with smallpox. This is in all probability depending on the reports that linked Śītalā with the illegal activities of the inoculators, and the belief that inoculation caused smallpox epidemics. Apart from that, this short piece is extremely accurate. It reports in an unbiased way the hygienic norms associated with various ritual practices, and gives an accurate translation of the ŚAS. One century later, the tone is dramatically different. The 19 April 1980 issue of BMJ discusses so Śītalā in relation to the eradication of smallpox:

> The smallpox goddess [...], Shitala Mata, will no longer have to be propitiated to save the people of India from the dreaded disease that she was said to scatter like grain from the basket balanced on her head, for, as doctors know, no case of smallpox has been reported since Saiban Bibi[53] was discharged from hospital on 4 July 1975. [...] Shitala Mata on her donkey may now merely be a pretty face, but Indians will be grateful that she no longer has the power to disseminate disease by a toss of her head. (BMJ 1980: 1081)

In this and similar reports, history from below continues to be ignored. In fact, the smallpox myth is so rooted that SEP in India has been called 'The War Against Sitala' (Shurkin 1979: 315–47), a struggle that ended when 'Saiban Bibi was released from the hospital and returned to her home in Bangladesh. She was the last human to suffer from the wrath of Sitala in India. [...] It was India which – for the first time in its history – was free of smallpox. Sitala had been vanquished and India was beautiful, misty and still' (ibid.: 347). Alternatively, the worship of Śītalā has been reduced to 'a pervasive fatalism about smallpox as an unchangeable fact of Indian life' (Tucker 2001: 92).

Smallpox medical narratives have often offered romantic and patronizing interpretations of the beliefs of Indians, just like *maṅgal* poems did. My discourse converges with Misnksy's argument against 'elite agency and cultural change that animate national and global histories of vaccination by demonstrating the importance of regional socio-environmental factors and the *creative, productive agency* of the agrarian lower classes' (ibid.: 167, emphasis added). The apotheosis of Śītalā in Bengali *maṅgalkāvya*s has been conducive to a restyling of the goddess and, in the long term, to the global consolidation of the 'goddess of smallpox' (cf. Shastri 2014: 29). Śītalā was made into an ambiguous heroine. Indigenous folk culture – with its natural fragmentations and contradictions – was filtered through the needs, expectations, fixations and fascinations of powerful internal and external agencies. The trend is not over. In 2010, Meryl Dorey, of the Australian Vaccination (Skeptics) Network, has suggested that: 'Measles in Sanskrit translates as "Gift from a Goddess" because huge developmental and growth spurts often followed infection' (Dorey n.d.: 26). The statement elicited outraged reactions, including a defence of Indian 'folk' culture and Śītalā (Gallagher 2011). In fact, this has led to a further confirmation of the disease-inflicting profile of the goddess, and her association with folk superstition: 'The World Health Organisation tells of a superstition in the Indian subcontinent that smallpox resulted from a wrathful kiss by the Goddess of Smallpox, Shitala Mata. That is quite the opposite to Dorey's claim' (McLeod 2010: 24).

Metamorphosis, monstrosity, ambiguity and the violent implementation of justice are all elements that continue to inform the dissemination and uncritical receptions of the goddess. The endurance of Orientalist fascination and ethnocentrism has eventually strengthened the reputation of Śītalā as the Indian smallpox goddess in contemporary culture.

Concluding remarks

From the seventeenth century, with the composition of the first ŚMK, the spectacular exploits of Śītalā as a capricious and violent goddess who demands to be worshipped are disseminated in north-eastern India, mostly by means of theatrical renditions (*yātrā*) of selected sections (*pālās*) of *maṅgal* poems. Self-proclaimed genuine folk narratives, the *Śītalāpālās*, and *maṅgal* poems in general, will be later estranged from their context by various figures of intellectuals and academics, and confirmed in India and abroad as authentic folk ballads, rather than premodern renditions of folk culture. In this chapter, I have argued that ŚMKs are in fact a commodification and a patronizing spectacularization of folk *bhakti*. The literature produced by *maṅgal* poets, some of whom were court poets of local *rājas* and *jamindār*s, and the way this has been managed after them, has contributed to a major change in public representations of Śītalā. Eventually the goddess became known as the angry smallpox-inflicting goddess of Bengali peasantry, first, and of Indians, later.

This process radicalized following the intervention of the IMS and the implementation of restrictive policies in matters of public health. With the aggravation of the smallpox emergency in nineteenth-century colonial Bengal, the British – in their effort to understand whether indigenous knowledge could be of any help in coping with, or preventing, smallpox epidemics – learnt about the worship of Śītalā. Early reports make reference to a system combining basic hygienic norms with religious beliefs revolving around rites informed by *bhakti*. The British also learnt, and approved, of the practice of inoculation, a non-ritual business associated with the *ṭikadār*s, a class of (mostly Brahman) 'marking doctors'. Yet following the success of Jennerian vaccination and its implementation in India (1802), inoculation was to be increasingly stigmatized and eventually, in 1880, outlawed.

Marking doctors, unwilling to give up economic gain and prestige, continued in their business and in order to defend their practice, they presented inoculation as

Śītalāpūjā. In response to that, *ṭikadār*s and their customers were considered by the British as state enemies, and were accused of being the cause of smallpox epidemics. The fact that inoculation was associated with Brahmans (i.e. 'priests', for the British) and that *Śītalāpūjā* used to be performed at the end of the operation, led to the conclusion that the problem had a 'religious' component. Controlling Śītalā, her ritualists, devotees and festivals became functional to colonial order. The worship of the goddess was monitored by officials of the IMS, and was publicly blamed as a sign of the superstition and backwardness typical of the Indian plebs, as opposed to the urban (Anglicized) gentry.

With independence, the myth of the dangerous goddess of smallpox of Indian folks is passed to, and uncritically received by, WHO SEP personnel operating in South Asia. Medical memoirs reporting on the struggle against smallpox show a fascination with Śītalā who, at that point, is globally advertised and celebrated as the deification of smallpox. The influential writings of medics involved more or less directly with the SEP and a growing corpus of academic works on the (mostly Bengali and *maṅgal-*) Śītalā would eventually establish the 'smallpox myth' globally. The final stage of this long process of cultural colonialism spectacularly emerges in contemporary narratives and new media, chiefly the internet.

Notes

1 The Niṣādas are known in relation to their kings and warriors. Particularly well known is the myth of Ekalavya, a Niṣādas prince who aspired to being admitted in the ashram of Droṇācārya and was eventually killed by Kṛṣṇa (MBh 1.61: 58; 1.123).

2 The presence of tigers, animals extraneous to Śītalā's mythology, is evocative of Durgā. In the Adalpura market, Śītalā is even more manifestly associated with the worship of Durgā. Her iconography merges with the latter at the point that she is represented as Mahiṣāsuramardiṇī ('Slayer of the Buffalo Demon', one of the most popular titles of Durgā).

3 Cf. H.ŚMK. 153, on Śītalā as a water goddess and her status among boatmen/fishermen.

4 In alternative variants, the boatman is indicated as the ancestor of all *mallāh*s, thus placing the episode in a more remote past, at the time of Niṣāda kingdoms.

5 Śītalā is occasionally identified with Sītā, or associated with vernacular versions of the story of Rāma and Sītā. In a women's folk song in Kannada (a major language of South India which is predominant in Karnataka), Sītā tries to convince Rāma of her purity. The final strophe reveals an unexpected association to Śītalā:

'The water-fed furrow in which Sītā was born
is the netherworld of Śītalā.
Sītā, who sank into a furrow twelve man-lengths,
that Sītā's virtue is true virtue.' (in Richman 2008: 56)

6 Besides widespread poverty and stories of violence and marginalization, informants refer to an on-going dispute with local Brahmans and temple authorities from Banaras. This conflict is evoked emphatically in a low-budget film production titled *Jai Mā Śītalā (Kahānī Adalpura Kī)* (see below, p. 166–7).

7 In turn, Nityānanda borrowed from the *Virāṭa Parvan* (Book 4) of *Mahābhārata* a variety of details and names of characters.

8 This entry is found more or less edited in an exponentially growing number of websites, blogs, tourist sites, Facebook pages, forums, Yahoo-answers and web pages on *vrata*s and local festivals. The list is too long to be included here. One just needs to type 'Sitala', 'Shitala', 'Sitla', 'Sheetla', etc. on any web search engine to appreciate the phenomenon.

9 The label persists not just in articles and books printed after 1979. At seminars, conferences and symposia, postgraduate research students and scholars continue to call Śītalā and Māriyamman 'goddesses of smallpox'.

10 Nicholas notes that ŚMKs 'contain little information of historical importance, are highly imitative of earlier *maṅgals* in style and content, and, generally, little can be said for them as literature' (2003: 195).

11 Translated by Stewart (1995: 397).

12 Chapal Bhaduri (b. 1938) is one of the last traditional interpreters of female roles. He is well known as Chapal Rani (Queen). With the slow erosion of Bengali *yātrā*, and possibly because he openly came out as a homosexual, he fell from grace. The 1999 documentary *Performing the Goddess. The Chapal Bhaduri Story*, produced by the Seagull Foundation for the Arts and directed by Naveen Kishore, has contributed to his newfound glory. Since then, he has appeared in various projects and in one television film. His major role – interpreting himself – is in the 2010 Bengali movie *Ārekṭi premer galpa* (Ben. 'Just another love story'), directed by Kaushik Ganguly. The movie – which was screened soon after the decriminalization of Section 377 on homosexuality in the Indian Penal Code – won the 2010 I-view Engendered Award for Outstanding Cinema.

13 The Aśvin twins are the physicians of the gods in Vedic literature. Dhanvantari is the god of health and medics, and is praised as the patron of Āyurveda.

14 *Śitalapālā*s may be inscribed in mass celebrations (such as *yātrā*, annual *pūjā*, etc.) (Curley 2008: 17). The practice of hiring actors on the occasion of festivals of the goddess is, however, neither customary nor mainstream.

15 Applying *sindūr* is culturally related to marriage. Women wear *sindūr* on their parted hair (*sīmanta; māṁg*) from the day of their marriage until they die, or are widowed.

16 Translated by Sarkar and Nicholas, in Nicholas (2003: 134).

17 Miraculous indeed, as the story contradicts at the same time the goddess's (alleged) low origin and the (alleged) euphemism of her name.

18 Translated by Rebecca Manring (2012).

19 Translated by Sarkar and Nicholas, in Nicholas (2003: 152–3).

20 McDermott has noted the same pattern in the representation of Kālī in *Kālikāmaṅgalkāvya*s (2011: 168). The grotesque here emerges in the sweetening of her fierce aspect (e.g. 'her corpse earrings are decorated with jewel') and her adaptation to *vaiṣṇava bhakti* standards.

21 Translated by Nicholas and Sarkar, in Dimock (1982: 194).

22 Translated by Stewart (2004: 196).

23 Kaviraj notes that: '*Maṅgalkāvya*s are primarily written in a rustic vernacular style, with a predominance of *deśi* vocabulary over *tatsama* words, matched by relatively unambitious, uncomplicated metric composition. Dialogues often approximate the grammatical laxity of ordinary conversation' (Kaviraj 2003: 516). In this case, however, we observe the typical hyperrealism that features public representations of *maṅgal* texts (cf. Curley 2008: 5).

24 In relation to that, we learn that: 'Kṛṣṇarāma, who collected and recorded no fewer than five maṅgala poems, explains that he has written it just as he heard it – a subtle caveat which hints that his fear of poetic failure could have personally disastrous results' (Stewart 1995: 391).

25 Most *maṅgal* narratives, but not ŚMKs, make ample reference to (animal and human) sacrifice, devotional austerities, possession, the presence of low-class *pūjārī*s and female ritualists, etc. See for instance *Dharmamaṅgalkāvyas* and their association with *gājan* culture (Ferrari 2010a).

26 But cf. Banerjee (1998: 94), who talks about the 'domestication of Hindu divinities' in works like *maṅgalkāvyas*.

27 On satire and didactics in *maṅgal* literature, see Curley (2008: 18–23).

28 Translated by Nicholas and Sarkar, in Nicholas (2003: 136).

29 The text has been translated by Sarkar and Nicholas, in Nicholas (2003: 148–65).

30 *Maṅgal* poets were very keen to sign their works, and regularly indicated their *gotra* and *jāti*. Information about patronage, however, is rare (Curley 2008: 13). Among the authors of *Śītalāmaṅgalkāvyas*, we know that Kavi Jagannāth was court poet of Kamalnārayaṇ Rāj, the *vaiṣṇava* king who ruled over Tamluk, and Nityānanda Cakravartī worked at the court of Rāja Rājnārāyaṇ of the Kāśījoṛa Pargana. Whether the poems were commissioned, it remains unclear.

31 Nicholas has reported exhaustively on the powerful impact of inexpensive printed booklets in disseminating an increasingly standardized version of the mythology of Śītalā. Borrowing heavily from Nityānanda's text, modified versions of the *pālā*s have been sold as a support to singers and actors (Nicholas 2003: 192–211). The trend continues today, with the viral dissemination of gratis *maṅgal* hyper-narratives throughout the internet.

32 Cf. McDermott on patronage of *Durgāpūjā* and the relations of the big families of Calcutta (Kolkata) with British residents (2011: 11–38).

33 Among other things, the Act encouraged the local population to inform authorities of the seditious nature of Bengali dramas (cf. Kundu 2013).

34 But cf. Arnold (1993: 183–9); Klein (1994: 502–9); Mukharji (2011: 183); Harrison (1994: 132) on quarantine as a means to contain cholera.

35 Variolation was well known in various Asian regions. It was first introduced in Europe by Lady Mary Wortley Montagu in 1721, after being inoculated herself in Constantinople (Brimnes 2004: 199).

36 This is confirmed in a series of Bengal Sanitary Reports from 1868 (OIOC V/24 series). I am thankful to Alex McKay for kindly sharing this material with me.

37 It has been noted that 'the case-fatality rate associated with variolation was ten times lower than that associated with naturally occurring smallpox' (Riedel 2005: 22–3).

38 There is evidence that, as early as the 1780s, British residents in Calcutta had their children, including infants, inoculated, and that this indigenous practice contributed to a sensible diminishing of fatalities (Brendon 2006: 30). The practice continued for the following century, especially among Indians. Though officially discouraged, and later forbidden, vaccination was impractical, whereas inoculation was believed a viable alternative. See, for instance, the reports of Dr W. Durrant from 'Noacolly' (Noakhali, Bangladesh) (BSR 1868: 159) and Dr A. Fleming from Berhampore (Murshidabad district, WB) (ibid.: 67).

39 The 1850 RSC informs us that 'very poor people pay about 2 rupees to the *Ticcadar* for inoculating 2, 3, 4 or 5 children at once in a group or family, which is the custom. The middle class people pay from 3, 4 to 10 rupees to the operator for a similar party' (1850: 36).

40 According to Suśruta, diseases are either treatable (*kr̥tya*) or untreatable (*akr̥tya*) (Sū. 10.6). *Vaidhyas* are expected to be realistic about the efficacy of medicine, and not to take advantage of the situation for personal gain. Other reasons, often related to prestige and reputation, concur. See Wujastyk 2012: 113–14.

41 It would be interesting to known whether such stories are taken from the *vrata* or *maṅgal* tradition. Wise says storytelling 'often occupies six hours' (cited in Risley 1998: 62, II).

42 H. *devlī*. Wise, reporting from the Dacca District and otherwise quite accurate in rendering the Bengali vernacular in phonetic English transliteration, here uses Hindustani terms (Hindi/Urdu) only.

43 The *godāna* is a non-compulsory and expensive ritual involving the donation (*dāna*) of a cow (Skt. *go*) for the acquisition of merit. In this case, the term is symbolic of an act of monetary retribution in exchange for the ritual service.

44 Nineteenth-century reports confirm the unsystematic patterns of indigenous resistance to vaccination. In some areas 'inoculation is almost universal' (Dr R. F. Thompson on Hooghly, in BSR 1868: 53), whereas in others it 'is dying out of itself' (Dr R. Bird on Howrah, ibid.: 26).

45 Marglin, whose vastly quoted 2001 study relies on Derrida's critique to logocentrism and is almost entirely dependent upon the essays (on ŚMKs) of Nicholas and the historical and medical sources quoted by him, rejects the idea that Śītalā is a goddess expressing herself through binary oppositions (hot/cold, disease/health, life/death, etc.) Though I agree that reasoning in such terms is often unsophisticated, one cannot deny evidence simply to fit powerful meta-theories. The devotees of the goddess do talk of her in terms of a 'cold' goddess who counters and destroys 'hotness', i.e. disease, misfortune, etc., pace Derrida.

46 Cf. Ainslie 1829: 64, where worship is virtually equated to medicine.

47 In his reply to the commission, Issurchunder Chuckerbutty, one of the inoculators interviewed, mentions that 'Ticcadars [. . .] are of the castes of Brahmin, Dybogya, Mauley, Tautee, Koomar and Napit' (RSC xxx).

48 The translation of 'Itsha' (B. *icchā*, lit. will, wish, desire, liking) as '*favourable* visitation' (emphasis added) is interesting as it is in conflict with Bengali expressions like *māyer icchā* (Mother's will) and *icchā vasanta* (spring's will), which in SMKs indicate the caprice of the goddess who manifests as smallpox.

49 It is worth remembering the intimidating climate surrounding interviews to inoculators. Though they offer a glimpse of the situation, one should be cautious about the information they deliver.

50 Another major problem with Marglin's argument is her paradoxically dichotomic (i.e. logocentric) reading of SEP vis-à-vis 'local knowledge' (2001: 122), as if in India there was one medical/healing system.

51 Some of the doctors operating in India and Bangladesh, including some at the apex of the Smallpox Eradication Commission, seem to have developed a fixation for Śītalā, the alleged deification of their specialism. I was informed that former officials involved with SEP have carved Śītalā statues in their US offices. Some were brought from temples in Bangladesh and India, others were presented to them. This seems to have been quite widespread in rural areas of north India – and naturally evokes the spectre of cultural ransacking. Sanjoy Bhatthacharya, email communications, 19/5/2013 and 10/12/2013.

52 Skt. *svastayana*: a wellbeing ceremony.

53 A 30-year-old migrant beggar, Saiban Bibi, originally from the Takoikona village (Beanibazar Upazila, Sylhet Subdivision), is the last known case of smallpox in India. She was found on a railway platform in the town of Karimganj (Assam, India). 'On 4 July 1975, Smt. Saiban Bibi, the last smallpox case, was discharged from the isolation ward of Karimganj Civil Hospital and the same day she departed to her own village Takoikona in Bangladesh. Surprisingly, the last known smallpox outbreak consisted only of a single case, thus bringing to an end in India, the death, blindness and disfigurement caused by the dreaded disease — smallpox' (Jezek et al. 1976: 6). The last known person in the world to have been naturally infected by *Variola major* was the then two-year old Rahima Banu Begum in Bhola Island (Barisal District) in Bangladesh. She survived.

5

The Legacy of Śītalā

In the previous chapter, I have discussed how the myth of a capricious and disease-provoking folk goddess of smallpox has emerged in premodern and, more convincingly, colonial Bengal. I have also demonstrated how this ideology has been disseminated within and beyond India by means of reports on policies in matters of public health and *maṅgal*-centric studies of the goddess. In fact, Indian texts and material culture, as well as rituals and devotional practices in north India, show that Śītalā is neither disease nor a fear-inspiring goddess. In order to support this, I have offered an alternative reading of the celebrated Bengali *Śītalāmaṅgalkāvyas*. These texts, I argue, are not folk poems. They are highly fictionalized narratives that stereotypically rendered the myths, beliefs and rituals of the Bengali peasantry. Tales of Śītalā in *maṅgal* poems, and even more in theatrical renderings of *Śītalāpālās*, are romantic yet patronizing fabrications whose monstrous imagery has been uncritically received – and edited – by Bengali gentry and intellectuals, British residents in colonial Bengal, the IMS, WHO personnel of the SEP, and finally a long list of scholars. After an examination of colonial and post-colonial medical literature, it does emerge that the aggressive side of Śītalā has served to fit the agendas (political, personal and academic) of various professional figures, including indigenous health specialists such as inoculators (*ṭikādārs*). A discourse on mythologization, rather than one on myth, has been decisive to reach this conclusion. Eventually, I have shown how the dynamics that led to the inculcation of the myth of the goddess of smallpox within India and beyond depend upon the uncritical passage of (often biased) knowledge from the first observers to medics, civil servants, international agencies, media and, last but not least, various figures of scholars and intellectuals. The latter, with very few exceptions, continue to rely heavily on studies on the Bengali ŚMKs and ethnographies written decades ago in 'Bengal'.[1] Further, we witness a proliferation of narratives that pathologize the nature of the goddess, or diminish the social and political complexities of ritual (*pūjā*, *ārti*, *vrata*, *balidāna*, *yātrā*, etc.) and devotional (*bhar*, *khelnā*, *gīti*, *kathā*, etc.) practices by liquidating them as 'folk/popular/village' Hinduism.

Indian myths and material culture have responded variously to the threat posed by disease. In so doing, they have contributed to redefining *āñcalik* knowledge, including ritual literature and literacy. The 'ritual Śītalās' of northern India have served to provide holistic responses to moments of crisis that continue to be transmitted by means of a series of meaningful acts and narratives aimed at wellbeing and relief. It is thus unsurprising that patients affected by relatively new diseases, such as for instance HIV/AIDS, have started to seek Śītalā *darśana* for protection. Scheduled ritual performances such as the *vrata*s and the annual *pūjā*s celebrated across north India continue to be socializing events as well as occasions to discuss, and argue over, therapeutic strategies, including national and regional policies. Annual festivals particularly provide an arena where celebration is also information exchange, and therefore they become an occasion to debate medical, ritual and devotional ways to cope with illness, discomfort, blame, pain and pollution.

Although the overwhelming majority of devotees continue to worship Śītalā in relation to fertility issues and the wellbeing of children, there is evidence of a growing awareness of, and concern about, new health and environmental threats. In the last few years, especially in response to dramatic media coverage, I have heard of and witnessed expensive, articulate and time-consuming *pūjā*s sponsored by wealthy devotees seeking protection against global pandemics (SARS, Avian Flu, Swine Flu), natural disasters (tsunamis, earthquakes, water and earth pollution) and Islamism.[2] Events like these, however, are sporadic, and should not be regarded as the norm. In addition, one should be aware that Śītalā is seldom worshipped solo. She is regularly included in rituals involving other goddesses (Vaiṣṇo Devī, Kālī, Durgā, Santoṣī Mātā, Ṣaṣṭhī, Caṇḍī, etc.) and gods (Gaṇeśa, Hanumān, Bhairava, Śani, Sūrya, etc.).

To date, this is an unexplored area, a gap dramatically marked by the lack of recent ethnographies.[3] In response to that, in the last ten years of fieldwork in north India (mainly in the states of West Bengal, Uttar Pradesh, Bihar, Haryana and, to a lesser degree, Rajasthan, Gujarat and Punjab), I have tried to understand how myths and rituals of Śītalā have responded to the eradication of smallpox. Further, I have tried to ascertain whether the goddess is included in current debates on health, as happened during the struggle against smallpox in colonial and post-colonial India.

I believe it is safe to say that there is no evidence that Śītalā is being regularly and consistently associated with new diseases, or is being used to convey particular messages in matter of health awareness or sanitation. In fact, I argue that the eradication of smallpox has been irrelevant to the worship of Śītalā. The goddess did not switch from smallpox to chickenpox, measles or other childhood illnesses, as some have argued. As I have demonstrated in the first two chapters of this book, she has always been invoked as a protector of children in general, and from diseases manifesting with boils (*sphoṭa*) and fevers (*jvara*), in particular. With this in mind, the following sections intend to illustrate two opposite patterns. On the one hand, I explore the enduring fascination with the myth of the disease goddess in contemporary culture. On the other, I discuss yet another transformation of Śītalā, i.e. the Durgāfication of the goddess in contemporary India.

After smallpox. The AIDS myth?

In 2003, after hearing a number of unconfirmed voices on Śītalā and HIV/AIDS patients, I found evidence of a few such cases in two medium-sized provincial towns in lower West Bengal.[4] In order to gain recognition as special devotees of Śītalā, a condition often associated with the belief that one could charismatically treat illness, a limited number of informants suggested they were immune to HIV, and willing to prove it. Many in the community considered these claims to be forms of attention-seeking, a way to justify a reprehensible habit (some interviewees were habitual IV drug users), or plain madness.[5] Initially I was sceptical about such stories. They might well have been attempts to attract social workers from a local NGO, medical personnel, charities and, since I did not pass unnoticed, a foreign researcher. I decided to continue the investigation due to the originality of the potential outputs, and the possibility of contributing to cultural studies on contagious diseases and their relation to 'religion'. In fact, I soon realized that rather than a discourse on disease and new pandemics, my informants seemed to be victims of poverty and marginalization. AIDS is at the centre of a heated debate in India, just like smallpox in the past. My informants were using it as a way to advertise a distress whose origin they imputed to society at large. I was however intrigued by the realization that disease (or the idea thereof) is not discussed as infirmity, but as a form of empowerment and a way out of misery.[6]

I attributed this view to the possible lack of awareness of the dangers of HIV/AIDS. Although the local populace demonstrated an overall good understanding of the nature of the virus,[7] HIV – which is sometime called, like other blood infections, *khārāp khun* (B. 'bad/damaged blood') – is believed by many to be a consequence of wrongdoing, impure action or shameful conduct. This should be paired with the belief in the reversibility of illness,[8] an ideology derived from a variety of narratives since Vedic times. Āyurveda too bears witness to such belief. Narrative sections of medical compendia highlight the relation between human long life (*āyus*) and action (*karma*). When diagnostic charts are not used, the compilers of medical texts refer to mythological tales illustrating how what we do in this or preceding lives impacts on how we live (CaS.Ni. 7: 19–23; cf. Mukharji 2013: 271; Cerulli 2013). As per ritual and devotional performances, they are not just ways to thank the goddess for protection, but means to make up for wrongdoing, whether deliberate or accidental. See, for instance, the refrain of a Hindi song:

> If one fell in disgrace because of wrongdoing,
> If one fell in disgrace because of causing endless pain
> She will be saved only by touching the dust of your [Śītalā's] feet.[9]

Singing, presenting offerings, repeating mantras, taking part in pilgrimage, fasting and fulfilling vows are aimed at attracting the attention of the goddess, and of the community, by means of presentations that are believed to be a compensation for protection. Yet in the case of HIV I discuss here, there is one major difference, i.e. the awareness of doing something wrong. This, however, is compensated by the belief that challenging rules and conventions is conducive to redemption. Just as inoculators and, later, medical personnel of SEP incorporated Śītalā in their practice to gain consensus and validation, the possibility of developing *khārāp khun* (HIV/AIDS, or hepatitis) is explained as a sign of ultimate devotion, or the willingness to surrender to the will of Śītalā.[10] In fact, invoking the protecting presence of Śītalā is a status-booster that can be turned into a business (*vyavasā*). This is not novel (cf. Harman on Māriyamma<u>n</u> 2011: 190–6). Some elements, however, are distinctively unique. First, procedures that might cause infection are non-ritual. Second, unlike devotional practices, including health-threatening performances, this is not a public event. Thought informants aim at public recognition, the actions that are supposed to prove their power are secretive (B. *cupcāp*). (Naturally, this adds up to the perception that the whole business may be pretence.) Communication of intentionality is privileged over accomplishment of service.

In 2011, I returned to the same towns I visited five years before. Of my initial set of respondents, I was able to meet only one. He was in a much better state, and mentioned he benefited from the help of social workers. He made a vow to Śītalā Mā to take good care of his health.

The relation between Śītalā and AIDS is a feeble one. My case study, though extremely limited and unsystematic, certainly cannot serve to prove or disprove the emergence of a new pattern. In the following years (up to 2014), I have continued to look for information on Śītalā and HIV/AIDS. Nothing emerged. Colleagues, occasional informants, local acquaintances and research assistants from various north Indian sites are not aware of Śītalā being worshipped as a protector from AIDS. Media too do not report of Śītalā and AIDS. The only source I am aware of comes from McDaniel's study on Śāktism in Bengal:

> Today, the *patua* artist-singers [who specialize in scroll-paints] write illustrating the adventures of Shitala as the AIDS goddess, traveling to different countries and spreading the disease. [...] she was shown both causing and curing AIDS. The victims were symbolised by weight loss – they were shown as thin and sticklike, being weighted on a scale, very light in one pan against the weight in the other pan. People who did not worship Shitala died miserably, while those who had faith were saved, and gained weight again. AIDS was brought by Shitala because people were neglecting her worship, and this was her divine revenge upon irreligious and secular people. (McDaniel 2004: 65)[11]

This seems an isolated occurrence.[12] In fact, the general tendency in AIDS-scrolls is to impute AIDS, and other diseases, to unspecified demons. Scroll painters know very well of the ubiquity of Śītalā in Bengal. If they do not include her in their performances, it may be for a number of reasons. It seems however relevant to mention that *pāṭuya*s are entrepreneurs.[13] They would paint whatever a customer asks for a fee.[14] Yet customers are not interested in Śītalā. Indian and Western collectors, folklorists and tourists are fascinated by AIDS-scrolls, which are sold at high prices, often in US dollars. The gory stories of demons infecting wrongdoers have become popular, and their echo reverberates across media, tourist offices, NGOs, charities, cultural events, university programmes, etc. Themes such AIDS, tsunamis, earthquakes, Islamist terrorism (including 9/11 and Osama Bin Laden scrolls) and nuclear disasters have become popular in India and abroad. In that, the *pāṭuya*s seem to replicate the process by which selected *pālā*s from *Śītalāmaṅgalkāvyas* have dramatized the deeds of the goddess by means of hyperbolic tales of horror, devotion and redemption.

With the exception of the very few cases I have identified between 2003 and 2004, I believe it is safe to say that Śītalā has very little to do with AIDS and PLWHAs (People Living With HIV/AIDS). In my original 2007 article, I have suggested that local Śītalās in rural Bengali villages 'started to be *sporadically* [emphasis added] worshipped to keep away AIDS from the mid-1990s' (Ferrari 2007: 95). The incidents I witnessed are not the norm. They are isolated, and numerically irrelevant. But news that AIDS could be the new specialism of Śītalā, as well as the birth of an Indian AIDS-goddess in Kerala,[15] alerted the academic community (Narayanan 2000: 774; Narayanan 2006: 66–7; Foulston and Abbott 2009: 222; Lipner 2010: 344; Zeiler 2008: 162; Nanda 2009: 89–90, Bass 2012: 121; Manring 2012) and media (e.g. Beary 1999; David 1999; Gewertz n.d.). It seems therefore that 'disease goddesses' continue to enjoy much popularity in contemporary culture. With smallpox gone, AIDS might have been the best candidate as Śītalā's next specialism. In fact, new diseases like HIV/AIDS but also Avian Flu, SARS, Swine Flu, etc. did not have the time to be absorbed into local mythology.

The dissemination of pharmacies, dispensaries and hospitals along with higher levels of literacy, the overall rise of GDP per capita and, perhaps most of all, wider accessibility to sources of information (press, radio, television, the internet) have contributed to a general growth in health awareness. Conditions such as poxes, cholera, malaria, exanthemata, leprosy, skin diseases, infertility, etc. are still alive in Indian mythology. New plagues, conversely, are explained from the very beginning in biomedical terms. They do not even have vernacular names. The only evidence of their expression in cultural terms is that of abstract, anonymous, demons who strike wrongdoers. When the narrative process that is core to mythologization – with all its political implications – is controlled by such pervasive, powerful and authoritative exegeses, internal and external logics are difficult to reconcile. If, conversely, story-telling and myth-making adhere to ancestral knowledge (as with 'old' diseases), then the therapeutic element survives. The next section intends to reflect on the latter aspect.

Śītalā's shade in Calcutta: On a contemporary *maṅgal* novel[16]

During one of my sojourns in Kolkata, I had the chance to re-read Amitav Ghosh's *The Calcutta Chromosome* (1995). The novel, written in English by a cosmopolite Bengali scholar and acclaimed novelist, explores the play of disease, health and medicine in colonial and contemporary Bengal in a way that is reminiscent of Bengali *maṅgal* narratives. The book, 'a novel of fevers, delirium and discovery', perpetuates the thaumaturgic aspect of verbal testimony, as well as the contagious nature of information exchange (cf. Dimock 1982: 187). *Maṅgalkāvyas* too, and more emphatically the theatrical renditions loosely based on Nityānanda's *pālās*, have served the purpose of alerting the population about the always-threatening menace represented by disease in general, and smallpox in particular. This is achieved by means of moralizing tales built on fictionalized renderings of local culture, and conveyed by portentous females, i.e. Śītalā and, in the case of CC, Mangala. In fact, CC and the ŚMKs converge on many aspects.[17] Here I use a simplified version of Propp's (1968: 25) model to summarize the main points:

> Śītalā and Mangala are offended by humans and/or gods [*villainy*] and marginalized [*lack*] because they have no economic, social or symbolic capital. They react to violence with contagion [*counteraction*]. Śītalā and Mangala move with their assistants (Jvarāsura and Laakhan respectively) into a new spatial and temporal reality [*departure to a new world*]. This is achieved by means of extraordinary displacement. Śītalā moves from the *devaloka* (realm of gods) to *nārāloka* (realm of humans), whereas Mangala has the power to control her reincarnations. While amongst human beings, Śītalā and Mangala give their helpers important tasks, i.e. to facilitate contagion and pave the path toward the final aim [*function of the donor*]. The two heroines act in disguise: they look poor, wretched and diseased. In fact, they are (like) goddesses [*hero's reaction and struggle*]. Deceit serves the purpose to deploy revenge and to affirm their power [*victory*]. After affirmation [*liquidation*], Śītalā and Mangala continue their existence elsewhere [*return*], while their deeds on earth are perpetuated by means of worship, iconography and the diffusion of (secret, devotional, ritual and medical) knowledge [*solution*].

The two narratives do not only share structural similarities. In fact – and more relevant to this study – they bear witness to revealing semantic analogies. First, there is a convergence of iconographic tropes. Just like the Śītalā of premodern Bengali narratives, Mangala is ambiguous. She is a 'witch', a 'magician', a goddess (CC 143) or a 'false prophetess' (CC 90). Like Śītalā, Mangala holds a *jhāṛū*, and is described as a sweeper. Like Śītalā, she has a royal attitude (CC 90, 92), and is followed by assistants and sick devotees (CC 90). Like Śītalā, she requires blood (CC 90–1). Like

Śītalā, she may appear in a brightly coloured sari or in ragged clothes (CC 85). She may look young and old, just like Śītalā, who has the power to transform herself from a beautiful young lady into a decrepit Brahman woman. Mangala has a *mūrti* too. Like many aniconic renderings of Śītalā, this 'was made of painted clay, and it was small enough to fit quite easily into the palm of his hand. [. . .] The central part of the figurine was a simple, semicircular mound, crudely modelled and featureless except for two large stylized eyes, painted in stark blacks and whites, on the baked clay' (CC 25). A further concordance emerges, i.e. the idea that disease is propagated by mean of an animal carrier. Just as the ass is a symbol of illness and quite literally a carrier, in CC this function belongs to pigeons, while anopheles are vectors. Iconographic elements confirm this. While Śītalā rides an ass, or asses are sculpted in relief at her feet or on her throne, Mangala Bibi is represented by means of 'a semicircular mound with two painted eyes. On one side of the mound was a tiny pigeon, and on the other a small semicircular instrument' (CC 132), i.e. a nineteenth-century microscope.

Second, just as Śītalā is accompanied by Jvarāsura, a horrendous three-headed, crippled and unruly creature 'who goes disguised as a young servant' (Nicholas 2003: 70), Mangala is attended by Laakhan (or Lutchman). This character is described as 'worse than untouchable; [. . .] he carried contagion; [. . .] he was probably the child of a prostitute; [. . .] his misshapen left hand was a mark of hereditary disease' (CC 163). In *maṅgal* culture, Jvarāsura is given to Śītalā, who brought him with her on earth, where they will ravage the land and its inhabitants. Laakhan too is removed from his homeland, Renupur (Odisha). He is 'stray, orphaned by famine, with a thin, wasted body and a deformed hand' (CC 164), and he always precedes Mangala's apparition.

Third, the performance of Śītalā in *maṅgal* culture has been famously discussed as *līlā*, divine play (Dimock 1982). It is, however, a game that human beings fail to understand, even though the message is straightforwardly clear. Śītalā is not mysterious. She is vengeful and merciless: failure to worship her would cause epidemics. Śītalā's oscillation from *sāmya* to *ugra*, and vice versa, reflects the conflation of mythical time with historical time. This results in a number of spectacular distortions. The dissemination of a rationale for disease requires monstrosity. Contagion is spread by means of (poisoned) food or malign – ferocious and ugly – agents that act to vindicate offence caused to the goddess, or to satisfy caprice. Disease and death, however, are reversible events. Fear motivates devotion, and when devotion is acknowledged, Śītalā heals/resurrects. This is echoed in Mangala's performance. The woman's control of disease is ultimately part of a greater game in which life eternal is the prize. In this big game, human beings are just guinea pigs:

> She [Mangala] is not in this because she wants to be a scientist. She's in this because she thinks she's a god. And what that means is that she wants to be the mind that sets things in motion. The way she sees it, we can't ever know her, or her motives, or anything else about her: the experiment won't work unless the

> reasons for it are utterly inscrutable to us, as unknowable as a disease. But at the same time, she's got to try and tell us about her own history: that's part of the experiment too. (CC 145–6)

The necessity to tell a story featured by pain, injustice, resurrection and eternity is core to the logics of *maṅgal* poems, and reverberates in CC. A further element emerges. Śītalā and Mangala play with humans but, at the same time, they need them. It is by means of the stories of human beings that their myth, or knowledge, is propagated. It is through humans' bodies that their existence is perpetuated. And it is because of humans' fear that they are worshipped. Ultimately, malaria and smallpox are not absolute negatives. Śītalā and Mangala are powerful because they can transcend weakness, infirmity, impurity and stigma, and are able to transform them into immortality.

Fourth, Śītalā and Mangala have the power to infect as well as to cure (CC 143). On virtue of such portentous skills, the two women demand to be worshipped. I have already discussed how Śītalā requests absolute surrender. As per Mangala, her knowledge makes her think she truly is a goddess (CC 146). Therefore she must be worshipped. A sharp critique of religion emerges. Health-seekers are described as devotees 'in various attitudes of supplication, some touching her [Mangala's] feet, others lying prostrate' (CC 90). But like in *maṅgal pālās* there are no indications about how to invite, or activate, the healing power of the trickster-female. Just as in ŚMKs folk culture is portrayed as a world deprived of knowledge, so CC reinvigorates the mystery and esotericism of knowledge. Ritual is ultimately absent because ritual activity requires critical skills and knowledge. Neither Śītalā nor Mangala want human beings to be critical subjects.

> Maybe this other team [Mangala's circle] started with the idea that knowledge is self-contradictory; maybe they believed that to know something is to change it, therefore in knowing something, you've already changed what you think you know so you don't really know it at all: you only know its history. Maybe they thought that knowledge couldn't begin without acknowledging the impossibility of knowledge. See what I'm saying? [...] if it's true that to know something is to change it, then it follows that one way of changing something – of effecting a mutation, let's say – is to attempt to know it, or aspects of it. Right? (CC 63)

Devotees are individuals deprived of knowledge who worship an intimidating goddess with the power to heal. Those who know how to counter the power of Mangala and Śītalā are killed, as Hirādhara the *kavirāja* in Jagannāth's *Bardhamānapālā* (J.ŚMK. 6), or infected, as Murugan in CC. What is left to humans is the duty to narrate: the only ritual allowed is the cyclical repetition and transmission of the stories of Śītalā and Mangala. In this way, the symbolism of infection is the means by which storytelling is established as myth.

Finally, in both narratives time is shaped by the deployment of terror in society, which in turn is the manifestation of trickster-characters (Śītalā and Mangala). As Dimock notes: 'Although the epidemic is a diachronic event, the *maṅgal* poems are meant to describe its synchronic source, the endemic goddess herself'. In a similar fashion, Nicholas observes that *maṅgalkāvyas*, 'like the deities they eulogize, [...] stand outside time, even though they register the transitory events of history' (Nicholas 2003: 132). As per Mangala, her persistence in time suggests how control over infection is the key to the extra-temporal dimension par excellence: immortality. Śītalā and Mangala are both oscillating presences (Dimock 1982: 195; cf. Paniker 2003: 10), whose incursions in history produce distortions. Disease and healing truly are *līlā*. Yet this game is an experiment (CC 147), and history is a site for manipulation.

The lesson transmitted by the Bengali myth of the disease goddess continues to be one revolving around basic dichotomies such as illness/health, contagion/remission, knowledge/ignorance, presence/absence and ultimately life/death (or mortality/immortality). The fascination with disease as a mystical condition allowing otherized forms of being and knowledge, as well access to non-ordinary reality, seems to be a dominating theme, especially when informed by folklore. Murugan, one of the main characters in CC, says that: 'A lot of people who've had malaria know that: it can be more hallucinogenic than any mind-bending drug. That's why primitive people sometimes thought of malaria as a kind of spirit-possession' (CC 144). Similar conclusions have been reached by a number of scholars, who have seen in smallpox and other conditions a form of possession, or a privileged site for experiencing the goddess (see above p. 94).

The narratives discussed here show how the mythology of Śītalā, in the guise promoted by *maṅgal* poets, conforms to *Lebensangst*, the existential fear of living that Blumenberg defines as the incapacity to respond to a crisis (1985: 6). This specific theme is found variously edited at many levels of contemporary culture, e.g. fiction, arts, scholarship, education, etc. Not only does it inform the debate on how and why cultural memory is preserved and passed on (cf. Guillén 1971: 39). It also confirms that what I called the 'smallpox myth' and the stories of the 'disease goddess' are something more than popular tales that have been variously edited and replicated. Both are a vibrant part of Indian, and now global, culture. Authenticity, or the pretence thereof, is eventually irrelevant, and conflicting versions do not seem to be a concern to audiences. Devotees of the goddess, including Bengalis, know the difference between the story of a theatrical *pālā* (entertainment) and *pūjā* or *vrata* (ritual), just like we are able to tell history from fiction in Ghosh's novel. The tension between such seemingly opposite trends seems however to be reconciled in the superstar Śītalā emerging in contemporary pop-bhakti.

The Durgāfication of the goddess. Śītalā in pop-devotional culture

Tales of the disease goddess recapitulate fiction, entertainment, history, fear/horror, devotion and a happy ending, or the illusion thereof. At the same time, they feed on a romantic idealization of folk life. The *maṅgal*-Śītalā is an Orientalist construction *ante litteram*. This, however, has not impacted on ritual practice. Conversely, gentrification has proved functional to major changes in ritual, iconographic and narrative culture across north India. Śītalā is now more than ever a transversal goddess. Her success among upper and middle class sectors is a significant one. But it comes with a price. The downgrading of ancestral ritual and devotional practices (e.g. animal sacrifice, possession and austerities) is an indicator of a process that, in the long run, has determined a considerable shift in the way devotees respond to, and represent, Śītalā. Worship is being adapted to global ethical discourses and the dominant *vaiṣṇava bhakti*. Vernacular ritual know-how is being eroded, and the intense physical devotion that still features scheduled celebrations (e.g. *daṇḍavat, bhar, khelnā*, etc.) is increasingly criticized. *Śītalāgān*s are being replaced by songs to Durgā, or other pan-Hindu goddesses (Sarasvatī, Gaṅgā Mā, Lakṣmī, Vaiṣṇo Devī, etc.). Śītalā's iconography too is dramatically changing. The goddess is regularly portrayed as an affluent young woman on a finely decorated (white) donkey. Alternatively, she stands up holding a trident and a broom. Her companions are not dangerous demons, as Bengali *maṅgal* poets told us, but the popular god Hanumān and, occasionally, a child-like plump Bhairava with his loyal dog. This recent yet widespread iconography deserves some attention.

Śītalā takes here the place of Vaiṣṇo Devī, 'the vegetarian aspect of the goddess [Durgā] who is auspicious, powerful, and sometimes fierce and punitive, but who accepts no animal sacrifice' (Erndl 1993: 5). Vaiṣṇo Devī is represented with two miniature guardians, or doorkeepers: Hanumān, holding a red banner with the slogan 'Jay Mātā Dī' ('Victory to the Mother!'), and a child Bhairava, with his dog.[18] Both *śaiva* and *śākta* myths converge in Vaiṣṇo Devī, and are further accommodated within Vaiṣṇavism by means of practice (vegetarianism) and myth (*Rāmāyaṇa*, evoked by Hanumān). The tactical substitution of Vaiṣṇo Devī with Śītalā reminds devotees of the greatness and pervasiveness of the Cold Lady.

Other factors are contributing to such changes. Upward social mobility in rural and urban India as well as an unprecedented availability of traditional media, the success of last-generation technological gadgets and computer literacy have impacted on many levels on contemporary Hinduism. The surge in the production of devotional material – including online *bhakti* resources – is a response to a growing demand. The serialization of Śītalā's merchandise, in line with the general trend, has gone viral. The internet (particularly websites allowing the uploading and sharing of audio-visual material, such as YouTube) is the new global site for the apotheosis of the goddess.

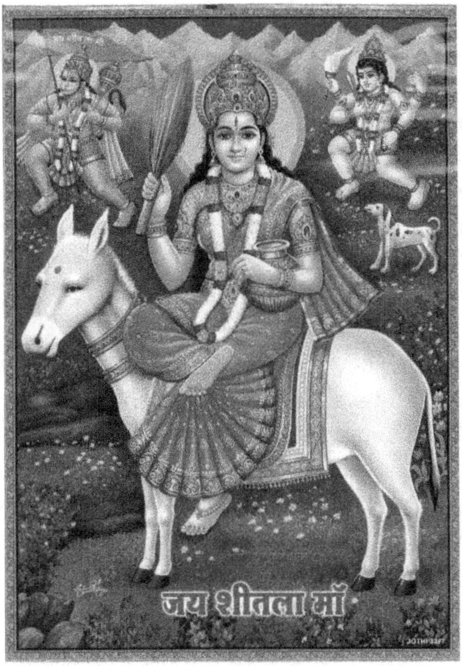

FIGURE 5.1 *Śītalā with Hanumān (top left) and Bhairava (top right), poster (author's collection).*

A cursory look at online material distinctly confirms the decline of Śītalā's traditional features. The goddess is advertised as an emanation of the pan-Hindu goddess Durgā, or her gentler forms (e.g. Vaiṣṇo Devī). The association of Śītalā with diseases is emphatically softened, if not obliterated. Temple committees, but also family-run shrines, are often willing to promote the goddess as an aspect of Mahādevī, especially if this confers on them authority, prestige and economic capital. Competition is a subsequent factor.

This transformation emerges dramatically in Hindi and Bhojpuri pop culture, particularly the celebration of the goddess in devotional songs (e.g. *devī pacrā*, *bhajan*, etc.). Songs like *Sītlā ghāṭ pe Kāśī meñ* (see above pp. 31–2) or the anonymous *pacrā* included in the *Dasāśvamedhamāhātmya* (see above p. 32–3) project the goddess in the global arena. Śītalā is neither praised as a healing goddess, nor are her traditional attributes/tools mentioned. Her inclusion in the Navadurgā tradition – often via the ass-riding Kālarātrī – confirms the trend of using popular Durgā devotional songs for the worship of Śītalā. Such is the case of the devotional hit *Baṛī śer par savār* (Bhp. 'Riding a big tiger').[19] The song, a popular Bhojpuri composition that celebrates Vaiṣṇo Devī in her form of Śeraṅvālī ('Rider of the Tiger/Lion'), is now sung or played loudly in most Śītalā temples across Uttar Pradesh, Bihar, Jharkhand and West Bengal. Strophes like *sonāke mukutoā sohe māike kapūr* (Bhp. 'a golden crown beautifully adorns the forehead of the Mother') or *lāl raṅg sarī māhe cāñdsī suratiyā* ('a red-coloured sari enhances the beauty of her moon-face') provide devotees with the grounds for visualizing Śītalā as a trident-armed (*triśūl hāth mẽ*), tiger-riding form of Durgā. Online video-clip culture emphatically bears witness to this phenomenon.

In Bhojpuri hits like *Jai ho Shitala bhabani* (H. 'Victory to Śītalā Bhavānī')[20] and *Sheetla maiya ke (dwar) chal* (H. 'Let's go to the gates of Mother Śītalā'),[21] the goddess is visually identified with Durgā, even though the devotional songs are associated with seats of power of the Cold Lady. Alternatively, if the lyrics do not suggest the restyling of Śītalā, the semantically charged images of video clips unmistakably point to her Durgāfication. Such is the case for *Saayar Sheetla Phoolmati*,[22] where devotees sing Śītalā's glory around a huge statue of Durgā. Although the Durgāfication of Śītalā seems now an established tendency, one can still appreciate the resistance of folk elements. It is the case of songs heavily relying on the charisma of selected shrines. The Śītalā-of-the-place is celebrated as the big-eyed protective goddess in *Sheetla maiya ke mandir mein hardam* (H. 'Always in the temple of Mother Śītalā'),[23] as the riverine goddess in *Adalpura Shitla Maiya Ke* (Bhp. 'Śītalā Mother of Adalpura')[24] and in the songs from Manoj Tiwari's album *Karuna Ke Khaan Sitla Maiya* (Bhp. 'Mother Śītalā is the source of grace').[25] A further confirmation of this trend is found in songs of the seven sisters, such as *Sitala sato re bahiniya ke*.[26] Along with the companion hit *Saato bahiniya jhula jhule* (Bhp. 'While the Seven Sisters swing'),[27] this song clearly advocates the worship of the goddess as the foremost representative of a group of seven sister virgins (*sāt kanyā*) traditionally associated with village culture. In the video, devotees offer them beautiful ornaments, bangles, clothes and perfume while Śītalā whispers through *nīm* branches and appears to them in dream visions. In the end, however, Śītalā and her sisters reveal themselves as a manifestation of the great goddess Durgā Śeraṅvālī or, alternatively, the Mahiṣāsuramardinī.

The stratification of new elements borrowed from the myth of Durgā or Vaiṣṇo Devī is accelerating the homogenization of *āñcalik* culture. The Hindi songs of albums celebrating the goddess of Gurgaon – e.g. *Maīyā Guṛgā̃v Vālī* (H. 'Mother of Gurgaon'), *Merī bigṛī banā do Mā Śītalā* (H. 'O Mother Śītalā, take me out of my misery') or *Mā Śītalā lā de paiso kī ḍherī* (H. 'O Mother Śītalā, let me have a lot of money') – and Bhojpuri VCDs with hymns in honour of the Adalpura Sitala Dhām – e.g. *Mahimā Adalpura vālī kī* – confirm such evolution.[28] In both cases, CD and VCD covers show the image of the local *mūrti* alongside that of the traditional ass-riding Śītalā. The lyrics of the songs reflect some vernacular features, but eventually there is commonality in describing Śītalā as the slayer of the buffalo demon, the one who holds a trident and rides a lion and even an aspect of Kāmākhyā Devī. Śītalā is worshipped according to the modes of northern Indian *bhakti*, but has taken the form of a powerful and benign Śakti.

What is perhaps the most distinctive feature of all these songs is the obliteration of Śītalā's power to heal. Not only are Śītalā's specific attributes (ass, winnowing fan, broom and pitcher) taken off the picture, but also any reference to protection from disease in general, and pustular diseases (measles, chickenpox, etc.) in particular, is omitted. One of the few exception is *Mai mori Sheetla* (Bhp. 'My mother Śītalā'),[29] the story of a crippled devotee who, after intense and continued worship, is healed by the goddess and walks again.

The serial production of devotional CDs, VCDs and DVDs, their affordable prices (recordings are sold from ₹25, around 27 pence) and the rise of internet channels specializing in devotional songs on free platforms have made it possible for new styles and trends to be conveyed fast at all levels. New means of expressions are not limited to songs and the video clips associated with them. The *Shitala Chalisa*, an iPhone and Android app powered by Transfer Junction and released on 11 September 2012, confirms what has been discussed so far. Along with the *cālīsā*, the app provides an audio file called 'Aarti Shitala Mata Ki' (H. 'the *ārti* of Mother Śītalā'). The melody is evocative of the popular 'Auṃ Jay Jagdīś Hare' ('Glory to the Lord of the Universe'), a *vaiṣṇava bhajan* in Hindi composed toward the end of the nineteenth century and featuring in Hindu global culture. The images accompanying the recitation are: 1) a Durgā Mahiṣāsuramardinī from a Bengali pavilion (B. *pāṇḍāl*); 2) a richly decorated and garlanded Śītalā on a grey-coated ass (the animal has a gold crown and gold reins); 3) the Śītalā *mūrti* of the Gurgaon *mandir*; and 4) the goddess Māriyammaṉ with lolling tongue, a trident and standing on fire.

The restyling of Śītalā in contemporary popular culture is not limited to *bhakti* songs. In 1981 – a few years after the eradication of smallpox – the Hindi movie *Śītalā Mātā* was released. The motion picture, directed by Ram Gopal Gupta, is now available in most markets outside Śītalā *mandirs*, and on a number of websites.[30] Here follows its synopsis:

> The story revolves around a poor widow, Kunti, who lives with her two sons and her daughters-in-law. Śītalā, as in most vernacular narratives, manifests in a dream vision, and tells Kunti that an old *pratimā* lies abandoned under the earth in the fields. It must be brought to light and installed in a temple that Kunti's sons are supposed to build. The owner of the land, emphatically called Zamindar Rana (King Landowner), refuses to grant Sarju and Bikhu (Kunti's sons) permission to dig his land. Meanwhile Bhagyawanti, Bikhu's wife, humiliates Kunti, and ridicules the idea of retrieving Śītalā's *mūrti* and building a temple. After Zamindar Rana's harsh refusal, Bikhu is convinced by the uncompromising words of Bhagyawanti and decides to give up. At nighttime, however, Sarju confides his intention to retrieve the *pratimā* to his heavily pregnant wife Dayawanti as well as to Kunti. The rich and arrogant landowner finds out what happened and, in consultation with his counsellor, Ram Bharose, forces Kunti, Sarju and Dayawanti out of the village. Desperate, penniless and hungry, they are hosted by a pious farmer who gives them shelter. Meanwhile Sarju decides that Śītalā deserves her temple. He finds the *pratimā* and wanders across nearby villages to collect money with the declared aim of building the *mandir*. The local farming populace is willing to help as soon as they know the story of the goddess's night visitation to Kunti and the

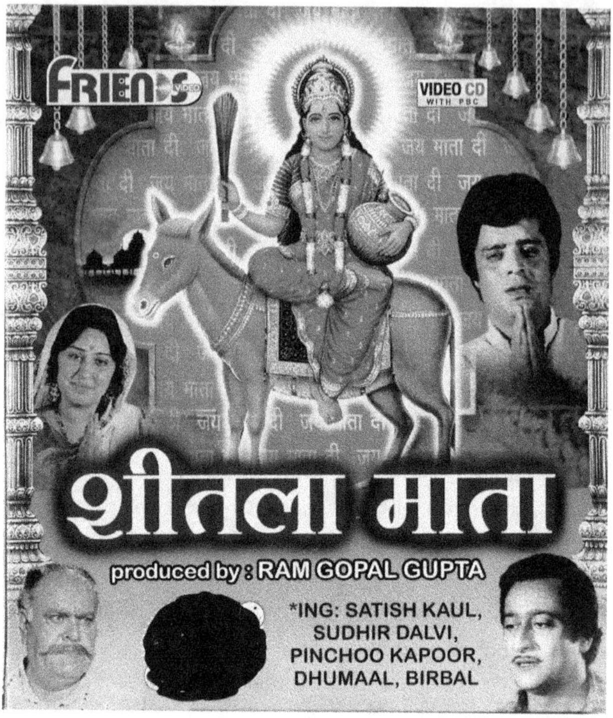

FIGURE 5.2 *Śītalā Mātā (1981), directed by Ramgopal Gupta, VCD cover (author's collection).*

tragic destiny of Sarju and his family. News of Sarju's entrepreneurial effort reaches Zamindar Rana's ears. Inspired by his *munim* (accountant), he decides to punish Sarju's hubris and to cleanse his tainted honour. When everybody is sleeping, the landowner steals the *mūrti* of Śītalā Mātā and throws it in a well. Meanwhile the lives of Kunti and Dayawanti become even more miserable. They struggle with their new life, and Dayawanti is forced to accept employment as a domestic labourer at her sister-in-law's. Bhagyawanti is cruel and humiliates in all possible ways Dayawanti, who keeps invoking Śītalā Mā. Sarju, who is robbed of his money, is eventually helped by a local outlaw, Sardar Phoolan, and the construction of the temple begins. A baby boy is born to Dayawanti and everything seems to go well. All the farmers go to Zamindar Rana and explain their intention to finish the temple on his land, as per Śītalā's wish. It will be a temple for all villages. The landowner pretends to give permission but at night destroys the *mandir* with dynamite. Śītalā becomes furious. She heats up and throws balls of fire toward the residence of Zamindar, who is badly hurt, and the rest of the village. Her fury knows no limits. A rain of fire destroys the village and causes the death of many innocent people. In the last scene of the movie, the survivors gather in the ruins of

> the temple to beg for forgiveness. Zamindar Rana too is present, urged by his wife. In front of the burnt corpses of the victims of Śītalā's wrath, the landowner repents. Sarju and Dayawanti pray to the goddess. In a moving singing performance, they celebrate the mother who gives life (*tu jivan detī hae, mātā*) and supplicate Śītalā not to abandon the village (*merī mātā nā toṛo nātā*, lit. 'my mother, don't break this bond'). Cold water is poured on the *mūrti* and from her celestial abode Śītalā starts crying, touched by the devotion of the villagers. Time goes backward and the dead are revivified. Śītalā descends to earth and gives *darśana* to the villagers. She promises to stay with them and asks the *mandir* to be rebuilt. After the reconstruction, Sarju takes responsibility for the new temple and Kunti, Dayawanti and the women of the village perform ritual worship. The song *Mātā kā vrat rakhne* (H. 'keeping the mother's vow') portrays an idyllic scenario, which includes a *pūjā* to Kunti's dog and a donkey. Stale edibles are presented to Śītalā (though the icon is actually Durgā) and a communal meal is offered to villagers, pilgrims, a heavily scarred Zamindar Rana, his wife and Ram Bharose. During the worship, the burns of the landowner and other villagers are finally healed.

The story is not striking in originality, yet some elements are of great interest. Smallpox (H. *cecak*) in 1981 is still a fresh memory. In the song *Suno suno jī* ('Listen, listen!'),[31] Kunti and Dayawanti urge villagers to follow Śītalā's rules (*Śītalā ke niyam*) for good health during the hot season (*garm mausam*). Children with chickenpox are fanned with branches of *nīm*, and pots of cold water are placed under their beds. Concerned relatives are asked not to give hot food to fevering patients, including *cāy*.[32] Rooms must be cleansed with a *jhāṛū* and the bodies of those around patients are expected to be clean. (Neither inoculators nor vaccinators are shown or mentioned.) Notwithstanding the association of Śītalā with smallpox, the movie is not about the healing power of Śītalā. The goddess is a protector and, it so seems, an agent of *dharma*. Śītalā is worshipped by peasants as a *patthar kā mūrti* ('[slab] stone icon'), but is visualized as a beautiful lady, wearing a red sari, a golden crown and holding a *triśula* (a trident, one of the weapons of Durgā). In her celestial abode, she sits on a huge golden throne and is constantly winnowed by two maidens with what appear to be *nīm* branches. At her feet are two prancing grey asses and in the background one can admire a huge golden *cakra*, a symbol of righteousness (*dharma*). The iconography of the goddess in *Śītalā Mātā* shows that as early as the beginning of the 1980s, the overlapping of Śītalā with the Great Goddess was already noticeable. This is particularly evident in the epilogue of the film. Śītalā's furious reaction is not vendetta. She is not retaliating because somebody offended her, or her devotees.[33] The goddess manifests among humans to counter *adharma*. This manifests as humiliation of righteous women, deceit, arrogance, violence, egoism, sycophancy, theft and irreligiosity. Yet Śītalā does not send diseases. She heats up and throws balls of fire, a consolidated pattern in narratives of angry goddesses (e.g. DBP 10: 1–16; on Durgā as fire in liturgy, see McDaniel 2004: 221; Rodrigues 2003: 63).

Śītalā is similarly portrayed in the short film *Jai Mā Śītalā (Kahānī Adalpura Kī)*.[34] The story is quite loyal to the foundation myth of Adalpura, and in that it distances itself from *Śītalā Mātā* and the many video clips in Hindi and Bhojpuri.

> The old mother of Adalpura is a riverine goddess who reveals herself to a poor *mallāh* while he is out fishing on the Ganges. The boatman is not convinced by the voice he heard, and so Śītalā appears to him again in a dream. The goddess is a young woman with a gold crown who stands at the feet of a huge *bargad* (banyan) tree holding her distinctive *jhāṛū* and a big metal pitcher on the crook of her arm. Her desire is to be worshipped. The next morning a group of fishermen sail to the river and perform *pūjā* to invite the goddess. Śītalā is pleased by the devotion of the *māṁjhī*s and descends from heaven on the back of her ass. The community establishes a *mūrti* of the goddess in a humble shrine on the banks of the river. Meanwhile the chief of the local Brahman *paṇḍits* learns that a new shrine has been erected and congratulates himself that his services will be soon required. Rage ensues when the Brahmans come to know that the *mallāhs* are acting as *pūjārī*s. During a confrontation, the chief of the Brahmans threatens the *mallāh* community to desist and throw them out of the shrine. The *mallāhs* resist and claim they are the custodians of a sacred spot that has been revealed to them directly by the goddess. They have the irrevocable right of care over the shrine as well as that of performing rituals, and sharing donations. Traditionally adverse to low class *pūjārī*s, the Brahmans appeal to scriptures and loudly proclaim they are the only *gaṅgāputra* (lit. 'sons of the Ganges', where the river is the goddess Gaṅgā). The right to perform rituals is theirs. The fisherman confesses Śītalā appeared to him in a dream. He is called a liar and cast out of the temple along with all other *mallāh*s. Later on, after a fight between the two parties, the poor *māṁjhī* is seriously injured. His furious wife loudly summons Śītalā Mā who, seeing her devotee badly hurt, takes revenge. Blazes, lightings and inundations strike the *āñcal*. After the storm, a *sādhu* explains to the chief Brahman he has to atone. He publicly repents in front of Śītalā at the Adalpura Mandir and begs forgiveness of the poor fisherman. From now on, the *mallāhs* are entitled to be the official *pūjārī*s of the temple. Śītalā, from her seat at the roots of the *bargad*, observes the Brahman imposing the *ṭīkā* on the fisherman's forehead.

In *Jai Mā Śītalā (kahānī Adalpura kī),* the goddess is not straightforwardly associated with Durgā. Although her standard iconography is easily distinguishable, Śītalā is emphatically associated with the river. She descends from heaven and emerges from the cold waters of the Ganges. As cold water, she is enshrined in a small earthen pot at the feet of a majestic *bargad*.[35] Only her *mallāh* devotees can see her *svarūpa* – the lady with the broom on an ass. In the case of Adalpura, as this short devotional film confirms, three different aspects converge: the fluvial goddess of the local boatmen community, the ass-riding Śītalā, and the pan-Hindu Mother Goddess Durgā. The latter aspect distinctively emerges in contemporary representations of the Śītalā Dhām as a powerful *saktipīṭha*, while the goddess is rendered as Mahiṣasuramardiṇī. All these aspects, as discussed above, are not in conflict. Baṛī Śītalā is primarily the protector of the *mallāh*s, irrespective of her form.

This is further confirmed by the story of the Śītalā Dhām as a disputed site of worship. By indicating the low status of the *mallāh*s and highlighting the greedy nature of *paṇḍit*s, the film bridges an ancestral myth into contemporary stories of social contrast. The dispute over the administration of the Śītalā Dham is not fictional. In the last few years, after a series of altercations, a fight ensued between Brahman *pūjārī*s and local *mallāh* ritualists. People were killed on both sides. The tragic event attracted the attention of local media and its discussion in the tribunal court of Varanasi contributed to further inflame the spirits. Not only was economic profit at stake; authority, charisma and tradition were being challenged. *Jai Mā Śītalā (kahānī Adalpura kī)* is not just the rendering of an ancient myth[36] that confirms the injustice suffered by a community chosen by the goddess. What I believe is worth considering is the politics behind myth-making. The narrative is not 'alternative' or 'dissident'. In fact, it seems appropriate to return to Barthes's comment that 'the fundamental character of myth is to be appropriated' (2009: 143). The core elements of the narrative are exactly the same as I encountered in several myths of foundations of various Śītalā *mandir*s across north India. Vernacular micro-myths are adapted to a consolidated frame to fit claims of power, and individual and community needs. If this is not enough, other means are found, including appeals to non-ritual authorities (e.g. local courts). Doron reports that: 'In 1968 the civil court of Banaras ruled in Manjhi's [a powerful *mallāh*] favour in a case brought by him against the ghat priests. This decision set a precedent by formally recognizing the boatmen's right as ritual specialists' (Doron 2008: 135).[37] The *mallāh*s of Adalpura do not see the divine origin of their claim as separate from the decision of the court which, incidentally, continues to be challenged by Brahman *pūjārī*s. In fact, the victorious struggle in the court has infiltrated the foundation myth of the Adalpura Dhām, thus proving that Śītalā continues to be the protector of the *mallāh*s.

Concluding remarks

Representations of Śītalā seem to follow two major trends. On the one hand, there is a continuation of the myth of the 'disease goddesses'. This is expressed in diverse yet mutually informing contexts such as media but also scholarly and fictional works. On the other, Śītalā is increasingly worshipped and represented as a gentle form of Durgā. In this chapter, I have decided to give some space to new forms of devotional expression, i.e. online and pop-*bhakti*. Considering the way India has developed in the last few decades, it would be unfair to ignore how new technologies are affecting everyday religion.

In response to Śītalā's growing popularity in global media as well as in all sectors of Indian society, ritual practices associated with folk or ancestral culture have been marginalized and discredited. Śītalā's inclusion in Durgā or Vaiṣṇo Devī's iconography shows not only how *bhakti* is developing within and beyond India, it also bears witness to its homogenizing tendency. Śītalā is no longer just a healing goddess. The goddess is now a global Devī. According to this process, she has converged in a hyper-model of benevolent mother, even though she continues to retain some of her most distinctive features. The only arena in which Śītalā is consistently a 'disease goddess' is that of fiction, or where the 'smallpox myth' is allowed to live.

Notes

1 The label is often used to indicate the Indian state of West Bengal. Though the homeland of c.ca 12 million Hindus, and a region where Muslims take part in public worship of goddesses like Śītalā, Bangladesh is often ignored in studies on Bengali Hinduism. This is a major problem in studies on Śītalā too, and a flaw affecting this work as well. The same applies to vast regions of Pakistan and Nepal, where the goddess is extensively worshipped. Such regions are virtually ignored in scholarly literature.

2 One such ceremony, in the form of *pūjā* and a conspicuous donation, was organized by a Bengali businessman in the aftermath of the 2010 Varanasi bombing on Śītalā Ghāṭ. On 7 December 2010, a bomb exploded during the evening *ārti*, killing a two-year-old girl and injuring 38 people including both Indians and foreign tourists. The Islamist group 'Indian Mujahideen' claimed responsibility for the attack. The ritual offering, as far as I am aware, is an isolated occurrence. It is however significant in that it bears witness to the consolidation of Śītalā as a form of protective Devī, rather than a minor healing goddess.

3 The last notable effort was Mukhopadhyay's analysis of the worship of the goddess in (West) Bengal (1994). The work draws extensively on the living *maṅgal* culture, to which Mukhopadhyay himself belongs. For shorter ethnographic accounts, see Mull 2005 (Pakistan); and Ferrari 2007 and 2010 (rural WB). Egnor's article (2005), often cited in relation to the role of Śītalā after the eradication of smallpox, actually reports on Māriyammaṉ in Madras (now Chennai), Tamil Nadu. I take the opportunity to note that the two goddesses are not the same, and should not be confused.

4 Fieldwork has been conducted between 2003 and 2004 and then between 2011 and 2012. I initially discussed my findings during a session of the 'Causes and Cures in Health Care in Asia' panel of the ICAS5 (International Convention of Asia Scholars) in Kuala Lumpur (2–5 August 2007). Reports from the initial phase of this research have been published in Ferrari 2007 and 2010b.

5 Informants were called *pāgal* (B. 'crazy', 'mad'), a colloquial term that has no medical implication.

6 The word 'liberation' (*mokṣa*, *mukti* or equivalent) was never used, tempting as it may be to read it in this way. Informants mostly indicated material gain as a way to escape from their present condition.

7 The majority of respondents indicated syringes infected by *junkies* and unprotected sex (rigorously outside marriage) as the principal causes of AIDS. Same-sex intercourse is emphatically mentioned. Blood transfusions and blood contact at birth-giving are discussed with great concern, as unrelated to actions that are considered infringements of *dharma*.

8 I heard similar discourses in relation to a wide range of diseases, such as cancer, leukaemia, cirrhosis, Alzheimer's disease, diabetes, etc. but also social diseases (alcoholism, drug dependence, violent behaviour – especially towards women and children) and 'blameful' behaviours (e.g. homosexuality, prostitution or being a client of prostitutes, and habits resulting in STDs). One should note that there is no moral judgement implied in these and other classifications. I am reporting the views of informants.

9 *maīyā tere caraṇõ kī dhūl jo mil jae*, recorded at Śītalā Mandir, Gurgaon, on 18 October 2012.

10 The ideology behind such claims evokes the dramatic exploits of heroes and heroines of *maṅgal* culture such as Behulā (in *Manasāmaṅgalkāvya*) and Rañjābatī and Lāusen (in *Dharmamaṅgalkāvya*). These and similar stories of extreme renunciation and self-sacrifice, including ritual suicide, did not emerge in the conversations with my informants. They are however well known in Bengali culture.

11 McDaniel confirms that at the beginning of the 1990s, while researching on Kālī in West Bengal, the *paṭuyā* with whom she spoke mentioned that there were storytellers singing Śītalā's story in relation to HIV/AIDS. 'Most people just described the goddess's old powers, but this particular scroll-painter was showing the goddess's new powers. The implication seemed to be that the more diseases a goddess can control, the more powerful she is. Such a goddess is thus reputed Mahādebī, and no longer just *grāmya debī*. Serving a more powerful version of the same goddess indicates a superior position for the *bhakta* himself' (McDaniel, email communication, 2/4/2013).

12 Apart from McDaniel's account, I have never heard of Śītalā in relation to Bengali scroll-painters. Frank Korom, who researched extensively on the subject (Korom 2006b), confirmed that he saw hundreds of AIDS scrolls, but never once did he notice a connection between AIDS and Śītalā (Frank Korom, email communication, 2/4/2013).

13 Following the surge of HIV/AIDS cases in India and the attention paid to this worrying scenario by national and global media, the *paṭuyā*s have started to exponentially produce scrolls on AIDS. The large majority of AIDS scrolls tell stories of demons punishing, for instance, intravenous drug users, homosexuals, prostitutes, people enjoying 'free sex' as well as cheating husbands and wives. *Materialists* are also favourite victims of the disease.

14 Frank Korom, email communication, 2/4/2013.

15 The event, witnessed by Anna Portnoy (2000; cf. Gewertz 2000), has attracted substantial media and scholarly attention. Eventually it proved to be an isolated incident.

16 An earlier and lengthier version of this section has appeared in Ferrari and Refolo 2005.

17 Amitav Ghosh has confirmed that *maṅgal* texts and the myths of Śītalā have indeed informed his work. Amitav Ghosh, email communication, 3/7/2013.

18 The goddess has been alternatively explained as a domesticated form of the demoness Laṅkinī, the guardian of Laṅkā who, in the *Rāmāyaṇa*, is defeated by Hanumān and follows him back to the north (Rāy 1976: 348).

19 http://www.youtube.com/watch?v=B22RS2sU-Ko

20 http://www.youtube.com/watch?v=UywE9kuBLCw

21 http://www.youtube.com/watch?v=-1rERbSMnm0

22 http://www.youtube.com/watch?v=tivJs-fKFkY

23 http://www.youtube.com/watch?v=dOwz8ATzm7Q

24 http://www.youtube.com/watch?v=Ix6CHlv6dlk

25 See for instance *Shitala Ke Laagal Kachahari Ho*, http://www.youtube.com/watch?v=p2D0xjOcLSA

26 http://www.youtube.com/watch?v=RFuFw3owPEw

27 http://www.youtube.com/watch?v=9h-j7pnGlD0&feature=youtu.be&a

28 See also the portrayal of the Adalpura Mandir in *Ek Tu Sacchi Daati*, http://www.youtube.com/watch?v=PWcnPaAdi6g

29 http://www.youtube.com/watch?v=4ZAOlOcdkb8

30 The movie features well-known actors of the 1970s, such as Sudhir Dalvi (Bhikhu), Satish Kaul (Sarju) and Pinchoo Kapoor (Zamindar Rana). Śītalā Mātā is played by Jaya Kausalya. This is not the only major motion picture. In 1958, the Bengali black-and-white movie *Śītalā Mā* was directed by Deb Narayan Gupta. The film did not achieve success. Unfortunately, I was not successful in finding a copy in the archives I consulted in India and abroad.

31 https://www.youtube.com/watch?v=9f-Bhto4tt0

32 The beverage, made of tea, whole milk, spices (notably ginger) and lots of sugar is not recommended for patients with very high temperatures.

33 Cf. KD.ŚMK. 283, when Śītalā causes leprosy and blindness to the sceptical *rāja* who is about to kill a merchant devoted to her.

34 The script of the movie, which features non-professional actors, is an adaptation of local folk tales by Candan Maurya. A short trailer is available for preview on http://www.youtube.com/watch?v=xFmUwYi_1oI

35 The site is currently occupied by a *mūrti* representing a *maithuna* couple – see above, Figure 2.4.

36 The story is said to be 'at least four hundred years old' (H. *kahānī kam se kam cār so sālõ ke purāṇī*).

37 Doron gives us the details of the lawsuit: 'The State v. Mata Prasad', Suit no. 323 (1968), the Court of the Civil Judge, Varanasi (Doron 2008: 135).

Concluding reflections

In the introduction to this book, a question was posed on the legitimacy of a consolidated myth, that of the 'disease goddess'. Over the preceding pages, I have argued the myth is by and large a fabrication. The study of Śītalā shows a considerable gulf between authoritative external claims and the beliefs and practices of devotees. This reminds me of Smith's words on the academic study of religions: 'The world is not given; it is not simply "there". We constitute it by acts of interpretation. We constitute it by activities of speech and memory and judgement. It is by an act of human will, through projects of language and history, through words and memory, that we fabricate the world and ourselves. But there is a double sense to the word *fabrication*. It means both to build and to lie' (2013: 125). With this in mind, claiming authenticity is a dangerous exercise. Śītalā's forms and personality had been informed across the centuries by a variety of myths and rituals, and by diverse worldviews. This is a natural process that works in both ways. The problem is when authoritative representations, especially in the current globalized epoch, ignore real people and their beliefs. Such is the case when Śītalā is ontologically explained as '[…] the disease and the absence of the disease, or the illness and its cure' (Marglin 2001: 123; cf. Harlan 1998: 238). Śītalā is neither disease, nor its absence. This is what the authors of ŚMKs have suggested, and many after them have reported as matter-of-factly. According to her devotees, Śītalā is Mā (but cf. Kolenda 1982: 240, who believes this title is 'ironic'). She is a mother goddess who – because of her cold nature (*śītala*) – has the power to vanquish heat (i.e. disease, disorder, injustice, etc.). The bottom line is: why should Hindu deities be called gods or goddesses *of* something? This logic, I believe, has perpetuated the otherization of Hinduism and, in the case of Śītalā, points to the enduring fixation and fascination with the 'smallpox myth'.

This book has argued otherwise. The culture revolving around Śītalā has been discussed from five different points of view, each informing the other. In Chapter 1, I have investigated textual sources ranging from *purāṇa*s, āyurvedic compendia, *tantra*s, law digests (*dharmanibandha*), stories of fasting (*vratakathā*), folk songs in Hindi and Bhojpuri, and the Bengali *Śītalāmaṅgalkāvya*s. This has permitted one to appreciate that, contrary to general opinion, there exists in Indian texts an overall uniformity in describing and worshipping Śītalā as a protector. The only exception is a bulk of narratives composed in West Bengal, the *Śītalāmaṅgalkāvyas*. Here the goddess is primarily a threatening, capricious and intimidating presence. One must worship her, or else be killed by poxes, plagues and other diseases.

In Chapter 2, I have examined the iconography of Śītalā. I discussed representations of the goddess by means of various *mūrtis*: aniconic, zoomorphic, phytomorphic, cephalomorphic and anthropomorphic. None is distinctive of Śītalā. Besides an analysis of the goddess's attributes (pitcher, broom and winnower), I have specifically investigated her mount, the ass. The *vāhana* has been neglected in previous studies. It has been simplistically argued that Śītalā rides an ass because it is a strong beast of burden. The animal is needed to carry the heavy load of poisoned pulses that (the *maṅgal-*) Śītalā uses to spread contagion. Others have pointed to the fact that the ass (in fact, a jenny) provides the milk to treat skin diseases. This is difficult for two reasons. First, there is no evidence the equid is a jenny. Second, the theory of 'jenny milk' as a remedy against smallpox is unconfirmed. I have thus suggested that the ass in Indian culture is an element of excess. The scary brayer of desert regions is traditionally associated with disease, drought and infertility. It is significant, I argue, that it is ridden – i.e. controlled – by a cold goddess known for her power to counter imbalances, including disease, infertility, droughts and famines. This confirms the power of Śītalā in restraining, or balancing, disorder.

The next three chapters examine changes in internal and external perceptions of Śītalā and her worship. In response to phenomena of upward mobility, gentrification and globalization, I have showed how consolidated ritual and devotional practices (possession, animal sacrifice and austerities) are currently challenged in contemporary India. This is particularly evident in ethical debates, as well as in the Indian and international press. It thus appears that a class-bound bias is impacting on public representations of the goddess. The trend, I argued in Chapter 4, is not novel. With the success of the *maṅgalkāvya* genre in premodern Bengal, a new chapter has emerged: the *Śītalāmaṅgalkāvyas*. These stories are not, as many have argued, folk poetry. They are fictional (and fashionable) narratives constructed by Brahman professional poets on the basis of their understanding (or that of their patrons/target audiences) of the culture of Bengali peasantry. ŚMKs are works specifically designed to entertain. Theatrical adaptations of their *pālās* have contributed to their diffusion and success by exalting dramatic, and gory, features. I have concluded that ŚMKs are *ante litteram* Orientalism. Their message has been uncritically received by powerful elites who passed it on to the British – by then scrutinizing indigenous medical knowledge – the myth of the 'goddess of smallpox'. This has been conveniently manipulated to counter the struggle against variolators and to implement mass vaccination. Little has changed with the advent of the WHO SEP. By the end of the 1970s, Śītalā was known globally as the Indian smallpox goddess. Her fame, as I discussed in the final chapter, lives on in contemporary academia, and in the texts they inform. Besides raising the issue of scholarly responsibility in representing other cultures, I showed that Śītalā continues to be worshipped as a protector and a caring mother. This is evident in contemporary Indian pop culture, e.g. cinema and music. A separate, yet significant, trend however emerges. Śītalā is slowly merging into the great mother goddess. She is no longer exclusively worshipped for protection from diseases, and her distinctive attributes are fading away. She is God, and her devotees proudly, and unproblematically, present her as an aspect of the benevolent, protective and vegetarian Durgā.

It is my hope this book will contribute to the debate on fair and ethical representations of other people's cultures. As the history of the study of Hinduism shows, there are various levels of scholarship. A plethora of interpretative essays – often built on a combination of personal fixations, politics, academic conventions and fashion – has contributed to create an alternative mythology, one that is meaningless, and sometimes offensive, to real people out there. With this in mind, I will conclude with the words of a beautiful song I heard one early morning in November 2011 in the Śītalā Mandir at Dāsāśvamedha Ghāṭ, Banaras:

Listen to this old lady, Mā
Listen to this old lady, Mā
I look at my sister-in-law, Mā
Please, give her children.
I look at the poor people, Mā
Please, give them money.
I look at that girl, Mā
Please, give her *darśan*
I look at your door, Mā
Please, keep it open
I look at myself, Mā
Please, cut my pain.
Listen to this old lady, Mā
Listen to this old lady, Mā.[1]

Notes

1 The song was sung for me by a middle-aged woman known as Mahārajī, one of my chief informants in the Banaras temple, and leader of the devotees at Causaṭṭī Yoginī Devī Mātā Mandir (cf. Ferrari 2013: 153–6). The performance was not part of a ritual. It was recited as a sample of a large repertoire in *Bānarsī bolī*.

Appendix A

Śrīśītalāsaptamīvratakathā (ŚVK 9–14)[1]

Invocation: auṃ guruve namaḥ; auṃ gaṇeśāya namaḥ; auṃ śrī śītalāyai namaḥ

Lord Sadāśiva said: 'O Sanatkumār! I will now tell you the story of *Śītalāsaptamīvrata*. A person should fast on the seventh day of the bright half of the month of Śrāvaṇa. First, draft a deep tank with steps (*bāvlī*) on a wall and in it, draw the seven divine, lightly-clothed incorporeal (*aśarīrī*) water gods (*jaladevatā*). Also draw a triad made of two boys, a woman and a man; a horse, an ox, a palanquin along with a cart. Then take the vow of worship and wear a thread with seven knots on the wrist after having worshipped it. For seven years fast on the seventh day of the bright half of every month. Worship the goddess Śītalā and the water gods in sixteen ways, and offer them cucumber (*kakaṛī*; *Cucumis utilissimus*) and a mix of yogurt and rice as food offering (*naivedya*). The *naivedya* should be then given to Brahmans. This fast should be observed for seven years, each year feeding seven women who must not be widows. Then one should put an end to it. Place the images (*pratimā*) of goddess Śītalā and the seven water gods on a golden plate and let your son worship them reverentially on the first day. On the second day, early in the morning, offer oblations to the fire to appease the planets (*grahahoma*) and make offerings of *khīr* (rice, milk and sugar).' Lord Sadāśiva said: 'O Sanatkumār! Now I will tell you about those who have first performed this fast, and the rewards that they got. Listen carefully: There was a town named Śobhan in the Saurāṣṭra region.[2] Therein lived a pious (*dharmik*) rich man. He financed the digging of a *bāvlī* in a forest without water. He spent a lot of money in getting firm and solid stairs [decorated with] precious stones to enable animals' access and also to provide drinking water to thirsty travellers. Alongside the *bāvlī*, he also arranged for a big garden for the benefit of exhausted travellers. But not a single drop of water was found in that *bāvlī*. The rich man was sad. He said: 'My money and my hard work have turned fruitless.' Afflicted with such thoughts, he fell asleep near the *bāvlī* that night. In the night, the water gods came to him in his dream and said: 'O rich man! Hear from us how to get water from the ground. If you respectfully sacrifice (*bali*) your grandson to us, the *bāvlī* will be filled with water right away.' After this vision, the rich man went home and told his committed-to-*dharma* son, Draviḍa, the whole dream. Having heard the story, his son said: 'Father! You are the person who gave birth to both me and my son. Besides, this is an act of *dharma*. What is there to think about? In fact, *dharma* is a permanent thing (*sthāyī*), and I have two sons, Śītāṃśu and Caṇḍāṃśu. Let's sacrifice my elder son Śītaṃśu without giving it a second thought. But Father! Keep this a secret from the women because my wife is pregnant and the time of delivery is near. She is about to go to her parents' place. My younger son will accompany her. After their departure, this task can be performed without any obstacle.' The rich man listened to his son's words and said: 'O Son! You are truly blessed, and since you're my son I too, am blessed. I consider myself the father of a son.' Meanwhile, [Draviḍa's] wife, Suśīlā, had received an invitation from her parents, and began to make preparations to visit them. Just then, Draviḍa said to his wife: 'The elder son will stay here with me and the younger one will go with you.' Obeying her husband's command, Suśīlā left her elder son with her husband and set off for her parents' place with her younger son. After she left, the father and son together gave Draviḍa's son a thorough bath. They massaged his body with oil, and dressed him up with expensive clothes and ornaments. When the day of *pūrvāṣāṛhā nakṣatra* (an auspicious asterism) presided by Varuṇa (Lord of the waters) arrived, they took him to the *bāvlī* and made him stand on its bank. They recited: 'May the water-gods be pleased with the sacrifice of this boy.' They had hardly sacrificed him when the *bāvlī* filled with nectar-like pure water. Both father and son were so happy to see the water, but returned home saddened at having sacrificed their son. Meanwhile, at her parents', Suśīlā gave birth to her third son. When the boy was three months old, she returned to her in-laws'. Along the road, she was amazed at seeing the *bāvlī* full of water. She happily bathed in it and said: 'My father-in-law's hard work and money paid off.' That day was the seventh day of the bright half of the month of Śrāvaṇa. After bathing, Suśīlā performed the auspicious fast for the goddess Śītalā. She had yogurt and rice delivered to the goddess right there, and prepared a delicious dish with them. Then she worshipped the water gods, presented them with rice, yogurt and cucumber as food, and offered it to the Brahmans. She, too, ate a meal consisting of yogurt, rice and cucumber along with those accompanying her. Suśīlā's village was approximately four *krośa* (circa eight miles) from that place. When Suśīlā set off for home from the *bāvlī* with her two sons, the Mother of the World, Śītalā Mātā, appeared before the water gods. The water gods, seeing the goddess Śītalā before them, sang her praises with extreme reverence:

> *vande'haṃ śītalāṃ devīṃ rāsabhasthāṃ digambarām /*
> *mārjanī kalaśopetāṃ śūrpālaṅkṛtamastakām* [3]

Pleased with their eulogy (*stuti*), the goddess blessed them and said: 'O water gods! Suśīlā has performed the fast for me with great diligence and reverence. Return her son to her.' The water gods joined their palms in supplication and said very politely to the goddess: 'O Jagadambā (Mother of the World)! Śītāṃśu has been sacrificed, so he has gone to the abode of Yama (*yamaloka*). It is not in our power to bring him back to life from there. But if you show mercy, Suśīlā's son will have his life back.' Then the goddess summoned Yamarāja. He arrived and worshipped the goddess Śītalā in various ways. Touched by her devotion, he sang her praise:

> *ekaveṇī japākarṇapūrā nagnā kharasthitā lamboṣṭhī karṇikākarṇā*
> *tailābhyaktaśarīriṇī / vāmapādollasallohalatā kaṇṭakabhūṣaṇā*
> *vardhanamūrdhadhvajā kr̥ṣṇā kālarātrībhayaṅkarī //* [*dhyānamantra* of Kālarātrī][4]

The goddess was very pleased at hearing Yamarāja's praises. She said: 'Give Suśīlā's son back to the water gods.' And Yamarāja, as per the Mother's command, handed over Śītāṃśu's life to the water gods. In turn, they brought Suśīlā's dead son out of the water alive and sent him on his way. The boy ran after the palanquin, shouting: 'Mother! Mother!' Hearing her son's voice, Suśīlā turned around and looked back. She was amazed to see him. She made him sit on her lap and blessed her son, but did not ask the boy any question. She thought: 'If I ask, he will be scared.' She began thinking: 'What if some thief had taken the precious ornaments he was wearing? If *piśācas* have abducted him from home, how could they possibly have let him go? What family members must have gone through upon being separated from him?' She arrived home with these thoughts. As soon as the father and son learnt she was arrived home, they thought: 'What will Suśīlā say to us now, and how will we answer her?' In the meantime, Suśīlā entered the house with her three sons. Her father-in-law and husband were astonished, but also pleased, at the sight of Śītaṃśu. They asked Suśīlā: 'O *subhadrā* (gentle lady)! Which *puṇya* (act of merit) or fast did you observed? O *bhāminī* (woman)! You must have earned merit (*puṇyavratā*). This boy Śītāṃśu has been dead for two months now. How did you get him back? And the *bāvlī* was filled with water. At the time of leaving you took one son from here. At your return, you brought back all three of them together. O *śubhrā* (pure one)! You have brought salvation to our family (*vaṃśa*). O *śubhānanā* (auspicious one)! How should I sing your praises?' Her father-in-law looked at her in admiration, and her husband with love. Her mother-in-law also sang her praises. Pleased at this, she said: 'All this is the fruit of sticking to the virtuous path (*sumārga*), and the grace and blessing of the water gods and Jagadambikā Bhagavatī Śītalā.' Suśīlā, along with her husband, sons and all of the family members, sang the praises of goddess Śītalā:

> *śītale tī purā khyātā yuge dvāparsaṅgīte /*
> *kalau punaḥ samākhyātā kaliduḥkhāntakāriṇīm //*[5]

All of them had a blissful life in this world by savouring the pleasure of all the things that they desired. Young one (*tāt*)! I told you about the *Śītalāsaptamīvrata*. The prescribed things are: yogurt, rice, cool cucumber, water from a *bāvlī*, and [the worship of] the water gods and of goddess Śītalā. Those who observe [this *vrata*] will be freed from the three heats (*tāptraya*, i.e. physical, spiritual and environmental afflictions). For this reason, the real name of the seventh day of the bright half of the month of Śrāvaṇa has become *Śītalāsaptamī*.

Appendix B

Śrīśītalāsaptamīvrata of *Skandapurāṇa* (VR 310–311)[6]

Now we tell you about the *Śītalāsaptamī* fast. This fast should be undertaken on the seventh day of the dark half of the month of Srāvaṇa – counting the beginning of the month from the bright half – when the seventh day happens to extend until afternoon. We get proof of this from the *Hārītasmṛtikā* in *Kālamādhava.*[7] [There it says that] it is acceptable for fasts that are predominantly worship-oriented to last until the afternoon. Now we tell you about the method of fasting: in the *Skandapurāṇa* it is written that first of all the worshipper should go in front of goddess Śītalā and pray to her with the hands in *añjali* pose:[8] 'I bow to the goddess Śītalā who is naked, rides an ass, holds a broom and a pitcher of water on her hands and is crowned with a winnowing basket.' Then install the image of the goddess described above on the pitcher (*kalaśa*) and have a bath while chanting her *nāmamantra*: '*Auṃ Śītalāyai namaḥ.*' Offer *naivedya* in the form of five kinds of cooked cereals, yogurt mixed with ghee and rice with the words: 'I humbly offer this *naivedya* to you. O Goddess! O Beautiful One! Consume this *naivedya*.' After offering the food in this way, present *dakṣiṇā* (ritual fee). Upon completing *pūjā*, pray: 'O Śītalā! Destroy my sins (*pāpa*). Grant me the pleasure of having sons and grandsons, the wealth of food and money. O Goddess! Accept my *pūjā*. I bow to you.' Then offer water (*arghyadāna*) and read aloud the verse 'Śītalā'. It means: 'O, you with a cool form (*śītalā ākāravālī*)! O you who grants the state of married woman (*saubhāgya*) and sons to women! O Śītalā! Accept this *arghya* on the seventh day of the dark half of Śrāvaṇa. I bow to you.' Worship lovingly seven young girls of the age of seven and feed them well. At the beginning of this fast, take the *saṅkalpa* (vow) and read aloud the words: '*Auṃ tat sat, Auṃ tat sat, Auṃ tat sat adyaitasya brahmaṇo* etc.' after mentioning the time of worship (i.e. the lunar month, bright or dark half of the month, time of the day), one's country, name and family (*gotra*), etc. This *saṅkalpa* is suitable for women only; its purport (*bhāva*) is: 'May I, of the so-and-so name and so-and-so *gotra*, get *saubhāgya* in this lifetime and in future lifetimes. May I get the pleasure of prolonged union (*akhaṇḍitasaṃyoga*) with my husband. May I get sons and grandsons and wealth of food and money. For this purpose, I shall undertake the *Śītalāsaptamīvrata* and worship Śītalā with all these ingredients that are assembled here.' The worshipper will spread a cloth (*vastra*) over a stool (*caukī*) and draw the shape of an eight-petal lotus using rice; she will place a clay pitcher that should not have any hole in the middle of this drawing; on top of this pitcher she will place a golden *mūrti* of Śītalā. Then she will meditate upon the form of the goddess and salute her with the aforementioned mantra *'Vandehaṃ Śītalāṃ'*. She will invoke the goddess with the *nāmamantra*: *'Oṃ Śītalāyai namaḥ avāhayāmi.'*[9] She will offer a seat (*āsana*) with the *nāmamantra*: *'Oṃ Śītalāyai namaḥ āsanasamarpayāmi, ihāgatya atrātiṣṭha.'*[10] Mentally repeating these words, the worshipper will give *pādya* (water to wash the feet), *arghya* (water to wash hands), *ācamana* (water for mouth rinsing), *snāna* (bath), *vastra* (clothes), *upavastra* (accessory clothing), *candana* (sandalwood paste), *alaṅkāra* (ornaments), *puṣpa* (flowers), *dhūpa* (incense) and *dīpaka* (ghee lamp). After offering the food with the mantra – *Śītalāy pañca …* – she will present in both palms of the hands fruits, betel leaves, *dakṣiṇā*, *ārti* and *puṣpāñjali*.[11] She should then complete circumambulation (*pradakṣiṇā*) repeating the *nāmamantra* of the goddess, humbly salute with the aforementioned mantra *'vandehaṃ Śītalāṃ'*, pray with the mantra *'Śītalāy daha pāpaṃ …'* and offer special *arghya* with the aforementioned mantra *'Śītalāe Śītalākāre.'* To obtain the reward of the fast, she will give food offerings (*vāyana*) to the Brahman. The mantra for that is *'dadhyannaṃ ….'* Its meaning is: 'For the sake of Śītalā's pleasure I hereby give you a *vāyana* consisting of yogurt, rice, fruit and the *dakṣiṇā*.'[12]

Appendix C

Śītalāsaptamīvratakathā of *Bhaviṣyapurāṇa* (VR 310–313)[13]

Lord Kṛṣṇacandra said: 'O King of Kings! Listen to this story. There is a famous city named Hastināpura. There was a king called Indradyumna, who was the protector of the three worlds. He had a faithful and popular wife named Dharmaśīlā. [1] She regularly observed many rituals (*anuṣṭhāna*) that yielded merit (*puṇya*), and was generous and sweet-talking. [2] First, she gave birth to a son. She named him Mahādharma. His father was very attached to [the child], who was always happy. Then, [Dharmaśīlā] gave birth to a daughter, [whom she] called Śubhakārī. This girl was also blessed with excellent qualities and auspicious signs. [3–4] The father made her happy too with his love. This girl was the best among girls for her physical beauty and other qualities. [5] She was blessed with all the auspicious signs mentioned in the *Sāmudrikaśāstra*;[14] she had a lotus sign in her palm and she was sweet talking. [6] In the city of Kauṇḍinya, there was a king by the name Sumitra. His son Gunavāṇ became Śubhakārī's husband. He was beautiful of body and excellent in qualities, good-looking and wealthy. [7] The *dharma*-abiding Gunavāṇ married Princess [Śubhakārī] in the proper ritual manner. After receiving a great dowry from his in-laws, he left for his father's capital city. [8] The princess, after staying there for some days, went back to her father's. Sometime later, the prince came to Hastināpura with his relatives from Kauṇḍinya for the *gaunā*.[15] [9] As soon as she saw him, the auspicious Śubhakārī's eyes became full with the joy of love. Then, eager to go to Kauṇḍinya with her husband, she began to laugh lightly with happiness. She went to her father, bowed to his feet and said: [10] 'O Father! I have come to know what Vidhātā (the creator and ordainer, i.e. Lord Brahmā) said about there being no *dharma* in all the three worlds equal to faithfulness toward one's husband (*pātivratya*). [11] To observe this, I will go to Kauṇḍinyapura. Please give me your permission with a blessing, so that I may go with my lord to my (new) home on a chariot. [12] King Indradyumna said to his daughter: 'O daughter! Stay one more day so that you may observe the

Śītalāvrata. [13] This fast enhances women's health and good luck. By observing it properly, one gets rid of the fear of widowhood (*vaidhavya*). This is my and your mother's advice.' [14] Having said so, he made her stay, had the *pūjā* tools prepared and told her that the place to worship Śītalā was on bank of a pond in the forest. Then the king gave [his daughter] the *pūjā* items and let [her] go to this pond to worship Śītalā. [15] He sent with her a Brahman knowledgeable in the Vedas, together with his wife. Śubhakārī ran ahead into the forest, overwhelmed with joy, [16] but did not find Śītalā's place. Eventually she became tired from wandering endlessly, although she continued to roam around looking for the pond [and] meditating on Śītalājī. [17] Then she saw a beautiful old lady. [Meanwhile] the Brahman who had been sent to perform the *pūjā* could not find the pond or the princess. He got tired of wandering aimlessly here and there, so he fell asleep. [18] His wife sat down next to him. An evil snake bit him and he died immediately. Near there, the old lady, moved to pity, said to Princess Śubhakārī: [19] 'O Princess! Your husband will live long; come with me for *pūjā*; I will show you that pond.' [20] Śubhakārī went to the pond with her; there she worshipped Śītalājī in the proper way [and] in a happy state of mind, so that Śītalājī was pleased (*santuṣṭha*). [21] Being content, the goddess Śītalā granted her a boon (*vara*). Upon receiving the boon, she got ready to go home. After walking some distance into the forest, she saw the Brahman who had died from snakebite. [22] His wife was weeping loudly, sitting next to his body. Seeing the condition of that young Brahman and his wife, Princess Śubhakārī, who had just received the gift of *saubhāgya* (marital felicity) due to goddess Śītalā being satisfied, began to feel grief and wept piteously. [23–4] The Brahman's *pativratā* wife consoled the princess and said: 'Please stay here until I enter the funeral pyre (Hutāśana, Skt. the 'destroyer', a title of Agni) with my husband. Don't go, stay. [25] By entering the funeral pyre with their husband women get heavenly pleasure.' Upon hearing the words of the Brahman's wife, Śubhakārī was moved even more to pity. [26] She began to concentrate on goddess Śītalā, who destroys the great suffering of widowhood. Goddess Śītalā, laughing lightly with happiness, came there to grant the boon [27] and said: 'O daughter! O dear daughter! Ask me for a boon. O Cāruhāsinī ('she of the lovely laughter')! What misery do you want to be vanquished, for which you have remembered me? If you are grieving from the suffering of this Brahman woman, give her the religious merit that you have earned from fasting for Śītalā. [28] Because of that merit, the snake venom will go away, and [her husband] will instantly come back to life and become conscious once again.' Lord Kṛṣṇa is saying to Yudhiṣṭhira that, having heard Śītalā's words, the princess compassionately gave away the merit of the *Śītalāvrata* that she had received. [29] Upon obtaining *puṇya*, the Brahman instantly became conscious, just as someone who has been sleeping for a long time wakes up. Seeing the effect of the merit, the loving desire to observe the *Śītalāvrata* also arose in the heart of the Brahman's wife. [30] Therefore, she too devotedly worshipped Śītalājī. Meanwhile, Princess Śubhakārī's husband Gunavāṇ was also coming there, out of his love for the princess, [but] on the road, [31] a snake bit him too. The *pativratā* princess was going home with Śītalā in the guise of an old woman and with the Brahmin's wife. When she saw her husband lying just as the Brahmin was earlier, she began to wail along with the Brahmin's wife. [32] Śītalā came there and said: 'O daughter! O Varabarṇini ('fine complexioned one')! O Sundari ('beauty')! Think back to what I said earlier. Any woman who observes the fast for Śītalā, never suffers widowhood. [33] So don't cry. Stand up and, by holding his hand, make him stand up too, just as one wakes up a sleeping man at home, standing by his bedside. And, O shy one, keep observing the fast for me, because it has the power to destroy the pain of widowhood.' [34] When the goddess Śītalā spoke so, Śubhakārī stood up and woke up her husband. He instantly rose. Her husband, Gunavāṇ, was happy upon seeing his beloved one, and his beloved was pleased too to see her husband alive. [35] People living there were amazed upon witnessing this miracle. The Brahman's wife was extremely happy [36] because her husband's life had been saved for she was a *pativratā*. She bowed to the old lady and said: 'O Mother! Grant me the boon that I never become a widow or be separated from my husband. [37] I also ask you the boon that whichever woman undertakes fast for Śītalā (i.e. for you) should also never become a widow, poor or separated from her husband.' [38] Just as that Brahman woman prayed, the old lady said: 'So be it.' Then she disappeared, because she was goddess Śītalā, who can take any form at will, like [that of] an old woman or any other woman. Upon receiving the boon from goddess Śītalā, the princess went to her father's along with her husband and the Brahman couple. [39] With the *prasād* of goddess Śītalā, she was blessed with a luxurious life full of wealth just like Pārvatī had gained all the pleasures of the world by worshipping goddess Śītalā, who is praised across the universe. [40] Thus ends the *Śītalāvrata* of *Bhaviṣyapurāṇa*.[16]

Appendix D

Śītalāpūjāpaddhati of *Picchilātantra*[17]

Auṃ. Obeisance to Gaṇeśa. Have a bath early in the morning. Make your daily mandatory rituals. Wear clean clothes. Install a well-built image of the deity on a wooden seat near a *snuhi* tree.[18] After sipping water, make the Brahmans recite: fortune (*svasti*), prosperity (*ṛddhi*) and auspiciousness (*puṇya*). Chant the above stated benedictory notes addressing your own *śākha* (branch of Brahmans). Recite mantras in honour of Sūrya, Soma, Yāma, Kāla, etc. Collect fruits, flowers, *tila* (black sesame seed) [and] *kuśa* grass. [Put] its blades on a copper vessel containing water and take the oath (*saṅkalpa*).[19] After invoking Viṣṇu [and uttering the mantra] '*auṃ tat sat*', [say] the name of the month, [the name of] the bright or dark fortnight (*pakṣa*), [the name of] the lunar day (*tithi*), [the name of your] family (*gotra*), [the name of] the one protected by the gods (i.e. the devotee's own name) and pray for the grace and love of Śrī Śītalā to calm down (*upaśamana*) pox (*visphoṭaka*) and various other diseases. Then after worshipping Gaṇeśa and various other deities, worship Ghaṇṭākarṇa along with Śrī Śītalā Devī as much as it is possible with animal sacrifice (*balidāna*). After taking the ritual oath, water should be dropped toward the north-eastern direction (*aiśana*) [Śiva's direction]. Give fruits and flowers to the Brahmans. In case of other *gotra*s, i.e. the *gotra* of a particular person, repeat the same.

The *sūkta* (hymn) of one's own lineage should be recited during the *cakṣurdāna*.[20] Take collyrium made of ghee on a leaf of *bel* (wood apple) and with the stalk of a *bel* leaf, [chant the *cakṣurdānamantra*]: 'Auṃ. May these three divine eyes shine with the effulgence of moon, sun and fire. May the goddess envision the three worlds.' Reading this aloud, chant the *mūlamantra* and invest sight with collyrium. Then, [uttering] the mantra of one's *śākha*, install the pitcher (*ghaṭa*) and cleanse the seat (*āsana*) with a small quantity of water. Then [say]: *gaṃ hṛdayay namaḥ* ...[21] Having done *karanyāsa* and *aṅganyāsa*,[22] pay homage to the guru tradition (*gurupaṅkti*). [By chanting the hymn beginning with] *kharvam* etc.,[23] invoke and meditate on Gaṇapati [saying]: *auṃ gaṇeśaya namaḥ*. [Then] worship with *pādya* (water for washing the feet) and other ingredients, [and] offer obeisance (*praṇām*) with the *ekadantam-[mantra]*,[24] etc. This should be followed by the offer of *pādya* to Śiva, the *pañcadevatā* (Gaṇeśa, Viṣṇu, Sūrya, Mahādeva, Durgā), the *navagrahas*, Indra, the *dikpālas* (holder of directions), the ten *avatāras*, Brahmā-Viṣṇu-Maheśvara, Gaṅgā, Yamunā, Lakṣmī and Sarasvatī.

Then follows the purification of the mortal body (*bhūtaśuddhi*), breath control (*prāṇāyāma*), placement of the letters (*mātṛkānyāsa*), of the syllables (*varṇanyāsa*) and seats [of the goddess] (*pīṭhanyāsa*) on the body. Pronounce the mantra: *śāṃ hṛdayāya namaḥ* [pointing to the heart] *śrīṃ śirase svāhā* [pointing to the head] *śūṃ śikhāyai vaṣaṭ* [pointing to the topknot] *śeṃ kavacāya huṃ* [embracing one's body] *śauṃ netratrayāya vauṣaṭ* [pointing at the three eyes] *śaḥ astrāya phaṭ* [slapping the palm of the hand] *tataḥ śāṃ aṅguṣṭhābhyāṃ namaḥ* [snapping fingers] *śrīṃ tarjjanībhyāṃ svāhā śūṃ madhyamābhyāṃ vaṣaṭ śaiṃ anāmikābhyāṃ huṃ śauṃ kaniṣṭhābhyāṃ vauṣaṭ śaḥ karatala pṛṣṭhābhyāṃ astrāya phaṭ* [slapping the palm of the left hand]. While doing *karanyāsa* and *aṅganyāsa*, meditate holding flowers in the fingers with the hands in *kūrmamudrā*.[25]

[*Dhyānamantra*:] 'Auṃ. White complexioned, sitting on an ass, holding a broom and a pitcher full [of water] in the palms of [her] two hands. With the broom [she] sprinkles the water of immortality (*amṛta*) from [her] pitcher and cools the heat. Naked, with a winnower on [her] head, the body adorned with gold and gems, and three eyes. I worship that Śītalā who heals poxes and intense heat.'

Meditating on this, place flowers on the worshipper's head, present offering mentally, offer water (*arghya*) and worship the seat (*piṭha*) [of the goddess]. Then, once again, perform *karanyāsa* and *aṅganyāsa*, meditate and offer flowers on the pitcher and say: 'Auṃ Śītalā Devī be gracious and come right here, stay right here and, once installed, please accept my worship.' Then make *mudrās* (gestures) like *āvāhānī-*, *sthāpanī-*, *yoni-mudrā* and install life (*prāṇapratiṣṭhā*) with *lelihānāmudrā* (sticking out the little finger). Then say: '*auṃ hrīṃ kroṃ yaṃ raṃ laṃ vaṃ śaṃ ṣaṃ saṃ hauṃ haṃ saḥ*. May the breath (*prāṇa*) of Śrī Śītalādevī be installed here, [may] life (*jīva*) be invested here, [may] all the sense organs and speech, eyes, ears, nose and *prāṇa* stay here happily forever. Svāhā. May the butter's rapid flow delight the spirit! May Bṛhaspati extend this act of worship and restore the sacrifice uninjured. Here let all gods rejoice. Auṃ. Step you forward.'[26] Investing life by chanting mantras such as this, [say]: '*Auṃ hrīṃ śrīṃ śītalāyai namaḥ*.' With this mantra, worship the goddess resolutely using ten or sixteen offerings (*upacāra*) [and say]: '*Auṃ namāmi śītalāṃ devīṃ rāsabhasthāṃ digambarīṃ mārjanīkalasopetāṃ sūrpālaṅkṛtamastakāṃ*.'[27]

Worshipping the *snuhi* plant, say [the mantra]: '*Auṃ ghaṇṭākarṇāya namaḥ*' and offer *pādya* and other ingredients. [Say]: 'Auṃ. O Ghantakarna [Gheṇṭu] Mahāvira, destroyer of all ailments, protect me from *visphoṭaka* and the fear of diseases, protect me, o mighty one!'

Now the worship of Jvarāsura. 'Auṃ He has a lean body, a blue and yellow coloured tongue and eyes darkened with black collyrium (*añjana*). I meditate on the god who roars as the waters would roar during *pralāya* ('dissolution'; the end of the world), dangerous as all dangers, having three legs, six hands, nine eyes, holding weapons that burn everything into ashes. This is his *dhyāna [mantra]*: *'auṃ jvarāsurayaḥ namaḥ.'* Worship [him] with *pādya* and various tools [and say]: *'auṃ* obeisance to Jvarāsura, the minister (*mantri*) of Śītalā. Obeisance to you, Jvarāsura, the controller of the *mahābhairava* gods.'[28] Then respectfully prostrate.

Now meditate on Raktāvati. 'Auṃ. Raktāvati, the one who is dear to Śītalā, is of the colour of blood and has two hands. She wears blue clothes, blood-coloured jewellery. She holds water in the cup of her left hand and a betel leaf in the right one. She smiles and is in the dancing posture. She is the destroyer of boils. I so meditate on Mahādevī who would shower grace on her devotees.' Worship should be offered with the chanting of mantra *'auṃ raktāvatya namaḥ'* along with five ingredients and the obeisance. 'Auṃ. Obeisance to Raktāpriyā, who destroys infants (*śiśusaṃhārakāriṇi*). Homage to you, Raktāvati Devī who holds a conch-shell in her hand in the pose of blowing it.' Then respectfully prostrate.

Now the worship of the ass [with the mantra]: *'auṃ gardabhāya namaḥ.'* Offer the five ingredients (*pañcopacāra*)[29] [and say]: 'Auṃ obeisance to the ass that always carries Śītalā. Salutations to the ass that always stays with the goddess.'

Collect some water for the offering of *arghya* and then chant with strength the *mūlamantra*: 'O Goddess, you keeper of the innermost intimate secrets, please accept my chanting as an offering. Give me perfection, o graceful one.'[30] Signing the *jāpa* in this way, perform *prāṇāyāma*, chant the hymns (*stava*) and offer as much as possible animal sacrifices (*balidāna*) and the fire oblation (*homayajña*). Then *dakṣiṇā* should be offered.

I present as *dakṣiṇā* money of this amount honouring the so-and-so Brahman by grace of God of the so-and-so lineage (*gotra*) for the service of worshipping Śītalā Devī who heals of various illnesses such as *visphoṭaka*, etc. The priest (*pūjaka*) will accept it saying '*svastī*'.

Auṃ. May this ritual called *Śītalādevīpūjā* be free from all lapses. Whatever faults have occurred, remember the name of Viṣṇu for peace, and offer all the ingredients for worship to the *ācārya* (instructor, teacher). This is the method of worshipping Śītalā as described in the *Picchilātantra*.[31]

Notes

1 This section is translated from Hindi. The text is taken from a booklet (Hindi and Sanskrit) called *Śrī Śītalā Vrata Kathā* (ŚVK). This is divided in the following sections: (1) *Bhūmikā*; (2) *Śrī Dakṣiṇī Ādi Śītalā (Buṛhiyā Māī) kā māhātmya* (pp. 79–80); (3) *Guphā kā prācīn itihās* (pp. 75–80); (4) *Saṅkalp*; (5) *Śrī Śītalā saptamī vrata kathā*; (6) *Śrī Śītalā saptamī vrata kathā sāmagrī*; (7) *Mā ke chaṭh pūjan kā vidhān* (pp. 13–14); (8) *Gīt*; (9) *Śrī Ādi Śītalā stotram* (18–9); (10) *Śrī Ādi Śītalā mātā kī vijay stuti* (p. 18); (11) *Śrī*; (12) *Bhagavatī kī stuti*; (13) *Bhagavatī Durgā ke nau nām*; (14) *Durgākavacam – Nārāyaṇ uvāc*; (15) *Daśāśvamedh (Rudratīrth) māhātmya* [from KKh 42] (pp. 32–3); and (16) *Śrī Śītalā mātāmāī kī ārtī* (pp. 17–8).

2 The name of a peninsula on the Arabian Sea in Western Gujarat.

3 BhPr.Ma. 60: 71 (see above p. 10).

4 ŚVK 4 (see above p. 79).

5 SkP 7.1.135: 1–2 (see above p. 8).

6 Original text in Sanskrit. Here I use the Hindi translation included in VR.

7 A thirteenth-century *dharmanibandha* authored by Mādhavācārya.

8 The cupped hands are placed together and raised on the forehead.

9 'Auṃ obeisance to Śītalā. I invite [you].' (Only the first words of mantras are given in the following text.)

10 'Auṃ obeisance to Śītalā. I offer the seat; come and sit here.'

11 Flowers or petals to be showered on the *mūrti*.

12 Wadley has included in her 1980 article a Gujarati version of the same *kathā* taken from Kr̥ṣṇaprasād Bhaṭṭa's *Vratasaṅgraha* (Ahmedabad: Mahadev Ramshandra Jagushte, 1975) (cf. Wadley 1980: 51–3).

13 Original text in Sanskrit. Here I use the Hindi translation included in VR.

14 The Indian system of physiognomy and body divination. The *Sāmudrikaśāstra* was compiled in the twelfth century by Durlabharāja and his son Jagaddeva. *Samudra* sections are included in a number of *purāṇa*s (Pingree 1981: 76–8).

15 According to this ritual, the groom comes to take his wife from her parents' and bring her to the new home permanently.

16 An alternative version of this tale from Gujarati is translated in Wadley (1980: 51–3). There, too, there is no mention of smallpox.

17 Original text in Sanskrit (Bengali script).

18 *Euphorbia antiquorum* or *E. neriifolia*, the Indian spurge tree.

19 A verbal testimony pronounced before any ritual act (e.g. *pūjā*, *balidāna*, *vrata*, etc.). The *saṅkalpa* formula commits the performer to the perfection of the ritual.

20 Ceremony of anointing the eyes of an image at the time of consecration; lit. 'gift of sight'.

21 The *vijayamantra* of Gaṇeśa.

22 The ritual of pronouncing mantras and imposing them onto the hands (*kara*) and the limbs (*aṅga*).

23 The *stuti* in honour of Gaṇeśa, the remover of obstacles.

24 The mantra to the 'One-toothed', one of the names of Gaṇeśa.

25 A particular position resembling the back of a tortoise.

26 *máno jūtír juṣatām ājyasya bŕ̥haspátir yajñám imáṃ tanotu \ áriṣṭaṃ yajñáṁ sám imáṃ dadhātu víśve devā́sa ihá mādayantām óṃ prá tiṣṭha* \\ (VS *Madhyandina* 2: 13).

27 'I bow to goddess Śītalā, seated on the ass, in nudity, holding the broom and the pot, wearing a winnower on the head.'

28 A different *dhyānamantra* is given in Basu 1405BS: 72. The source is not indicated.

29 A ritual offering of *gandha* (fragrant oils), *puṣpa* (flowers), *dhūpa* (incense), *dīpa* (lamp), *naivedya* (stale vegetarian edibles).

30 *guhyātiguhyagoptrī tvaṃ gr̥hāṇāsmatkr̥taṃ japaṃ siddhirbavatu me devi tvatprasādānmayi sthitā* (*Śrīmahālakṣmīhr̥dayam* 117).

31 The ŚAS now follows (see above p. 10–11). Here too, the *stotra* ends with the line '*iti skandapurāṇe śītalā stotraṃ samāptaṃ*', thus pointing to *Skandapurāṇa* as the original source.

Bibliography

Primary sources

Ācāradinakara of Vardhamāna Sūri (two vols.). Edited by Kamalāsūri. (1922–1923). Bambaī: Śrī Kharataragaccha Granthamāla Samiti.

Āgamatattvavilāsa of Raghunātha Tarkavāgīśa. Edited by Pañcānana Śāstri (1985). Kalikātā: Navabhārata Pābliśārs.

Agnikāryapaddhati. Manuscript no. 781 Research Library Jammu and Kashmir Government, Shrinigar, p. 72b. E-text available from the digital library of the Muktabodha Indological Research Institute, http://muktalib5.org/digital_library.htm (accessed 12/05/2014).

Ananga Ranga (The). Translated by R.F. Burton and F.F. Arbuthnot. (1885). London and Varanasi: Kama Shastra Society

Aṣṭāṅgahṛdayasaṃhitā: Vāgbhaṭa's Aṣṭāṅga Hṛdayam (three vols.). Translated by K.R. Shrikantha Murthy (2011). Varanasi: Chowkhamba Sanskrit Series Office.

Atharvaveda. Inni magici. Edited and translated by C. Orlandi and S. Sani. (1992). Torino: UTET.

Āvantyakhaṇḍa, Revākhaṇḍa. The Skanda Purāṇa, Part XIV, trans. G.V. Tagare. (1999). Delhi: Motilal Banarsidass.

Bandopādhyāy, N. (1923). *Śītalā Sambhāva Kāvya*. Kalikātā: Bradākānta Cakravartī.

Berā, Ś. (2001). *Kavi Nityānander Śītalāmaṅgal. Madhyayuger ek nava-āviṣkṛta pūthi*. Pūrva Medinīpur: Sahajiyā.

Bhāvaprakāśa of Bhāva Miśra (two vols.). Translated by K.R. Shrikantha Murthy. (2008). Varanasi: Chowkhamba Sanskrit Series Office.

Bhaviṣya Purāṇa (1959). Bambaī: Śrīveṅkaṭeśvara Sṭīm Pres.

Caraka Saṃhitā, based on Cakrapāṇi Datta's Āyurveda Dīpikā (six vols.). Edited and translated by R.K. Sharma and B. Dash. (2011). Varanasi: Chowkhamba Sanskrit Series Office.

Caturvarga Cintāmani of Hemādri, vol. 2, *Vrata-khaṇḍa* (1871–1911). Calcutta: Asiatic Society of Bengal.

Devī Purāṇam. First Critical Devanāgarī Edition. Edited by Pushpendra Kumar Sharma. (1976). New Delhi: Kendriya Sanskrit Vidyapeeth.

Devībhāgavatapurāṇa (Śrīmaddevībhāgavatam). Text with English translation by Swami Vijayananda. (2008). Varanasi: Chaukhamba Sanskrit Pratisthan.

Devīnāmavilāsa by Sāhiba Kaula. Edited by Madhusūdana Kaula Śāstri. (1942). Śrīnagar: Kaśmīra Saṃskṛta Granthāvali.

Dīkṣāprakāśaḥ of Maithili Paṇḍit Jīvanāth Śarma. Edited by Rāmatejaśāstrī Pāṇḍeya and Raghunandanaprasāda Śukla. (1934). Banāras: Saṃskṛtapustakālaya Kacauṇīgalī.

Dvyāśrayakāvya of Hemacandra, with a commentary by Abhayatilakagaṇi. Edited by Ābājī Viṣṇu Kāthavaṭe. (1915–1921). Bombay: Government Central Press.

Gerson da Cunha, J. (ed.) (1877). *The Sahyadri-khanda of the Skanda Purana: a Mythological, Historical and Geographical Survey of Western India*. Bombay: Thacker, Vining and Co.

Govindadāsa (1951). *Bhaiṣajya Ratnāvalī, with Vidyotinī Bhāshā-tikā*. Edited by Ambikādatta Śāstrī. Varanasi: Kashi Sanskrit Series.

Griffith, R.T.H. (trans.) (1916). *The Hymns of the Atharvaveda*. 2 vols. Benares: E.J. Lazarus and Co.

Griffiths, A. (2009). *The Paippalādasaṃhitā of the Atharvaveda. Kāṇḍas 6 and 7. A New Edition with Translation and Commentary*. Leiden: Brill.

Harivaṃśa (The): being the khila or supplement to the Mahābhārata. Edited by P.L. Vaidya. (1969–1971). Poona: Bhandarkar Oriental Research Institute.

Hitopadeśa. Translated by A.N.D. Haksar. (2006). New York: Penguin Books.

Kalkipurāṇa, edited by B. Miśra. (1954). Bambaī: Śrīveṅkaṭeśvara Chāpākhānā.

Kāśī Khaṇḍa. The Skanda Purāṇa, Parts X and XI, trans. G.V. Tagare. (1996). Delhi: Motilal Banarsidass.

Kriyākālaguṇottara. Manuscript NGMCP 3/392 reel number B 25/32. Catalogue number: M00278. E-text: Muktabodha Indological Research Institute, 2011 (Text revised December 16, 2013), http://muktalib5.org/digital_library.htm (accessed 12/05/2014).

Kṛṣṇarām Dās (1958). 'Śītalā Maṅgal'. In S. Bhaṭṭhācārya (ed), *Kavi Kṛṣṇarām Dāser Granthāvalī*. Kalikātā: Kalikātā Biśbābidhyālay, pp. 251–285.

Kubjikāmatatantra, The. Edited by T. Goudriaan and J. A. Schoterman. Leiden: E. J. Brill, 1988.

Kulārṇavatantra. Translated by R.K. Rai. (1983). Varanasi: Pracya Prakashan.

Mahābhārata. Critical Edition (nineteen vols.). Edited by V.S. Sukthankar et al. (1927–59). Poona: Bhandarkar Oriental Research Institute.

Mahākālasaṃhitā (Kāmakalākālīkhaṇḍa) with the Jñānavatī Hindi commentary. Commented and edited by Radeshyam Chaturvedi. (2009). Vārāṇasī: Caukhambā Subhāratī Prakāśan.

Maṇḍal, P. (ed.) (1960). *Haridever Racnāvali: Rāymaṅgal o Śītalāmaṅgal*. Śāntiniketan: Viśvabhārati Viśvavidyālāya.

Maṇḍal, P. (1966). *Dvādas Maṅgal*. Sahityā Prakāśika (vol. 5). Śāntiniketan: Viśvabhārati Viśvavidyālāya.

Mānikrām Gāṅguli (1966). 'Śītalā-maṅgal', in P. Maṇḍal (ed), *Dvādās Maṅgal* (five vols.). Śāntiniketan: Viśvabhārati Viśvavidyālāya, pp. 283–294.

Mañjuśrīmūlakalpa (three vols.), edited by M.M.T. Ganapati Shastri. (1989). Delhi: Sri Satguru (reprint, 1925).

Merutantra, edited by Śrī Ragunāthaśāstri. (1908). Mumbayyāṃ: Śrivenkaṭeśvara Pres.

Mūlasarvāstivādavinaya, in Dutta, N. (ed.) (1984), *Gilgit Manuscripts*. Vol. 3. New Delhi: Sri Satguru Publications.

Nārada Purāṇa (five vols.). Translated and annotated by G.V. Tagare. (1980–1982). Delhi: Motilal Banarsidass.

Nidāna. Mādhava Nidānam (Roga Viniścaya) of Mādhavakara. Text with English translation of K.R.S. Murthy. (2011). Varanasi: Chaukhambha Orientalia.

Nityānanda Cakravartī (1879). *Śītalā Jāgaraṇa Pālā*. Kalikātā: Trailokyanāth Datta.

Nityānanda Cakravartī (1339 BS). *Bṛhat Śītalā Mangala vā Śītalār Jāgaraṇa Pālā; Arthāt Śītalār Janma, Indrālaye devatāder Śītalāpūjā, Śītalār bandanā, Nimājagātirpālā, Virāṭapālā, Gokulapūjārpālā evaṃ Aṣṭamaṅgal*. Kalikātā: Tārācād Dās and Sons.

Pañcatantra (The): The Book of India's Folk Wisdom. Translated by P. Olivelle. (2009). Oxford: Oxford University Press.

Prabandhacintāmaṇi of Merutuṅga Ācārya. Translated by C.H. Tawney. (1901). Calcutta: Gilbert and Rivington for the Asiatic Society.

Prabhāsakhaṇḍa. The Skanda Purāṇa, Part XX. Translated by G.V. Tagare. (2003). Delhi: Motilal Banarsidass.
Prāṇatoṣinītantra of Rāmatoṣaṇa Vidyālaṃkāra. Edited by S. Nāth (1991). Kalikātā: Navabhārata Pābliśārs.
Pratiṣṭhālakṣanasārasamuccaya, edited by B. Śarmā (1967). Kāṣṭhamaṇḍapaḥ (Kathmandu): Vīrapustakālaya.
Puraścaryārṇava of Pratāp Siṃha Sāhadev Bahādur, edited by M. Jhā. (1901). Banāras: Prabhakari and Co.
Rāmāyaṇa (The Vālmīki-Rāmāyaṇa). General editor G.H. Bhatt. (1963–1975). Baroda: Oriental Institute.
Rudrayāmalam. Uttara Tantra. Edited by a team of scholars at Yogatantra Department. (1980). Vārāṇasī: Sampūrṇānanda Saṃskṛta Viśvavidyālaya.
Śāktapamodaḥ of Deva Nadan Singh. Edited by M. Khanna (2013). New Delhi: D.K. Printworld.
Śaṅkarabhaṭṭa (1937) [1881]. *Vratārka: Jismeṅ Parevāse Pūrṇamāsī tak Sāl Bhar ke Sab Vrat aur Unkī Pūjāvidhi Udyāpan Kathā Bhakshyā Vastu*. Lakhnaū : Naval Kishaur.
Sarvadevadevīpūjāpaddhati. Compiled by Śyāmācaraṇ Kaviratna, Surendranāth Bhaṭṭācāryya, Rāmdev Bhaṭṭācāryya. (n.d.). Kalikātā: Rājendra Lāībrerī.
Sarvollāsatantra of Sarvavidyāsiddha Sarvānandanātha. Edited by R. Cakravartti, G. Kavirāja, D. Bhaṭṭācāryya (1953). Kalikātā: Śrī Herambacandra Bhaṭṭācāryya.
Śītalacālīsā. Compiled by Śrī Rupeś Ṭhākur Prasād. (n.d.). Vāraṇāsī: Bhārat Pres.
Smṛtitattva of Mahāmahopādhyāya Śrī Raghunandanabhaṭṭācāryya. Edited by Śrī Jīvānanda Vidyāsāgar. (1895). Kalikātā: Nārāyaṇa Yantre Mudritaḥ.
Śrī Śītalā Vrat Kathā. Compiled by Śrī Śiv Prasād Pāṇḍey and Śrī Śrīyantra Pīṭham Samiti (fourth edition). (2012). Vāraṇāsī: Grāphics Lāin.
Śrītattvacintāmaṇi of Pūrṇānanda. Edited by Chintamani Bhattacharya. (1937). Calcutta: Metropolitan Printing and Publishing House.
Śrītattvanidhi of Krishnaraja Wodeyar (1908). Bombay: Shri Venkateshvar Press.
Śūnya Purāṇa of Rāmāi Paṇḍit. Edited by Nagendranāth Basu. (1314 BS). Kālikātā: Baṅgiyā Sāhitya Pariṣad.
Suśruta Saṃhitā, 3 vols. Translated by Kaviraj Kunjalal Bhishagratna and edited by Laxmidhar Dwivedi. (2003). Varanasi: Chowkhamba Sanskrit Series Office.
Tantrasadbhāva. Partially and provisionally edited by M.S.G. Dyczkowski. E-text available from the digital library of the Muktabodha Indological Research Institute, http://muktalib5.org/digital_library.htm (accessed 12/05/2014).
Tantrasāra of Kṛṣṇānanda 'Āgamavāgīśa' Bhaṭṭācārya. Edited by Sādaśiva Śarmā Jośi. (1938). Vāraṇāsī: Caukhambā Saṃskṛta Granthamālā.
Tantra-Sāra-Saṅgraha of Nārāyaṇa (Tāntric) of Śivapuram. Edited with English and Sanskrit introductions by Vaidyaratna Pandit M. Duraiswami Aiyangar. (1950). Madras Government Oriental Series 15. Madras: University of Madras.
Tārābhaktisudhārṇava of Narasiṃha Ṭhākur, edited by P. Bhaṭṭacarya. (1940). Calcutta: Sanskrit Book Depot.
Viṣṇupurāṇa, with the commentary of Śrīdhara (1967). Bombay: Veṅkaṭeśvara Press.
Viśvanātha (2011). *Śrīvratarāja*. Bombay: Shri Venkateshvar Press.
Yāmunāchāryaswāmin (1937). *Āgamaprāmāṇyam*. Edited by Rāmamiśraśāstri. Banāras: Rāmeśvara Pāṭhakena Tārāyantrālaya.
Yoginīsaṃcāratantram with Nibandha of Tathāgatarakṣita and Upadeśānusāriṇīvyākhyā of Alakakaśala. Edited by J.S. Pandey. Rare Buddhist Texts Series no. 21. Sarnath: Central Institute of Higher Tibetan Studies.

Unpublished archival records

Bengal Sanitary Reports, from OIOC (Oriental and India Office Collection, British Library) V/24 series, 383.

Published archival records

Bengal Legislative Department (India) (1902). *The Bengal Vaccination Act, 1880: (Bengal Act V of 1880), as modified up to the 1st June, 1902*. Calcutta: Bengal Secretariat Press.

Bengal Sanitary Commission (1866). *First Annual Report of the Sanitary Commission for Bengal, 1864–65*. London: Presented to Parliament by Her Majesty's Command; Ordered by the House of Commons.

Central Government Act (1876). 'The Dramatic Performances Act, 1876', http://indiankanoon.org/doc/1511172/ (accessed 12/05/2014).

Central Government Act (1880). 'The vaccination act, 1880. Act no. 13 of 1880 1 [9 July, 1880]', http://indiankanoon.org/doc/318197/ (accessed 12/05/2014).

Coady, D. (2008). 'Davida Coady Oral History.' Interview by Chris Zahbhiser, 20008–07–11. *The Global Health Chronicles*, http://globalhealthchronicles.org/items/show/3533 (accessed 12/05/2014).

Emory Global Health Institute. (2012). *The Global Health Chronicles. A Collection of Material on Public Health Efforts to Prevent, Control and Eradicate Global Disease*, http://globalhealthchronicles.com (accessed 12/05/2014).

Jezek, Z., M.N. Das, A. Das, M.L. Aggarwal and Z.S. Arya (1976). 'The Last Known Outbreak of Smallpox in India', *World Health Organization*, Document no. WHO/SE/76.85, from IRIS (Institutional Repository for Information Sharing) http://apps.who.int/iris/ (accessed 12/05/2014).

Shoolbred, J. (1805). *Report on the Progress of Vaccine Inoculation in Bengal from the Period of its Introduction, 1802, to the end of the Year 1803: with an Appendix, submitted to the Medical Board at Fort William*. Calcutta: Honorable's Company Press.

Stewart, D. (1844). Report on small-pox in Calcutta, 1833–34, 1837–38, 1843–44; and vaccination in Bengal, from 1827 to 1844. Calcutta: Huttmann.

Watson, W. (1870). *Returns of Vaccination for the Season 1869–70. North-Western Provinces*. Allahabad: Government Press.

Secondary sources

Agrvāl, R.C. (1958). 'Rājasthān kī pracīn mūrtikalā meṅ gardabhā-vāhanā Śītalā', *Śodha Patrikā (Udaipur)*, 9(4): 1–14.

Ainslie, W. (1813). *Materia Medica of Hindoostan and Artisan's and Agriculturalist's Nomenclature*. Madras: Government of Madras Press.

Ainslie, W. (1829). 'Observations Respecting the Small-Pox and Inoculation in Eastern Countries; With Some Account of the Introduction of Vaccination into India', *Transactions of the Royal Asiatic Society of Great Britain and Ireland*, 2(1): 52–73.

Allocco, A. (2009). 'Snakes, Goddesses, and Anthills: Modern Challenges and Women's Ritual Responses in Contemporary South India.' Unpublished PhD dissertation, Emory University.

Allocco, A. (2013). 'Fear, Reverence and Ambivalence: Divine Snakes in Contemporary South India', in F.M. Ferrari and T. Dähnhardt (eds), *Charming Beauties and Frightful Beasts. Non-Human Animals in South Asian Myth, Ritual and Folklore*. Sheffield: Equinox, pp. 217–235.

Amin, S. (2005). *A Concise Encyclopaedia of North Indian Peasant Life: Being a Compilation from the Writings of William Crooke, J.R. Reid, G.A. Grierson*. Delhi: Manohar.

Anderson, M. (1988). *The Festivals of Nepal*. Calcutta: Rupa & Co.
Anita (2009). 'Children Subjected to Piercing to Appease Sheetla Mata,' *The India Post*, 16 August 2009, http://www.theindiapost.com/nation/chandigarh/children-subjected-to-piercing-to-appease-sheetla-mata/ (accessed 12/05/2014).
Anonymous. (2006). 'Pox in Calcutta.' *Chikitsak-o-Samalochak*, Phalgun (February-March), B.S. 1301 (1894), in P.K. Bose (ed), *Health and Society in Bengal. A Selection from Late 19th-Century Bengali Periodicals*. New Delhi: Sage Publications, pp. 245–346.
Apte, V.S. (1965). *The Practical Sanskrit-English Dictionary*. Revised and Enlarged Edition. Delhi: Motilal Banarsidass.
Arnold, D. (ed) (1988). *Imperial Medicine and Indigenous Societies*. Manchester: Manchester University Press.
Arnold, D. (1993). *Colonizing the Body: State Medicine and Epidemic Disease in Nineteenth-Century India*. Berkeley: University of California Press.
Arnold, D. (2004). *The New Cambridge History of India. Science, Technology and Medicine in Colonial India*. Cambridge: Cambridge University Press.
Arya, U. (1968). *Ritual Songs and Folksongs of the Hindus of Surinam*. Leiden: Brill.
Attewell, G. (2007). *Refiguring Unani Tibb. Plural Healing in Late Colonial India*. New Delhi: Orient Longman.
Babb, L. (1975). *The Divine Hierarchy. Popular Hinduism in Central India*. New York: Columbia University Press.
Babu, D.S. (1990). *Hayagrīva. The Horse-Headed Deity in Indian Culture*. Tirupati: Oriental Research Institute, Sri Venkateswara University.
Bahulkar, S.S. (1994). *Medical Ritual in the Atharvaveda Tradition*. Tilak Maharashtra Vidyapeeth: Pune.
Bakker, H. (1986). *Ayodhyā. Pt. 1. The History of Ayodhyā from the 7th century BC to the middle of the 18th century. Its development into a sacred centre with special reference to the Ayodhyāmāhātmya and the worship of Rāma according to the Agastyasaṃhitā*. Groningen: Forsten.
Bakker, H. and A.W. Entwistle (eds) (1983). *Devī. The Worship of the Goddess and its Contribution to Indian Pilgrimage: a Report on a Seminar and Excursion*. Groningen: Institute of Indian Studies, State University of Groningen.
Bandyopādhyāy, H. (2001). *Baṅgīya Śabdakoṣa*, 2 vols. (fifth edition). Dillī: Sāhitya Akādemi.
Banerjee, S. (1998). *The Parlour and the Streets. Elite and Popular Culture in Nineteenth Century Calcutta*. Calcutta: Seagull Books.
Banerjee, S. (2002). *Logic in a Popular Form: Essays on Popular Religion in Bengal*. Calcutta: Seagull Books.
Bang, B.G. (1973). 'Current Concept of the Smallpox Goddess Sitala in Parts of West Bengal', *Man in India*, 53(1), 79–104.
Banthia, J. and T. Dyson (1999). 'Smallpox in Nineteenth-century India,' *Population and Development Review*, 25(4), 649–680.
Barāṭ, R. (1915). *Śītalā Bhakti*. Pābanā: Bhakti Enḍ Kaṃpanī.
Barrett, R. (2008). *Aghor Medicine. Pollution, Death, and Healing in Northern India*. Berkeley: University of California Press.
Barthes, R. (2009). *Mythologies* (reprint, 1957). London: Vintage Books.
Bass, D. (2012). *Everyday Ethnicity in Sri Lanka: Up-Country Tamil Identity Politics*. New York: Routledge.
Basu, G. (1405 BS). *Bāṁlār Laukik Devatā*. Kalkātā: Dej Pābliśiṅg.
Basu, R.N., Z. Jezek and N.A. Ward (1979). *The Eradication of Smallpox from India*. New Delhi: World Health Organization, South-East Asia Regional Office.

Bauman, M. (2006). 'Performing Vows in Diasporic Contexts: Tamil Hindus, Temples, and Goddesses in Germany,' in W. Harman and S. Raj (eds), *Dealing with Deities. The Ritual Vow in South Asia*. Albany: State University of New York Press, pp. 129–145.

BBC. (2003). 'Donkey Wedding Staged to Bring Rain.' *BBC News*, http://news.bbc.co.uk/1/hi/world/south_asia/2998872.stm (accessed 12/05/2014).

Beary, H. (1999). 'India's Temple to the AIDS goddess,' *BBC News*, 2 December 1999, http://news.bbc.co.uk/1/hi/world/south_asia/545405.stm (accessed 12/05/2014).

Beck, B.E. (1969). 'Color and Heath in South Indian Rituals', *Man, New* Series, 4(4), 553–572.

Behbehani, A.M. (1983). 'The Smallpox Story: Life and Death of an Old Disease', *Microbiological Reviews*, 47(4): 455–509.

Behera, P.R. (2013). 'Cult of Sitala Mata in Indian Folklore', *Journal of Odisha History Congress*, 26: 185–191.

Bhabha, H. (2007). *The Location of Culture*. London and New York: Routledge.

Bhaṭṭācārya, A. (1998). *Bāṁlā Maṅgalkāvyer Itihās* (eighth edition). Kalikātā: A. Mukhārjī.

Bhaṭṭācārya, H. (1997). *Hinduder devadevī*, vol. 3 (reprint, 1980). Kalkātā: Phirmā KLM.

Bhattacharya, F. (2000). 'Rūparām's *Dharma maṅgal*: An Epic of the Low Castes?', *Archiv Orientální* 68(3), 359–386.

Bhattacharya, S. (1998). 'Re-Devising Jennerian Vaccines?: European Technologies, Indian Innovation and the Control of Smallpox in South Asia, 1850–1950', *Social Scientist*, 26(11/12): 27–66.

Bhattacharya, S. (2006). *Expunging Variola. The Control and Eradication of Smallpox in India 1947–1977*. New Delhi: Orient Longman.

Bhattacharyya, A. (1952). 'The Cults of the Goddess of Smallpox in West Bengal', *The Quarterly Journal of the Mythic Society*, 43, 55–69.

Bhattacharyya, A. (1955). 'The Cult of the Village Gods of West Bengal', *Man in India*, 35(1): 19–30.

Bhattacharyya, B. (1989). *An Introduction to Buddhist Esoterism*. Delhi: Motilal Banarsidass.

Bhattacharyya, N.N. (2000). *Indian Demonology: The Inverted Pantheon*. Delhi: Manohar.

Bhattasali, N.K. (1972). *Iconography of Buddhist and Brahmanical Sculptures in the Dacca Museum* (reprint, 1929). Varanasi: Indological Book House.

Biardeau, M. (2004). *Stories about Posts. Vedic Variations around the Hindu Goddess*. Chicago: The University of Chicago Press.

Blumenberg H. (1985). *Work on Myth*. Cambridge, MA: MIT Press.

BMJ (1980). 'Uplift for the Spirit', *British Medical Journal*, 280(6221): 1081–1082

Board of Directors, American Academy of Religion. (2014) 'Updated: Academic Freedom and the Work of Professor Wendy Doniger. A Statement Adopted by the Board of Directors of the American Academy of Religion', March 3, 2014, https://www.aarweb.org/about/updated-academic-freedom-and-the-work-of-professor-wendy-doniger (accessed 12/05/2014).

Boddy, J. (1994). 'Spirit Possession Revisited: Beyond Instrumentality', *Annual Review of Anthropology*, 23: 407–434.

Bose, P.K. (ed.) (2006). *Health and Society in Bengal. A Selection from Late 19th-Century Bengali Periodicals*. New Delhi: Sage Publications.

Brendon, V. (2006). *Children of the Raj*. London: Phoenix.

Brighenti, F. (2012). 'Hindu Devotional Ordeals and Their Shamanic Parallels', *International Journal of Vedic Studies*, 19(4): 103–175.

Brilliant, L.B. (1985). *The Management of Smallpox Eradication in India*. Ann Arbor: University of Michigan Press.

Brilliant, L.B. and C. White Conrad (2000). 'The Eradication of Smallpox from India', in Bhattacharya, S. and S. Messenger (eds.), *The Global Eradication of Smallpox*. Hyderabad: Orient BlackSwan, pp. 61–83.

Brimnes, N. (2004). 'Variolation, Vaccination and Popular Resistance in Early Colonial South India', *Medical History*, 48, 199–228.

British Library, The (2009). 'Ancient Female Statue Now Called Agam Kua, Patna', Photograph by Alexander E. Caddy, 1895. *Online Gallery, Asia, Pacific and Africa Collections*, http://www.bl.uk/onlinegallery/onlineex/apac/photocoll/a/019pho000001003u0210c000.html (accessed 12/05/2014).

Brodbeck, S. (2009). 'The Bhāradvāja Pattern in the *Mahābhārata*,' in P. Koskikallio (ed), *Parallels and Comparisons. Proceedings of the Fourth Dubrovnik International Conference on the Sanskrit Epics and Purāṇas*. Zagreb: Academia Scientiarum et Artium Croatica, pp. 137–179.

Brown, P. (1965). *Indian Architecture: Buddhist and Hindu Periods*. Bombay: D.B. Taraporevala.

Buchanan, F. (1833). *A Geographical, Statistical and Historical Description of the District, or Zila, of Dinajpur, in the Province, or Soubha, of Bengal*. Calcutta: Baptist Mission Press.

Bühneman, G. (ed) (2003). *The Hindu Pantheon in Nepalese Line Drawings: Two Manuscripts of the Pratiṣṭhālakṣaṇasārasamuccaya*. Varanasi: Indica Books.

Carrin, M. (1999). 'Reasserting Identity Through Suffering: Healing Rituals in Bengal and Karnataka', in M. Carrin (ed), *Managing Distress. Possession and Therapeutic Cults in South Asia*, Delhi: Manohar, pp. 90–115.

Catanach, I.J. (1986). 'Plague and the Indian Village, 1896–1914', in P. Robb (ed), *Rural India: Law, Power and Society under the British Rule*. New Delhi: Oxford University Press, pp. 216–243.

Chakravorty Spivak, G. (2001). 'Moving Devi', *Cultural Critique*, 47, 120–163.

Chatterjee, S. (2012). 'Śrī Śrī Choṭa Śītalā Mā Snān Yātrā,' *Blogspot*, http://shitalamata.blogspot.co.uk/2012_01_01_archive.html#.U29-HShZh8E (accessed 12/05/2014).

Chatterji, R. (2003). 'The Category of Folk', in V. Das (ed), *The Oxford India Companion to Sociology and Social Anthropology*. Oxford: Oxford University Press, pp. 567–597.

Caudhurī, M.K.K. (2000). *Āñcalik Devatā Lokasaṃskṛti*. Bardhamān: Bardhāman Viśvavidyālay.

Chaudhuri, N. (1939). 'Cult of the Old Lady', *Journal of the Royal Asiatic Society of Bengal, Letters*, 5(14), 417–425.

Cohen, J. (2004). 'HIV/AIDS: India's Many Epidemics', *Science*, 304(5670), 508–514.

Collins, E.F. (1997). *Pierced by Murugan's Lance. Ritual, Power, and Moral Redemption among Malaysian Hindus*. DeKalb: Northern Illinois University Press.

Cossio, C. (1987). *Il Romanzo Anchalik Hindi*. Milano: Cesviet.

Craddock, E. (2001). 'Reconstructing the Split Goddess as Śakti in a Tamil Village,' in T. Pintchman (ed), *Seeking Mahādevī. Constructing the Identities of the Hindu Great Goddess*. Albany: State University of New York Press, pp. 145–170.

Crooke, W. (1978). *The Popular Religion and Folklore of Northern India* (reprint, 1894). Delhi, Munshiram Manoharlal.

Curtin, P.A. and T.K. Gaither (2006). 'Contested Notions of Issue Identity in International Public Relations: A Case Study', *Journal of Public Relations Research*, 18(1), 67–89.

Damodaran Nambiar, K. (1979). *Nārada-Purāṇa: a Critical Study*. Varanasi: All-India Kashiraj Trust.

Das, R.P. (2000). 'Notions of "Contagion" in Classical Indian Medical Texts', in L.I. Conrad and D. Wujastyk (eds), *Contagion. Perspectives from pre-Modern Societies*. Aldershot: Ashgate, pp. 56–78.

David, S. (2009). 'Prayer and Precaution. Aidsamma: A Temple for Goddess or 'Amma' of AIDS in Karnataka,' *India Today*, 10 May 1999, http://indiatoday.intoday.in/story/aidsamma-a-temple-for-goddess-or-amma-of-aids-in-karnataka/1/253925.html (accessed 12/05/2014).

Davidson, R.M. (2002). *Indian Esoteric Buddhism. A Social History of the Tantric Movement*. New York: Columbia University Press.

De Chowdhuri, R. (2009). 'West Bengal Farmers Fight Bad Monsoon with Frog Marriage.' *Reuters*, http://in.reuters.com/article/2009/07/21/idINIndia–41204820090721 (accessed 12/05/2014).

Dehejia, V. (1986). *Yoginī Cult and Temples: A Tantric Tradition*. New Delhi: National Museum.

Deva, R. (1967). *Śabdakalpadruma*, re-edited by Varadāprasāda Vasu and Haricaraṇa Vasu, 5 vols. (Third edition) Varanasi: Chaukambā Saṃskṛta Sīrīj Āphis.

Dhaky, M.A. (1961). 'The Chronology of Solanki Temples of Gujarat', *Journal of the Madhya Pradesh Itihāsa Pariṣad*, 3: 1–83.

Dharmapal (ed.) (2000). *Indian Science and Technology in the Eighteenth Century. Some contemporary European accounts* (reprint, 1971). Goa: Other India Press.

Dhavalikar, M.K. (1965). '"Eye goddesses" in India and their West Asian Parallels', *Anthropos*, 60, 533–540.

Dimock, E.C. Jr. (1963). *The Thief of Love. Bengali Tales from Court and Village*. Chicago: The University of Chicago Press.

Dimock, E.C. Jr. (1982). 'A Theology of the Repulsive: the Myth of the Goddess Śītalā', in J.S. Hawley and D.M. Wulff (eds), *The Divine Consort. Rādhā and the Goddesses of India*. Berkeley, University of California Press, pp. 184–203.

Dorey, M. (2010).' Compulsory Vaccination: It's Here!', Australian Vaccination Network, *Informed Voice Magazine*, http://loveforlife.com.au/files/Compulsory%20Vaccination%20.pdf (accessed 12/05/2014).

Dwyer, G. (2003). *The Divine and the Demonic. Supernatural Affliction and its Treatment in North India*. London and New York, Routledge.

Egnor, M.T. (1984). 'The Changed Mother or What the Smallpox Goddess Did When There Was No More Smallpox', *Contribution to Asian Studies*, 18: 24–45.

Elamon, J. (2005). 'A Situational Analysis of HIV/AIDS-related Discrimination in Kerala, India', *AIDS Care*, 17 (Supplement 2), 141–151.

Elmore, W. T. (1995). *Dravidian Gods in Modern Hinduism* (reprint, 1913). New Delhi: Asian Educational Services.

Erndl, K.M. (1993). *Victory to the Mother: the Hindu Goddess of Northwest India in Myth, Ritual, and Symbol*. Oxford: Oxford University Press.

Fenner, F., D.A. Henderson, I. Arita, Z. Ježek, I.D Ladnyi. (1988). *Smallpox and its Eradication*. Geneva: World Health Organization, http://whqlibdoc.who.int/smallpox/9241561106.pdf (accessed 12/05/2014).

Ferrari, F.M. (2007). '"Love Me Two Times." From Smallpox to AIDS: Contagion and Possession in the Cult of Śītalā,' *Religions of South Asia*, 1(1), 81–106.

Ferrari, F.M. (2010a). *Guilty Males and Proud Females. Negotiating Genders in a Bengali Festival*. Calcutta, London, New York: Seagull Books.

Ferrari, F.M. (2010b). 'Old Rituals for New Threats. The Post-smallpox Career of Śītalā, the Cold Mother of Bengal,' in C. Brosius and U. Hüsken (eds.), *Ritual Matters*. London and New York: Routledge, pp. 144–171.

Ferrari, F.M. (2012). 'Mystic Rites for Permanent Class Conflict: The Bāuls of Bengal, Revolutionary Ideology and Post-capitalism,' *South Asia Research*, 32(1): 28–38.

Ferrari, F.M. (2013). 'Alternative Yoginīs with Alternative Powers. Singing the Blues in the Cauṣaṭṭī Yoginī Devī Mandir of Vārāṇasī,' in I. Keul (ed.), *Yoginī in South Asia. Alternative Approaches*. London and New York: Routledge, pp. 148–162.

Ferrari, F.M. (2013). 'The Silent Killer. The Ass as Personification of Illness in Northern Indian folklore', in F.M. Ferrari and T. Dähnhardt (eds), *Charming Beauties and Frightful Beasts. Non-Human Animals in South Asian Myth, Ritual and Folklore*. Sheffield: Equinox, pp. 236–257.

Ferrari, F.M. (2015). 'Devotion and Affliction in the Time of Cholera: Ritual Healing, Identity and Resistance among Bengali Muslims,' in I. Vargas-O'Bryan and X. Zhou (eds), *Disease, Religion and Healing in Asia. Collaborations and Collisions*. London and New York: Routledge, pp. 38–53.

Ferrari, F.M. (ed) (2011). *Health and Religious Rituals in South Asia. Disease, Possession and Healing*. London and New York: Routledge.

Ferrari, F.M. and M. Refolo. (2005). 'Mito e contagio: per un'analisi comparativa dei *Śītalāmaṅgalkābya* e de *Il Cromosoma Calcutta*', *Annali di Ca' Foscari*, 44(3), 139–163.

Filippi, G.G. (2002). 'Il movimento della Devī: un'epidemia di possessione collettiva', *Annali di Ca' Foscari*, 41(3), 191–210.

Filliozat, J. (1937). *Étude de Démonologie Indienne: le Kumāratantra de Rāvana et les Textes Parallèles Indiens, Tibétains, Chinois, Cambodgien et Arabe.* Paris: Imprimerie Nationale.

Flueckiger, J. (2006). *In Amma's Healing Room. Gender and Vernacular Islam in South India*. Bloomington: Indiana University Press.

Forbes, A.K. (1856). *Râs Mâlâ: Or, Hindoo Annals of the Province of Goozerat, in Western India*, vol. 2. London: Richardson Brothers.

Foster, S. (1977). 'Smallpox Eradication: Lessons Learned in Bangladesh', *WHO Chronicle*, 31, 245–247.

Foster, S. (1978). 'Participation to the Public in Global Smallpox Eradication', *International Health*, 93(2), 147–149.

Foulston, L. (2003). *At the Feet of the Goddess. The Divine Feminine in local Hindu Religion*. Delhi: Adarsh Books.

Foulston, L. and S. Abbott (2009). *Hindu Goddesses. Beliefs and Practices.* Eastbourne: Sussex Academic Press.

Freed, R.S. and S.A. Freed (1985). 'The Psychomedical Case History of a Low-caste Woman of North India', *Anthropological Papers of the American Museum of Natural History*, 60(2): 1–326.

Freed, R.S. and S.A. Freed. (1993). 'Ghosts: Life and Death in North India', *Anthropological Papers of the American Museum of Natural History*, 72: 1–396.

Freed, R.S. and S.A. Freed. (1998). 'Hindu Festivals in a North Indian Village', *Anthropological Papers of the American Museum of Natural History*, 81: 1–326.

GAIN (Global Alliance for Improved Nutrition). (2012). 'Shitala Mata Self Help Group: Mothers take the Lead in the Fight against Malnutrition', http://www.gainhealth.org/photo-essay/shitala-mata-self-help-groups-interaction-board (accessed 12/05/2014).

Gallagher, P. (2011). 'Measles: A Gift from a Goddess?', *Losing In The Lucky Country. Skeptical Musings on the Denial of Evidence*, http://luckylosing.com/2011/11/13/measles-a-gift-from-a-goddess/#comments (accessed 12/05/2014).

Gelfand, H.M. (1966). 'A Critical Examination of the Indian Smallpox Eradication Program', *American Journal of Public Health*, 56(10): 1634–1651.
Gewertz, K. (2000). 'Undergraduate Witnesses Birth of a Goddess', *The Harvard University Gazette*, February 24, http://www.news.harvard.edu/gazette/2000/02.24/AIDS.html (accessed 12/05/2014).
Gewertz, K. (n.d). 'Hinduism's AIDS-amma: Deity vs. Disease', *Beliefnet. Inspiration, Spirituality, Faith*, http://www.beliefnet.com/Faiths/2000/06/Hinduisms-AIDS-Amma-Deity-Vs-Disease.aspx?p=2 (accessed 12/05/2014).
Ghatak, P. (2013). 'The Sitala Saga: A Case of Cultural Integration in the Folk Tradition of West Bengal', *Ropkatha Journal of Interdisciplinary Studies in Humanities*, 5(2): 119–131.
Ghatak, P. (2013). 'Sitala Worship: The Continuing Story of Vulnerability, Protection and Fortune in the Social Fabric of the Savaras of West Bengal', *The Asian Man*, 7(1–2): 154–159.
Ghosh, A. (1995). *The Calcutta Chromosome*. New York: Avon Books.
Girard, R. (2011). *Sacrifice*. East Lansing: Michigan State University Press.
Giri, K., M. Tivāri and V.P. Siṃha (n.d.). *Kāśī ke Mandir aur Mūrtiyā̃*. Vārāṇasī: Jilā Sāṃskr̥tik Samiti.
Gold, A.G. (2002). 'Counterpoint Authority in Women's Ritual Expressions. A View from the Village', in L. Patton (ed), *Jewels of Authority. Women and Textual Tradition in Hindu India*. Oxford and New York: Oxford University Press, pp. 177–201.
Gold, A.G. (2008). 'Deep Beauty: Rajasthani Goddess Shrines Above and Below the Surface', *International Journal of Hindu Studies*, 12(2): 153–179.
Gopalan, G.V. (1978). 'Vrat: Ceremonial Vows of Women in Gujarat, India', *Asian Folklore Studies*, 37(1): 101–129.
Goudriaan, T. (1978). *Māyā. Divine and Human*. Delhi: Motilal Banarsidass.
Goudriaan, T. and S. Gupta. (1981). *A History of Indian Literature: Hindu Tantric and Śākta Literature*. Wiesbaden: Otto Harrassowitz.
Gramsci, A. (2007). *Quaderni del carcere*, 4 vols. Valentino Gerratana (ed.). Turin: Einaudi.
Greenhough, P. (1980). 'Variolation and Vaccination in South Asia c. 1700–1865: A Preliminary Note', *Social Science and Medicine*, 14, 345–347.
Griffiths, A. and J.E.M. Houben (eds) (2004). *The Vedas. Text, Language and Ritual*. Leiden: Brill.
Guillén, C. (1971). *Literature as System: Essays towards the Theory of Literary History*. Princeton: Princeton University Press.
Hahn, R.A. (1984). 'Rethinking "Illness" and "Diseases"', *Contribution to Asian Studies*, 18, 1–23.
Handa, D. (1984). *Osiañ: History, Archaeology, Art and Architecture*. Delhi: Sundeep.
Hāphij, A. (1978). *Laukik Saṃskār o Bengali Samāj*. Ḍhākā: Muktadhār.
Harlan, L. (1998). 'Satī. The Story of Godāvarī', in J.S. Hawley and D.M. Wulff (eds.), *Devī. Goddesses of India*. Delhi: Munshiram Manoharlal, pp. 227–249.
Harman, W. (2004). 'Taming the Fever Goddess: Transforming a Tradition in Southern India', *Manushi*, 140, 2–15.
Harman, W. (2011). 'Possession as Protection and Affliction: The Goddess Mariyamman's Fierce Grace', in F.M. Ferrari (ed), *Health and Religious Rituals in South Asia. Disease, Possession and Healing*. London and New York: Routledge, pp. 185–198.
Harman, W. (2012). 'From Fierce to Domesticated: Mariyamman Joins the Middle Class', *Nidan : International Journal for the Study of Hinduism*, 24: 41–65.
Harman, W.P. (1989). *The Sacred Marriage of a Hindu Goddess*. Delhi: Motilal Banarsidas.

Hauser, B. (2012). *Promising Rituals. Gender and Performativity in Eastern India*. New Delhi: Routledge.
Hazra, R.C. (1987). *Studies in the Puranic Records on Hindu Rites and Customs* (reprint, 1940). Delhi: Motilal Banarsidass.
Henderson, D.H. (1980). 'A Victory for All Mankind'. *World Health*, 3–5.
Hiebert, P. (1989). 'A Sacrifice to the Smallpox Goddess', in P. Hiebert and F.F. Hiebert (eds), *Case studies in Missions*: Grand Rapids, MI.: Baker Book House.
Hiltebeitel, A. (1991). *The Cult of Draupadī, 2: On Hindu Ritual and the Goddess*. Chicago: University of Chicago Press.
Holwell, J.Z. (1971). 'An Account of the Manner of Inoculating for the Smallpox in the East Indies (reprint, 1767)', in Dharmapal, *Indian Science and Technology in the Eighteen Century: Some Contemporary European Accounts*. Delhi: Impex India, pp. 143–163.
Hopkins, D.R. (1983). *Princes and Peasants: Smallpox in History*. London and Chicago: University of Chicago Press.
Hopkins, D.R. (1988). 'Smallpox: Ten Years Gone', *Public Health Then and Now*, 78(12): 1589–1595.
Hora, S.L. (1933). 'Worship of the Deities Olā, Jholā and Bon Bībī in Lower Bengal', *Journal of the Asiatic Society of Bengal, New Series*, 29: 1–4.
Humes, C.A. (1993). 'The Goddess of the Vindhyas in Banaras', in B.R. Hertel and C.A. Humes (eds), *Living Banaras. Hindu Religion in Cultural Context*. Albany: State University of New York Press, pp. 181–204.
Hunter, W.W. (1996). *The Annals of Rural Bengal* (reprint, 1868). Calcutta: West Bengal District Gazetteers.
International Congress of Medicine, 17th, 1913, London (1914). *The History of Inoculation and Vaccination for the Prevention and Treatment of Disease: Lecture Memoranda*. London: Burroughs Wellcome.
Jain, J. (1999). *Kalighat Painting. Images fron a Changing World*. Ahmedabad: Mapin Publishing.
James, S.P. (1909). *Smallpox and Vaccination in British India*. Calcutta: Thacker, Spink and Co.
Jamison, S.W. and M. Witzel (2003). 'Vedic Hinduism,' in A. Sharma (ed), *The Study of Hinduism*. Columbia: University of South Carolina Press, pp. 65–113.
Jest, C. and G. Ravis-Giordani (1985). 'L'âne au Tibet,' *Ethnozootechnie*, 37: 15–20.
Jones, C.A. and J.D. Ryan (2007). *Encyclopedia of Hinduism*. New York: Infobase Publishing.
Junghare, I.Y. (1975). 'Songs of the Goddess Shitala. Religio-cultural and Linguistic Features', *Man in India*, 55(4), 298–316.
Kaimal, P. (2013). 'Yoginīs in Stone. Auspicious and Inauspicious Power', in I. Keul (ed.), *'Yoginī' in South Asia. Interdisciplinary Approaches*. London and New York: Routledge, pp. 97–108.
Kane, P.V. (1958). *History of Dharmaśāstras* (five vols.). Poona: Bhandarkar Oriental Research Institute.
Kattimani, B.F. (2011). 'Donkey Wedding Staged to Bring Rain', *The Times of India*, 10 August 2011, http://timesofindia.indiatimes.com/city/hubli/Donkey-wedding-staged-to-bring-rain/articleshow/9557694.cms?referral=PM (accessed 12/05/2014).
Katyal, A. with N. Kishore (1991). 'Performing the Goddess: Sacred Ritual into Professional Performance', *The Drama Review*, 45(1): 96–117.
Kāvirāj, G. (1972). *Tāntrika Sāhitya*. Vārāṇasī: Bhārgav Bhūṣaṇ Pres.
Kaviraj, S. (2003). 'The Two Histories of Literary Culture in Bengal', in S. Pollock (ed), *Literary Cultures in History: Reconstructions from South Asia*. Berkeley: University of California Press, pp. 503–566.

Kelton, P. (2004). 'Avoiding the Smallpox Spirits: Colonial Epidemics and Southeastern Indian Survival', *Ethnohistory*, 51(1), 45–71.

Keul, I. (2012). 'Blending into the Religious Landscape: The Yoginīs in Benares', *Numen*, 59(4): 366–402.

Kim, J. (2013). 'Demons and Humans with Pockmarks, Goddesses with Healing Powers: Images of Sickness and Healing in Pre-modern South Asia', unpublished paper presented at the AAS (Association for Asian Studies) Annual Conference, March 21–24, 2013, San Diego (CA).

Kinsley, D.R. (1997). *Tantric Vision of the Divine Feminine. The Ten Mahāvidyās*. Berkeley: University of California Press.

Kolenda, P. (1982). 'Pox and the Terror of Childlessness: Images and Ideas of the Smallpox Goddess in a North Indian village', in J.J. Preston (ed.), *Mother Worship*. Chapell Hill: University of North Carolina Press, pp. 227–250.

Korom, F.J. (2006). *South Asian Folklore. A Handbook*. Westport. CT and London, Greenwood.

Korom, F.J. (2006). *Village of Painters. Narrative Scrolls from West Bengal*. Santa Fe: Museum of International Folk Art.

Kumar, M. (2010). 'Pumpkins, Cucumbers Replace Animal Sacrifice in Puja', *The Times of India*, 16 October 2010, http://timesofindia.indiatimes.com/city/patna/Pumpkins-cucumbers-replace-animal-sacrifice-in-Puja/articleshow/6756355.cms (accessed 12/05/2014).

Kumar, S.V. (1983). *The Purāṇic Lore of Holy Water-Places*. Delhi: Munshiram Manoharlal.

Kundu, M. (2013). 'The Dramatic Performances Act of 1876: Reactions of the Bengali Establishment to its Introduction', *History and Sociology of South Asia*, 7(1): 79–93.

Lambert, H. (1997). 'Illness, Inauspiciousness and Modes of Healing in Rajasthan', *Contribution to Indian Sociology*, 31(2): 253–271.

Lambert H. (2015). 'The Management of Sickness in an Indian Medical Vernacular,' in I. Vargas-O'Bryan and X. Zhou (eds), *Disease, Religion and Healing in Asia. Collaborations and Collisions*. London and New York: Routledge, pp. 9–21.

Leslie, J. (1991). 'Śrī and Jyeṣṭhā: Ambivalent Role models for Women', In J. Leslie (ed), *Roles and Rituals for Hindu Women*. London: Pinter, pp. 107–128.

Lipner, J. (2010). *Hindus: Their Religious Beliefs and Practices* (second edition). London and New York: Routledge.

Lobo, W. (1982). *The Sun-Temple at Modhera. A Monograph on Architecture and Iconography*. München: C.H. Beck.

Lochtefeld, J.G. (2001). *The Illustrated Encyclopedia of Hinduism* (vol. 2). New York: The Rosen Publishing Group.

Lotman, J. (2005). 'On the Semiosphere', *Sign Systems Studies*, 33(1): 205–229.

Manring, R.J. (2012). 'Śītalādevī', in K.A. Jacobsen, H. Basu, A. Malinar and V. Narayanan (eds), *Brill's Encyclopedia of Hinduism*. Leiden: Brill Online.

Marglin, F.A. (1985). 'Types of Oppositions in Hindu Culture', in J.B. Carman and F.A. Marglin (eds), *Purity and Auspiciousness in Indian Society*. Leiden: Brill, pp. 65–83.

Marglin, F.A. (1986). 'Eradication of Smallpox, the Cult of Sitala, and Ecological Politics', *Suomen Antropologi*, 11(4): 160–181

Marglin, F.A. (2001). 'Smallpox in Two Systems of Knowledge', in F.A. Marglin and S.A. Marglin (eds.), *Dominating Knowledge: Development, Culture, and Resistance* (reprint, 1990). Oxford: Clarendon Press, pp. 102–144.

Mather, R.J. and T.J. John (1973). 'Popular Beliefs about Smallpox and Other Common Infectious Diseases in South India', *Tropical and Geographical*, 25, 190–196.

Mc Gregor, R.S. (1997). *The Oxford Hindi-English Dictionary*. Delhi: Oxford University Press.

McDaniel, J. (2003). *Making Virtuous Daughters and Wives. An Introduction to Women's Brata Rituals in Bengali Folk Religion*. Albany: State University of New York Press.

McDaniel, J. (2004). *Offering Flowers, Feeding Skulls. Popular Goddess Worship in West Bengal*. Oxford and New York: Oxford University Press.

McGee, M. (1991). 'Desired Fruits: Motive and Intention in the Votive Rites of Hindu Women', in J. Leslie (ed.), *Roles and Rituals for Hindu Women*. London: Pinter, pp. 71–88.

McLeod, K. (2010). 'Meryl Dorey's Trouble with the Truth. Part 3', http://luckylosing.com/2011/10/11/meryl-doreys-trouble-with-the-truth-part–3-lies-and-fraud/ (accessed 12/05/2014).

Meister, M.W. (1986). 'Regional Variations in Mātr̥kā Conventions', *Artibus Asiae*, 47, 233–262.

Meister, M.W. (1991). 'Amber's Antiques: Text and Context', in C. Singh, and N. Vashishtha (eds), *Pathways to Literature Art and Archaeology. Pt. Gopal Narayan Baura Felicitation Volume. Volume II*. Jaipur: Publication Scheme, pp. 192–195.

Meister, M.W. (1998). 'Sweetmeats or Corpse. Community, Conversion, and Sacred Places', in J. Cort (ed.), *Open Boundaries: Jain Communities and Cultures in Indian History*. Albany: State University of New York Press, pp. 111–138.

Meulenbeld, G.J. (1999–2002). *A History of Indian Medical Literature* (five vols.). Groningen: E. Forsten.

Mevissen, G.J.R. (2000). 'Īṣat-paṅgu Śanaiścara, The Lame Planetary God Saturn and his Vāhanas', *South Asian Archaeology 1997. Proceedings of the Fourteenth International Conference of the European Association of South Asian Archaeologists, Rome, 7–11 July 1997*, vol. 3: 1267–1297.

Minsky, L. (2009). 'Pursuing Protection from Disease: The Making of Smallpox Prophylactic Practice in Colonial Punjab', *Bulletin of the History of Medicine*, 83(1): 164–190.

Mishra, P.K. (ed.) (1999). *Studies in Hindu and Buddhist Art*. Delhi: Abhinav Publications.

Mishra, S. and N. Kumar (2011). 'Shaking the Roots of Western Science in Amitav Ghosh's The Calcutta Chromosome', *Asiatic*, 5(1), 78–85.

Misra, B. (1969). 'Sitala: The Small-pox Goddess of India', *Asian Folklore Studies*, 28(2): 133–142.

Mitter, S. (1996). 'Customs that Can Kill Women', in *Times Higher Education*, 27 May 1996, http://www.timeshighereducation.co.uk/books/customs-that-can-kill-women/163281.article (accessed 12/05/2014).

Monier-Williams, M. (1995). *Sanskrit-English Dictionary* (reprint, 1899). Delhi: Motilal Banarsidass.

Moreno, M. and Marriott, M. (1989). 'Humoral Transactions in Two Tamil cults: Murukan and Mariyamman', *Contributions to Indian Sociology* (New Series), 23(1): 149–167.

Mukhopadhyay, S.K. (1994). *Cult of Goddess Sitala in Bengal. An Enquiry into Folk Culture*. Calcutta: Firma K.L.M.

Mull, D.S. (2005). 'The Sitala Syndrome: The Cultural Context of Measles Mortality in Pakistan', in M.C. Inhorn and P.J. Brown (eds), *The Anthropology of Infectious Disease. International Health Perspectives* (reprint, 1997). Amsterdam: Routledge, 299–330.

Nabokov, I. (2000). *Religion Against the Self. An Ethnography of Tamil Rituals*. New York: Oxford University Press.

Nagar, S.L. (1988). *Mahisasuramardini in Indian Art*. New Delhi: Aditya Prakashan.

Nahar, P.C. (1983). *Jaina Inscriptions: Containing Index of Places, Glossary of Names of Shrāvaka Castes, and Gotras of Gachhas, and Achāryas with Dates* (reprint, 1918). Delhi: Indian Book Gallery.

Nalin, D.R. (2004). 'The Cover Art of the 15 June 2004 Issue', *Clinical Infectious Diseases (Correspondence)*, 39(11): 1741–1742.

Nanda, M. (2009) *God Market: How Globalization Is Making India More Hindu*. London: Random House Publishers.

Naraindas, H. 'Preparing for the Pox: A Theory of Smallpox in Bengal and Britain', *Asian Journal of Social Sciences*, 31(2), 304–339.

Narayanan, V. (2000). 'Diglossic Hinduism. Liberation and lentils', *Journal of The American Academy of Religion*, 68(4), 761–779.

Narayanan, V. (2006). 'Shanti: Peace for the Mind, Body, and Soul', in L.L. Barnes and I. Talamantez (eds), *Teaching Religion and Healing*. Oxford and New York: Oxford University Press, pp. 61–82.

Navaljī (1994). *Nālandā Viśāl Śabd Sagar*. Dillī: Nyū Impirīal Buk Ḍipo.

Neog, M. (1984). *Religions of the North-East*. Delhi, Munshiram Manoharlal.

Nicholas, R. (2003). *Fruits of Worship: Practical Religion in Bengal*. New Delhi: Chronicle Books.

Nirmalānanda (Svami). (1413 BS). *Devadevī o Tā̃der Vāhan* (seventh edition). Kolkātā: Bhārat Sevāśram Saṅgha.

Oberoi, H. (1992). 'Popular Saints, Goddesses, and Village Sacred Sites: Rereading Sikh Experience in the Nineteenth Century', *History of Religions*, 31(4): 363–384.

Obeyesekere, G. (1978). 'The Fire-walkers of Kataragama: The Rise of Bhakti Religiosity in Buddhist Sri Lanka', *Journal of Asian Studies*, 37: 457–476.

Obeyesekere, G. (1987). *The Cult of the Goddess Pattini*. Delhi: Motilal Banarsidass.

Oddie, G.A. (1995). *Popular Religion, Elites and Reform: Hook-Swinging and Its Prohibition in Colonial India, 1800–1894*. New Delhi: Manohar.

Offredi, M. (1974). *Il Romanzo Hindi Contemporaneo*. Milano: Cesviet.

OIE (Office International des Epizooties). (2009) 'Trypanosoma evansi infections (including surra).' *World Organization for Animal Health*, http://www.oie.int/fileadmin/Home/eng/Animal_Health_in_the_World/docs/pdf/TRYPANO_EVANSI_FINAL.pdf (accessed 12/05/2014).

Pallikadavath, S., C. Sreedharan and R.W. Stones (2006). 'Source of AIDS Awareness among Women in India', *AIDS Care*, 18(1), 44–48.

Pāṇḍey Ārya, L. (2037 VS; 1980/1981 CE). *Hindū Devatāõ ke Vividha Rūpa aur Vāhana*. Vārāṇasī.

Parpola, A. (2004–2005). 'The Nāsatyas, the Chariot and the Proto-Aryan Religion', *Journal of Indological Studies*, 16/17: 1–63.

Parpola, A., and J. Janhunen. (2011). 'On the Asiatic Wild Asses and their Vernacular Names', in T. Osada and H. Endo (eds), *Linguistics, Archaeology and the Human Past*. Occasional Paper 12: 59–124. Kyoto: Indus Project – Research Institute for Humanity and Nature, pp. 59–124.

Pati, B. (2002). 'Negotiating with *Dharma Pinnu*: Towards a Social History of Smallpox in Colonial Orissa', *Canadian Bulletin of Medical History*, 19(2): 477–492.

Pati, B. and M. Harrison (eds) (2001). *Health, Medicine and Empire: Perspectives on Colonial India*. New Delhi: Orient Longman.

Patton, L.L. (2005). *Bringing the Gods to Mind. Mantra and Ritual in Early Indian Sacrifice*. Berkeley: University of California Press.

Pearson, A.M. (1996). *'Because it Gives Me Peace of Mind': Ritual Fasts in the Religious Lives of Hindu Women*. Albany: State University of New York Press.

Pingree, D. (1981). *Jyotiḥśāstra. Astral and Mathematical Literature*. Wiesbaden: Otto Harrassowitz.

Pollock, S. (2006). *The Language of the Gods in the World of Men. Sanskrit, Culture, and Power in Premodern India*. Berkeley: University of California Press.

Portnoy, A. (2000). 'A Goddess in the Making. A Very Hard-to-find Town in India Builds a Shrine to a Goddess for AIDS', *Whole Earth*, http://www.findarticles.com/p/articles/mi_m0GER/is_2000_Fall/ai_66240450 (accessed 12/05/2014).
Pringle, R. (1868). 'On the Possibility of Stamping-out Smallpox', *The Lancet*, 92(2358): 597–599.
Pringle, R. (1885). 'Ancient and Modern Methods of Treating Small-pox Epidemics in India', *Journal of the Royal Society of Arts*, 33: 737–739.
Propp, V. (1968). *Morphology of the Folktale*. Austin: University of Texas Press.
Raghunath, D. (2002). 'Smallpox Revisited', *Current Science*, 83(5), 566–576.
Raj, S.J. and W. Harman (eds) (2006). *Dealing with Deities: The Ritual Vow in South Asia*. Albany: State University of New York Press.
Ram, K. (2013). *Fertile Disorder. Spirit Possession and its Provocation of the Modern*. Honolulu: University of Hawaii Press.
Rao, A. R. (1972). *Smallpox*. Bombay: Kothari Book Depot.
Rau, W. (2012). 'A Note on the Donkey and the Mule in Early Vedic Literature.' In K. Klaus, and J.F. Sprockhoff (eds), *Wilhelm Rau. Kleine Schriften*. Vol. 2. Wiesbaden: Otto Harrassowitz, pp. 987–997.
Rāy, G. (1976). *Hanumān ke Devatva tathā Mūrti kā Vikās*. Prayāg: Hindī Sāhitya Sammelan.
Raza, G., B. Dutt and S. Singh (1997). 'Kaleidoscoping Public Understanding of Science on Hygiene, Health and Plague: A Survey in the Aftermath of a Plague Epidemic in India', *Public Understanding of Science*, 6, 247–267.
Reddy, G. (2005). *The Third Sex. Negotiating Hijra Identity in South India*. Chicago and London: The University of Chicago Press.
Riedel, S. (2005). 'Edward Jenner and the History of Smallpox and Vaccination', *Baylor University Medical Centre Proceedings*, 18(1): 21–25.
Risley, H.H. (1998). *The Tribes and Castes of Bengal*, 3 vols. (reprint, 1891). Calcutta: Firma KLM.
Rodrigues, H.P. (2003). *The Liturgy of the Durgā Pūjā with interpretations*. Albany: State University of New York Press.
Rose, H.A. (1916). *A Glossary of the Tribes and Castes of the Punjab and North-West Frontier Province*, vol. 1. London: Macmillan and Co.
Roy, S.N. (1927). 'Popular Superstitions in Orissa about Small-pox and Cholera', *Man in India*, 7, 200–208.
Sahani, J. (2011). 'Ma Sheetla Adalpur Wali,' *Adalpura Śītalā Dhām*, http://adalpura.blogspot.co.uk/2011/01/ma-sheetla-adalpur-wali.html (accessed 12/05/2014).
Samuel, G. (2008). *The Origins of Yoga and Tantra. Indic Religions to the Thirteenth Century*. Cambridge: Cambridge University Press.
Śaṅkar, H. (1996). *Kāśī ke Ghāṭ. Kalātmak evaṁ Sāṃskr̥tik Adhyayan*. Vārāṇasī: Viśvavidyālay Prakāśan.
Sankalya, H.D. (1948). *Winnowing Basket and the Cult of Sitala*. Poona: Aryatohushan Press.
Sanyal, H. (1982). *Literary Sources of Medieval Bengali History. A Study of a Few Mangalkavya Texts*. Calcutta: Centre for Studies in Social Sciences.
Saraswati, D. (n.d.). *The Light of Truth (The Satyarth Prakash)*, http://www.aryasamajjamnagar.org/satyarth_prakash_eng.htm (accessed 12/05/2014).
Sarkar, B.K. (1972). *The Folk Element in Hindu Culture* (reprint, 1917). New Delhi: Oriental Reprint.
Śarmā, V. (2012). *Śītalā Saptamī par Pāe kā Sitala kī Kr̥pā*, http://www.youtube.com/watch?v=0KUE2qa_U48 (accessed 12/05/2014).
Sastri, H. (1897). *Discovery of Living Buddhism in Bengal*. Calcutta: Sanskrit Press Depository.

Sax, W. (2009). *God of Justice: Ritual Healing and Social Justice in the Central Himalayas*. New York and Oxford: Oxford University Press.

Schmidt, H.P. (1973). 'Vedic Pathas', *Indo Iranian Journal*, 15(1): 1–39.

Schröder, U. 2012. 'Hook-swinging in South India: Negotiating the Subaltern Space within a Colonial Society,' in U. Hüsken and F. Neubert (eds.), *Negotiating Rites*. New York: Oxford University Press, 215–235.

Seely, C. (2000). 'Secular and Sacred Legitimation in Bharatcandra Ray's *Annada-mangal* (1752 C.E.)', *Archiv Orientální*, 68(3), 327–358.

Sharma, P.V. (ed) (1992). *History of Medicine in India: from Antiquity to 1000 A.D.* New Delhi: Indian National Science Academy.

Sharma, R.C. (1989). 'The Cult of Śītalā in Uttar Pradesh', in B. Chatterjee et al., *History and Archaeology. Prof. H. D. Sankalia Felicitation Volume*. Delhi: Ramanand Vidya Bhawan, pp. 66–73.

Sharma, R.C. and P. Ghosal (eds) (2006). *Śākta Contribution to Varanasi*. Delhi: D.K. Printworld.

Shastri, S. (2014). 'The Deadly Hemorrhagic Form of Smallpox: An Epidemic Disease in British Colonial India', *IOSR Journal Of Humanities And Social Science*, 19(2): 28–31.

Shaw, M.E. (2006). *Buddhist Goddesses of India*. Princeton, NJ: Princeton University Press.

'Shitala' (n.d.). In *Wikipedia*. Retrieved April, 13th 2014, http://en.wikipedia.org/wiki/Shitala (accessed 12/05/2014).

Shulman, D. D. 1989. 'Outcaste, Guardian, and Trickster: Notes on the Myth of Kāttavarāyan', in A. Hiltebeitel (ed.), *Criminal Gods and Demon Devotees: Essays on the Guardians of Popular Hinduism*. Albany: SUNY Press, pp. 35–67.

Shurkin, J.N. (1979). *The Invisible Fire. The Story of Mankind's Victor over the Ancient Scourge of Smallpox*. New York: G.P. Putnam's Sons.

Siṃha, R.P. (1990). *Caũsaṭh Yoginiyā̃ evaṃ Unke Mandir*. Dillī: J.P. Pabliśiṅg Hāus.

Siṃha, S. (2000). *Bhojpurī Lokgāthā*. Ilāhābād: Hindustānī Ekeḍemī.

Singh, R.P.B. (2002). *Towards the Pilgrimage Archetype. The Pañcakrośī Yātrā of Banāras*. Indica Books: Varanasi.

Singh, R.P.B. (2010). *Sacred Geography of the Goddess in South Asia. Essays in Memory of David Kinsley*. Newcastle-upon-Tyne: Cambridge Scholars Publishing.

Singh, R.P.B. and P.S. Rana (2006). *Banaras Region. A Spiritual and Cultural Guide*. Indica Books: Varanasi.

Sircar, J. (2005). *The Construction of the Hindu Identity in Medieval Western Bengal. The Role of Popular Cults*. Kolkata: Institute of Development Studies.

Smith, B.K. (1994). *Classifying the Universe. The Ancient Varṇa System and the Origins of Caste*. New York: Oxford University Press.

Smith, F.M. (1994). 'Purāṇaveda', in L. Patton (ed), *Authority, Anxiety, and Canon: Essays in Vedic Interpretation*. Albany: State University of New York Press, pp. 97–138.

Smith, F.M. (2006). *The Self Possessed: Deity and Spirit Possession in South Asian Literature and Civilization*. New York: Columbia University Press.

Smith, F.M. (2010). 'Possession, Embodiment, and Ritual in Mental Health Care in India', *Journal of Ritual Studies*, 24(2), 35–50.

Smith, J.Z. (2013). *On Teaching Religion*. New York: Oxford University Press.

Sonnerat, P. (1782). *Voyage aux Indes Orientales et à la Chine*, 2 vols. Paris: Chez l'Auteur.

Staal, F. (2008). *Discovering the Vedas. Origins, Mantras, Rituals, Insights*. New Delhi: Penguin Books.

Stewart, T.K. (1995). 'Encountering the Smallpox Goddess: The Auspicious Song of Śītalā', in D.S. Lopez Jr. (ed), *Religious of India in Practice*. Princeton, NJ: Princeton University Press, 389–397.

Stewart, T.K. (2004). *Fabulous Females and Peerless Pīrs. Tales of Mad Adventure in Old Bengal*. New York: Oxford University Press.
Sujatha, V. (2007). 'Pluralism in Indian Medicine: Medical Lore a Genre of Medical Knowledge', *Contribution to Indian Sociology*, 41(2): 169–202.
Svoboda, R.E. (1997). *The Greatness of Saturn. A Therapeutic Myth*. Twin Lakes, WI: Lotus Press.
Tewari Jassal, S. (2012). *Unearthing Gender. Folksongs of North India*. Durham, NC and London: Duke University Press.
Thanindian News. (2009). 'Old Dailt Woman Accused of Witchcraft Stripped and Beaten.' *Thaindian News*, http://www.thaindian.com/newsportal/india-news/old-dailt-woman-accused-of-witchcraft-stripped-and-beaten_100196466.html (accessed 12/05/2014).
Thurston, E. (1912). *Omens and Superstitions of Southern India*. New York: McBride, Nast and Co.
Times of India (The). (2001). 'Donkey Milk to Be Tried on Humans.' *Times of India*. Lucknow, 26 September 2001, http://articles.timesofindia.indiatimes.com/2001-09-26/lucknow/27233965_1_donkey-milk-human-body-trials (accessed 12/05/2014).
Times of India (The). (2009). 'Woman Stripped, Paraded for 'witchcraft'.' *The Times of India*. http://timesofindia.indiatimes.com/city/nagpur/Woman-stripped-paraded-for-witchcraft/articleshow/4573434.cms (accessed 12/05/2014).
Times of India (The). (2012). 'Anima Sacrifice Still in Vogue,' *The Times of India*, 23 October 2012, http://timesofindia.indiatimes.com/city/patna/Animal-sacrifice-still-in-vogue/articleshow/16922845.cms (accessed 12/05/2014).
Tiwari, M.N. (1996). 'Śītalā on Indian Art and Tradition', *Berliner Indologische Studies*, 9(10), 451–462.
Tod, J. (1920). *Annals and Antiquities of Rajasthan or the Central and Western Rajput States of India*, 3 vols. London: Oxford University Press.
Tucker, J.B. (2001). *Scourge: The Once and Future Threat of Smallpox*. New York: Grove Press.
Upadhyaya, H.S. (1967). 'Some Annotated Indian Folk Songs', *Asian Folklore Studies*, 26(1): 63–98.
Vidyarthi, L.P. (2005). *The Sacred Complex of Kashi: A Microcosm of Indian Civilization* (reprint, 1979). Delhi: Concept Publishing.
Waddell, L.A. (1903). *Reports on the Excavations at Pataliputra (Patna), the Palibothra of the Greeks*. Calcutta: Bengal Secretariat Press.
Wadley, S.S. (1980). 'Śītalā: The Cool One', *Asian Folklore Studies*, 39: 33–62.
Wadley, S.S. (2003). 'Śītalā', in M.A. Mills, P.J. Claus and S. Diamond (eds), *South Asian Folklore. An Encyclopaedia*. London and New York: Routledge, pp. 561–562.
Wadley, S.S. (2007). 'Grāma', in S. Mittal and G. Thursby (eds), *The Hindu World*. London and New York: Routledge, pp. 429–445.
Wallis, G. (2002). *Mediating the Power of Buddhas. Ritual in the Mañjuśrīmūlakalpa*. Albany: State University of New York Press.
Ward, W. (1822). *A View of the History, Literature, and Mythology of the Hindoos: Including a Minute Description of Their Manners and Customs, and Translation from Their Principal Works*, Vol. 1. London: Kingsbury, Parbury, and Allen.
White, D.G. (2003). *Kiss of the Yoginī: "Tantric Sex" in Its South Asian Contexts*. Chicago and London: University of Chicago Press.
WHO (2009). 'Safety of Smallpox Vaccine: Questions and Answers,' *Global Vaccine Safety*, http://www.who.int/vaccine_safety/committee/topics/smallpox/questions/en/ (accessed 12/05/2014).

Witzel, M. (1997). 'The Development of the Vedic Canon and its Schools: The Social and Political Milieu', in M. Witzel (ed), *Inside the Texts, Beyond the Texts. New Approaches to the Study of the Vedas*. Cambridge: Harvard Oriental Series, Opera Minora 2, pp. 257–346.

Witzel, M. (2003). 'Vedas and Upaniṣads', in G. Flood (ed), *The Blackwell Companion to Hinduism*. Oxford: Blackwell, pp. 68–101.

Woodroffe, J. (2009). *Śakti and Śākta* (third edition). Leeds: Celephaïs Press.

Wujastyk, Dagmar and F.M. Smith (eds) (2008). *Modern and Global Ayurveda: Pluralism and Paradigm*. Albany: State University of New York Press.

Wujastyk, Dagmar. (2012). *Well-Mannered Medicine. Medical Ethics and Etiquette in Classical Ayurveda*. Oxford and New York: Oxford University Press.

Wujastyk, Dominik (1999). 'Miscarriages of Justice: Demonic Vengeance in Classical Indian Medicine', in J.R. Hinnells and R. Porter (eds), *Religion, Health and Suffering*. London: Routledge, pp. 256–275.

Wujastyk, Dominik. (2001). 'A Pious Fraud: The Indian Claims for Pre-Jennerian Smallpox Vaccination', in G.J. Meulenbeld and D. Wujastyk (eds), *Studies on Indian Medical History*. Delhi: Motilal Banarsidass, pp. 121–154.

Wujastyk, Dominik. (2003a). *The Roots of Āyurveda. Selection from Sanskrit Medical Writings*. New Delhi: Penguin Books.

Wujastyk, Dominik (2003b). 'The Science of Medicine', G. Flood (ed.), *The Blackwell Companion to Hinduism*. Oxford: Blackwell, pp. 393–409.

Younger, P. (1980). 'A Temple Festival of Mariyamman', *Journal of the American Academy of Religion*, 48(4): 493–517.

Zeiler, X. (2008). *Die Göttin Dhūmāvatī. Vom tantrischen Ursprung zur Gottheit eines Stadtviertels in Benares*. Unpublished PhD dissertation, Universität Heidelberg.

Zysk, K.G. (1993). *Religious Medicine. The History and Evolution of Indian Medicine*. New Brunskick and London: Transaction Publishers.

Zysk, K.G. (2000). 'Does Indian Medicine Have a Theory of Contagion?', in L.I. Conrad and D. Wujastyk (eds), *Contagion. Perspectives from pre-Modern Societies*. Aldershot: Ashgate, pp. 79–95.

Zysk, K.G. (2002). '*Mantra* in *Āyurveda*: A Study of the Use of Magico-religious Speech in Ancient Indian Medicine', in H.P. Alper (ed), *Understanding Mantras* (reprint, 1989). Delhi: Motilal Banarsidass, pp. 122–143.

Zysk, K.G. (2009). *Medicine in the Veda. Religious Healing in the Veda*. Delhi: Motilal Banarsidass.

Zysk, K.G. (2010). *Asceticism and Healing in Ancient India. Medicine in the Buddhist Monastery*. Delhi: Motilal Banarsidass.

Documentaries

Bearing the Heat: Mother Worship Goddess in South India. A film by Kristin Oldham. (1995). Madison: Centre for South Asia, University of Wisconsin.

Performing the Goddess. The Chapal Bhaduri Story (1999). A film by the Seagull Foundation for the Arts directed by Naveen Kishore.

Shuva and Me. A Journey with Shuvaprasanna. (2013). A film by Gautam Ghose. An Image Kraft Production.

Sitala in Spring: Festival of the Bengali Goddess of Health and Illness. A film by Joseph Elder and Aditi Nath Sarkar. (1986). Madison: Centre for South Asia, University of Wisconsin.

Śītalā Gājan. A documentary by Manojit Adhikary. (2013). Produced by: Shilparghya, http://www.youtube.com/watch?v=_cUlW9thgmo (accessed 12/05/2014).

Discography

Baghwa Banal Ba Hero. Voice: Naval Kumar Yadav and Sapna. Label: Sapna Cassettes, New Delhi.

Bāṛī Śer par Savār. Voice: Manoj Tivārī 'Mṛdul'. Label: T-Series, Super Cassettes Industries Limited, New Delhi.

Dai Ke Navkalsha (Chhattisgarhi Devotional Songs). Voice: Alka Chandrakar. Label: Shemaroo Entertainment.

Dhai Dihni Kalsha. Voice: Kuslesh, Radha. Label: Megna Music Records.

Jai Bol Sheetla Maa Ki. Voice: various. Label: Supertone VCDs.

Karuna Ke Khaan Sitla Maiya. Voice: Manoj Tivārī 'Mṛdul'. Label: T-Series, Super Cassettes Industries Limited, New Delhi.

Mā Śītalā Lā De Paiso kī Ḍherī. Voice: Satpāl Rohaṭiyā and Hemaltā Śarmā. Label: Supermax Cassette Industries, Rohtak (Haryana).

Mahimā Adalpur Vālī Kī. Voice: Dīpamālā Siṅh 'Jogan'. Label: Sonotek Cassette, New Delhi.

Maīyā Māph Karīñ. Bhojpurī Devī Gīt. Voice: Manoj Tivārī 'Mṛdul'. Label: T-Series, Super Cassettes Industries Limited, New Delhi.

Merī Bigṛī Banā Mā̃ Śītalā. Voice: Rāmāvatār Śarmā and Vandanā Bhārdvāj. Label: Raja Cassette Industries, New Delhi.

Navrat Ke Najar. Voice: Neeraj Nirala. Label: Angel Music.

Sheetala Maiya Ke Kamal. Voice: various. Label: Supertone VCDs.

Sheetla Maa Ka Danka Baaje. Voice: various. Label: T-Series, Super Cassettes Industries Limited, New Delhi.

Sheetla Mata Ke Ladu Batugi. Voice: Rajesh Singh Puriya, Upasna Sharma. Label: Spicebhakti Channel.

Filmography

Arekṭi Premer Galpa (Arekti Premer Golpo; Just Another Love Story) (2010). A film by Kaushik Ganguly. Bengali; colour.

Jai Mā Śītalā (kahānī Adalpura kī) (c.ca 2012). Directed by Candan Maurya. Hindi/ Bhojpuri; colour.

Mā Sitala (Maa Shitala) (1958). Directed by Deb Narayan Gupta. Bengali; black and white.

Śītalā Mātā (Sheetla Mata). (1981) Directed by Ram Gopal Gupta. Hindi; colour.

Index

Ācāradinakara 37n. 47
Adalpura 28, 40nn. 76, 78, 53, 114–18, 145n. 2, 146n. 6, 162, 166–8, 170n. 28
adharma (injustice, disorder) xxiiin. 5, 21, 165
adhiṣṭhātrī (controller) 3, 74
Ādinātha 7, 19
Agam Kuāṅ 6, 52–4, 107n. 5, 111n. 46,
āgama 19
Aghorā 7
Agnikāryapaddhati 19
Ahmedabad (Ahmadābād) 88, 100, 102, 109n. 35
AIDS goddess 154–5 *see* HIV/AIDS
ākanda (*Calotropis gigantean*) 50, 58
Alakṣmī 67, 84n. 52
alaku (devotional austerity involving piercing) 101–4
ambiguity xix, 24, 34, 50, 88, 119–21, 130, 143–4, 156
Anaṅgaraṅga 70–1
āñcal (hem [of the sari]; peripheral territory) xx, 88, 95, 101, 129, 166
āñcalik (regional, vernacular) xx, 3, 23, 28, 99–100, 114, 130, 151, 162
annakūṭ (festival of the 'heap of rice') 14–15, 37n. 38, 103 *see Govardanapūjā*
Annapurṇā 14, 32
Ārekṭi premer galpa (Bengali movie) 121, 146n. 12
Arka 58
artha (advantage, utility; aim) 8, 13, 18
ārti (< Skt. *ārātrika* ritual worship) 16, 17, 67, 105, 131, 151, 163, 168n. 2, 180, 187n. 1
aruḷ (grace) 100
aruḷvākku (oracular speaking) 101
Arya Samaj 40n. 80
āsana (sitting posture) 35n. 11, 60–1, 180, 185
ass 1, 7, 9–11, 16, 18, 21–2, 25–6, 34, 36n. 28, 39n. 67, 41, 59–63, 65, 67–75, 79–80, 84nn. 43, 48, 50, 85nn. 52, 61, 62, 66, 99, 115, 117–18, 138, 142, 157, 161–3, 166, 172, 179, 186–7, 188n. 27
  Indian Wild Ass 73 *see khara and* khur
  Tibetan Wild Ass 85n. 56 *see* kiang
  names of 11, 16, 18, 85n. 66
aṣṭamī (eighth day of half a lunar month) 9, 12, 52, 78
Aṣṭāṅgahṛdayasaṃhitā xxi, 10, 72–3
Aśvin xxiiin. 2, 67, 85n. 61, 146n. 13
Atharvaveda xx–xxiii, xxiiin. 2, 71, 74, 132
austerity xxii, 3, 24, 78, 87, 100, 101–6, 109n. 27, 111n. 42, 112n. 52 *see tapasyā*
Avanti 36n. 21, 37n. 35
Āvantyakhaṇḍa 8–9
Avian Flu 152, 155
Āyurveda xix, xxi–xxii, xxiiinn. 2 and 4, 5, 10, 45, 58, 69n. 5, 72–3, 118, 132, 153, 171

Bakker, Hans T. 8, 25n. 12, 36n. 15
Bakkhali (Bakkhāli) 26
balidān (animal sacrifice) 24, 57, 87–93, 96, 98, 104–6, 107n. 10, 108n. 17, 111n. 46, 131, 151, 185, 187, 188n. 19 see *paśubali* and sacrifice (animal)
Banaras xxii, 6, 7, 8, 13–14, 17, 31, 35n. 14, 36n. 25, 40nn. 77, 83, 43, 74–9, 86n. 71, 107n. 5, 114, 116–17, 146n. 6, 167, 173, 173n. 1 *see* Kāśī, Vārāṇasī
bandhya 16 *see* infertility
Bandī (Bandīdevī) 8, 35n. 14
Bangladesh xix, 40n. 80, 61, 63–4, 82n. 22, 105, 106n. 2, 113, 143, 148n. 38, 149nn. 51, 53, 168n. 1

barber 44, 133 *see nāpit/nāī*
Baṛī Śītalā Mandir (Adalpura) 40nn. 76, 78, 53, 114–18
Baṛī Śītalā 115–16, 167
Baṛo Mā 55–7, 88–93, 107n. 6, 107nn. 6 and 10, 108n. 17
barrenness 16–7, 27 *see bandhya*; infertility
Barthes, Roland 129–30, 167
baval (*Prosopis juliflora*) 58
Bengal Vaccination Act 139
Bengal 11, 13, 25, 26, 27, 39n. 67, 39nn. 87, 94, 113, 119–20, 131–6, 144, 151, 154, 156, 159, 172
bhadralok (gentry) 65, 89, 131
bhagat (healer) 46
Bhagavatī 3, 46, 79, 177, 187n. 1
Bhairava 6, 21–2, 31, 40n. 80, 52, 78, 152, 160–1, 187
Bhairo see Bhairava
Bhaironāth (Skt. Bhairavanātha) 16 *see* Bhairava
Bhaiṣajya Ratnāvalī 72
bhajan (devotional song) 14, 161, 163
bhakta (devotee) 28, 116, 169n. 11
bhakti (devotion) xx, xxii, 1, 10–11, 13, 27, 37n. 40, 81, 94, 102, 104–5, 121, 126–7, 130–1, 144, 146n. 20, 159, 160, 162–3, 167, 168
bhakti gīti/gān (devotional song) 27–33, 114
bhaṅgī (class of sweepers) 46, 48, 50
bhar (lit. weight; possession) 24, 94–9, 104–6, 107n. 10, 109nn. 26, 30, 33, 112n. 52, 151, 160
Bhārata 37n. 35, 71
Bhaṭṭācārya, Āśutoṣ 20, 38n. 61, 127
Bhattasali, Nalini K. 63–5
bhāva (emotion, mood; disposition; meaning) 97–8, 179
Bhāvamiśra xxi–ii, 5
Bhavānī 15, 36n. 23, 43, 138, 162
Bhāvaprakāśa xxi, 5, 10–11, 20, 87, 137, 188n. 3
Bhaviṣyapurāṇa 10, 13, 33, 36n. 22, 181–3
bhiṣáj (Vedic medicine man) xxi, xxiiin. 2
bhūt (being; ghost) 5, 92, 109n. 25, 126 *bhūtādhiṣṭha* (presence of spirits) 5; *bhūtaśuddhi* (purification ceremony) 186; *bhūtavidya* ("demonology"; psychiatry) 69
Bihar 27, 41, 51, 52, 96, 98, 106n. 2, 111n. 46, 152, 161
Bollywood 105
bourgeoisie 89, 99
Brahmā 7, 32, 35n. 11, 36n. 16, 39n. 64, 117, 123, 181, 186
brahmacāri.ī 48
Brahman/Brahmin (Skt. *brāhmaṇa*; Hindu ritual specialist) 3, 5, 8–9, 12, 16–17, 22, 25, 30, 37n. 46, 49, 80, 81nn. 10, 11, 89, 100, 110n. 39, 111n. 50, 116, 123, 126, 132, 134, 139, 142, 144–5, 146n. 6, 148n. 47, 157, 166, 167, 172, 175–6, 180, 182–3, 185, 187
British Medical Journal 142–3
broom 1, 7, 9–10, 16, 18, 21–2, 26, 34, 35n. 1, 41, 43, 50–1, 59, 61, 63, 65, 78, 80, 84n. 42, 114, 117–18, 122, 138, 142, 156, 160, 162, 166, 172, 179, 186, 188n. 27 see *jhāṛū* and *mārjana*
buhārī/buhāranī (brush) 50

Calcutta Chromosome (The) 156–9
Calcutta *see* Kolkata
cālīsā ([hymn in] forty [verses]) 67, 163
camar (flywhisk) 82n. 22, 122
Cāmuṇḍā (alt. Caṇḍamārī) 65, 68, 84n. 43
Caṇḍī/Caṇḍīkā 3, 23, 42, 43, 52, 58, 60, 70, 81nn. 2, 5, 94, 152
Candra 17, 33
Carakasaṃhitā xxi–xxii, xxiiinn. 2 and 6, 10, 153
cattle xxi, 1, 47, 83n. 34, 136
caturdaśī (fourteenth day [of half a lunar month]) 9
Caturvargacintāmani 37n. 33
Cauk Mātā 46
Caurāhā Mātā 43, 46
cecak (smallpox) 17, 165
Central Government Vaccination Act 139
chāg utsarga (consecration of the goat) 90
Chandigarh (Caṇḍīgaṛh) 88, 100, 102, 109n. 35
Chapal Kumar Bhaduri 108n. 21, 121–2, 146n. 12
Chaṭhpūjā 13, 187n. 1

chickenpox 54, 59, 100, 152, 162, 165
cholera 26, 39n. 72, 70, 118, 132, 147n. 34, 155
Choṭa Mā 54–7, 88, 97
Choṭa Mā Yātrā 54–7, 88, 95, 97, 109n. 25
contagion 50–1, 106n. 1, 124, 156–7, 159, 172
contagious diseases 2, 10, 34, 132, 153
Coult, Oliver 133
Cuḍakīdevī 8

Daivakīnanda 24 *see* Kavi Vallabha
ḍākinī (witch) 46, 123
dakṣiṇā (ritual fee) 12, 80, 90n. 2, 179–80, 187
Dakṣiṇāśītalā 6–7, 107n. 5
Ḍalhaṇa 5
daṇḍavat ('lying as a stick') 95, 101–2, 104, 160
daṇḍīkāṭā 95, 104 *see daṇḍavat*
darśana (vision) 3, 32, 75, 80, 101–2, 122, 152, 165, 173
Dāsāśvamedha Ghāṭ 35n. 14, 40n. 77, 43, 74, 78, 173
Dasāśvamedhamāhātmya 32, 161
Dayāmāyī 3
death 10, 11, 24, 39n. 64, 46, 48, 67, 68n. 3, 71, 107n. 14, 123, 125, 128, 148n. 45, 149n. 53, 157, 159, 164
Delhi (Dillī) 35n. 6, 43–4, 46–8
demon xxi, 2, 6, 16, 25, 39nn. 64, 67, 46, 65, 68–9, 70, 72, 117–19, 123, 125–6, 128, 145n. 2, 154–5, 160, 162, 169n. 13, 170n. 18
Devīmāhātmya 18
Devīnāmavilāsa 20–1
Dhaka (Ḍhākā) 61, 63–5, 84n. 43
Dhanvantari 128–9, 133, 146n. 13
dharma (order, justice, righteousness) xxi, 13, 18, 48, 88, 165, 176, 181
Dharma Ṭhākur 26–7 *see* Dharmarāj
dharmanibandha xix, 8, 11–12, 19, 34, 36nn. 20, 27, 37n. 33, 127, 171, 188n. 7
Dharmarāj 23, 26–7, 39n. 67, 55, 58, 81n. 2, 83n. 33, 39n. 67, 106n. 3
ḍheñki (husking pedal) 58, *ḍhenkimaṅgal* 83n. 33
Dhenuka 69, 71
Dhṛtarāṣṭra 48, 82n. 18
Dhumāvatī 80, 82n. 14, 84n. 52
diarrhoea 6, 26, 39n. 72, 43
digambara (lit. sky clad; naked) 1, 25, 65, 122, 176
Dīkṣāprakāśa 22
Dimock, Edward C. Jr. 4, 23, 119, 124, 126, 146n. 21, 156–7, 159
disease goddess xx, 4, 41, 113, 118, 155, 159–60, 167–8, 171
dolpūrṇimā 26 *see* Holi
donkey (*Equus asinus*) xxiiin. 6, 12, 22, 35n. 1, 36nn. 27, 28, 51, 67, 68–70, 72–3, 75, 78, 84nn. 48, 49, 85nn. 58, 59, 64, 114, 116–17, 125, 143, 160, 165
doṣā (failure, blemish; disease) 73
doṣa (humor) xxi, 73
dPal-ldan Lha-mo 70
Dramatic Performances Act 132
dream 3, 42, 46, 48, 70–1, 98, 114–15, 123, 133, 162–3, 166, 176
Droṇa (or Droṇācarya) 48, 145n. 1
drought 1, 42, 74, 85n. 58, 172
duḥkha (pain, sufferance, misery) 8, 31–2, 94, 177
Durgā 3, 15, 18–19, 32, 40n. 83, 42–3, 60, 68, 78, 80, 81n. 5, 100, 104–5, 108n. 17, 117, 145n. 2, 152, 160–3, 165–8, 173, 186, 187n. 1
Durgāfication 152, 160–7
Dvija Harideva 24, 26

elephant xxiiin. 6, 47, 57–8, 85n. 62, 125
epidemics 3, 26, 42, 52, 64, 67, 100, 108n. 23, 118, 124, 130, 132, 134, 137, 143–5, 157, 159
equestrian *mūrti* 41, 59–67
ethics 87–8, 92, 102–4, 140, 160, 172–3
ewer 50, 147n. 24
exanthemata xix, 1, 44, 106, 155
exorcism xxi, 94, 108n. 16

famine 1, 157, 172
fertility xix, 1, 6, 10, 19, 26–7, 50, 58, 72, 83n. 33, 85n. 58, 93, 96, 100, 108n. 19, 116, 152
fever xix, 1, 3–5, 10, 17–18, 21–3, 25–6, 35nn. 5, 9, 44, 46, 59, 61, 64, 73–4,

79, 84n. 41, 85n. 59, 86n. 70, 94, 100, 118, 128, 133–5, 138, 142, 152, 156, 165 Fever Demon: see Jvarāsura
fire-walking 101
folklore 5, 39n. 67, 46, 50, 71, 83n. 33, 98–9, 105, 110n. 38, 118–20, 126, 129, 151, 155, 159 folk *bhakti* 131, 144 folk god/dess xx, 40n. 80, 151 folk healing/healers 31, 40n. 80, 51 folk literature 2, 113, 117, 151, 144, 170n. 34, 172 folk medicine 72 folk poetry 2, 151, 172 folk songs 145n. 5, 171 folk theatre 121, 132 see *yātrā*
Forbes, Alexander Kinloch 22, 67
fortune 14, 16, 32–3, 58, 68, 79–80, 81n. 9, 84n. 52, 115

gādhā (ass) 73, 115
Gajalakṣmī 58
gājan (Bengali festival) 27, 110n. 40, 111n. 44, 147n. 125
galagaṇḍa (goitre) 11, 124
Gāndhārī (wife of Dr̥tarāṣṭra) 48, 82n. 18
Gāndhārī (*yoginī*) 68
Gaṇeśa 58, 63–4, 94, 152, 175, 185–6, 188nn. 21, 23, 24
gaṅgājal (Ganges water) 49, 80, 90, 117
Gaṅgā 3, 100, 160, 166, 186
garbhagr̥ha (inner sanctum) 44, 53, 89
gardabha (ass) 11, 16, 18, 71–4, 187
gardabha (type of skin disease) 73, 86nn. 67, 70 Gardabha (*yakṣa*) 69 *gardabhaka* 73, 85n. 65 *jālagardabha* 73, 86n. 67 *jvālāgardabha(ka)* 73, 85n. 66 *kīṭagardabhaka* 86n. 67 *pāṣāṇagardabha* 85n. 67
Gardabhadvādaśanāma 73, 85n. 66
gardabhī (eruption) 73
gardabhī (jenny) 72
ghaṭ (pitcher) 49–50, 128, 185
ghaṭ sthāpana (installation of the pitcher) 49, 128
ghāṭ (steps) 44, 53–4, 74, 96, 109n. 27, 161, 167
Ghenṭākarṇa *see* Ghenṭu
Ghenṭu 27, 94, 118, 186
Ghenṭudevatā *see* Ghenṭu
Ghosh, Amitav 156, 170n. 17
gīti (song) 11, 27–33, 131, 151
gotra (clan, family) 52, 74, 78, 131, 147n. 30, 179, 185, 187
Goudriaan, Teun 6–7, 38nn. 51, 55
Govardanapūjā 14
graha (grasper; asterism; planet) 6, 108n. 20 *grahahoma* (fire sacrifice to appease the planets) 175 *grahapīḍā* (planetary affliction) 9 *graharāja* (king of graspers, i.e. Śani) 69 *graharoga* (planetary affliction; malignant form of possession) 11, 106, 108n. 20 *grahī* (female of *graha*) 6, 35n. 8 *navagraha* (nine planets) 186
grahaṇ (grasping; possession) 109n. 25
grāmya (pertaining to a village) xx, 57, 73, 83n. 35, 106n. 3, 130, 169n. 11
Gujarat (Gujarāt) xxiiin. 1, 36n. 27, 37n. 46, 58, 61, 73, 86n. 79, 88, 100–2, 106n. 2, 111n. 46, 152, 188n. 2
guphā (grotto) 75, 78, 86n. 74, 187n. 1
Gurgaon (Guṛgā̃v) 44–9, 81n. 9, 162–3, 169n. 9

hāḍikāṭh (Y-shaped sacrificial stake) 89, 91, 107n. 15
Hanumān 32, 40n. 82, 78, 94, 128–9, 152, 160–1, 170n. 18
harā pattā ('green leaves') 49, 115 *see nīm*
Hārītī 6, 35n. 10
Hastināpura 13, 37n. 35, 181
haṭhayoga 19
Hayagrīva 63–5, 84n. 41
Hemādri 37n. 33, 68
Henderson, Donald 140
Heruka 69–70
hijṛā 89–90, 93, 96–7, 107nn. 10, 11
Hitopadeśa 71
HIV/AIDS 512–5, 169nn. 7, 11–3
Holi 26
Holwell, John 132
horse 31, 47, 57–8, 61, 72–3, 175
horse-headed 63, 65
hygiene xix, 1, 5, 23, 37n. 46, 44, 50, 87, 119, 127, 134, 140, 143–4

iconography xx, 1, 3, 6, 7, 9, 21, 41, 46, 48, 50–2, 59, 61, 65, 67, 69n. 5, 75, 80, 81n. 1, 84n. 50, 101, 105, 114–16, 121, 145n. 2, 156, 157, 160, 165–6, 168, 172
ilāj (remedy, cure, medicine) 44
illness xix, xxi, 2, 4, 54, 71, 79, 86n. 67, 93–5, 106, 116, 130, 152–3, 157, 159, 171, 187
immortality 19, 38n. 48, 158–9, 186
Indian Medical Service (IMS) 81n. 8, 132, 137, 139, 140, 144–5, 151
Indra 17, 32, 67, 186
Indradyumna 13, 37n. 35, 181
infertility 74, 106, 136, 155, 172
injustice xix, 67, 81, 96, 106, 158, 167, 171
inoculation 38n. 63, 113, 130, 132–40, 143–5, 148nn. 38, 44 *see ṭikā*; variolation
inoculator 132–41, 143, 148n. 47, 148n. 49, 151, 154, 165 *see mālākār*; *nāī*; *nāpīt*; variolator, *mālin*
insect 73–4, 86n. 67
internet 118–19, 145, 147n. 31, 155, 160, 163
Islamism 40n. 80, 105, 152, 155, 168n. 2
Iṭu 58

jādūṭonā (sorcery, evil spell) 6
Jagannāth (Kavi) 24, 147n. 30
Jāgatrānī 3
Jai Mā Śītalā (Kahānī Adalpura Kī) (Hindi/Bhojpuri movie) 146n. 6, 166–7
Jammu (Jammū) 88, 100–1, 109n. 35
Jammu and Kashmir (Jammū aur Kaśmīr) 85n. 56, 88, 100
jāpa (repetition of a mantra or the name of a deity) 142, 187
jāti (social class) 46, 74, 94, 114, 133, 147n. 30 *strījāti* (women's class) 28 *upajāti* (upper class) 126, 129
Javāhar Siṃha 47–8, 82n. 16
Jenner, Edward 133
jenny 67, 72, 172
Jharkhand (Jhārkhaṇḍ) 106n. 2, 161
jhāṛū (broom) 50, 75, 122, 156, 165, 166
jhulāi (swinging) 51, 108n. 16
Jvara-Jvarī 39n. 66
Jvarapātra 25 *see* Jvarāsura
Jvarāsura 25–6, 39nn. 64, 65, 67, 65, 69, 118, 128, 156–7, 186–7
Jyeṣṭhā 67–8, 80, 84n. 52

Kāl Bhairo (Skt. Kālabhairava) Mandir 6, 7, 107n. 5
Kāl Bhairo/Bhaironāth (Skt. Kālabhairava) 16, 78
kalā (point [of the body]) 19–20
Kālarātrī 3, 68, 78–80, 100, 161, 177
kalaśa (pitcher) 16, 49, 61, 179
kalāvā (red cotton thread) 42 *see mauli*
Kali 69
Kalighat paintings 65–6, 84n. 44
Kālikāpurāṇa 65, 69, 107n. 7
kalsi (water pitcher) *see kalaśa*
kāma (physical pleasure; erotic love) 13
Kāmakalākālī 7
Kāmākhyā Devī 111n. 48, 162
Kamalakārabhaṭṭa 37n. 33
kāmana (desire, wish) 82n. 19, 103
karma (action) xxi, 48, 153
Karuṇamāyī 3
Kashmir (Kaśmīr) 19–20, 85n. 56
Kāśī xxii, 8, 31, 86n. 75, 161
Kāśīkhaṇḍa 5, 8, 35n. 14, 86n. 72, 187n. 1
kathā (story) 10–11, 14, 34, 36n. 19, 37n. 46, 67, 127, 151
Kavirāj, Gopīnāth 20
kavirāja (āyurvedic physician) 39n. 64, 132, 134, 158
khaḍga (blade) 15, 91
khara (ass) 11, 16, 18, 70, 73, 85n. 63 *kharasthitā* (sitting on an ass) 68, 79, 177
Khara (demon chief) 69
khārāp khun ('bad blood', blood disease) 26, 153–4
Khecarīvidyā 19–20
khelā 94 *see khelnā*
khelnā (lit. to play; possession) 94, 99, 112n. 52, 151, 160
Khrag 'Thung (Tib.) 69 *see* Heruka
khur *see khara*
kiang (*Equus kiang*) 85n. 56 kiang mule 70
Kim, Jinah 7, 84nn. 42, 43, 50
Kolkata (Kalkātā) 25, 39nn. 67, 70, 43, 65–6, 83n. 32, 111nn. 47, 51, 118, 131, 134, 137–9, 148n. 38, 156

kōvil (temple) 101
Kriyākālaguṇottaratantra 35n. 8, 73, 85n. 66
kṛmi (worm) 74
Kṛpī 48–9
Kṛṣṇarāja Oḍeyar (Krishnaraja Wodeyar) III 21
Kṛṣṇarām Dās 24, 147n. 26
Kṛtyatattva 36n. 27, 137
Kṣetrapāla 60, 81n. 2
kṣudraroga (minor disease) 10, 86n. 67
Kubjikāmātātantra xxii, 23
Kumāratantra 6
kumkum (powder from saffron or turmeric) 42, 52
kumṛā bali (sacrifice of the cucumber) 91, 108n. 17
kuṇḍa (pool) 44, 47, 49

Laakhan/Lutchman (character from CC) 156–7
Lakṣmī 3, 18, 21–2, 36n. 23, 52, 58, 100, 160, 186
Lalitā 46, 82n. 14
laukika/laukik (popular) xx, 98, 130
Lavakuśapālā 128–9
lentils 4, 9, 21–2, 84n. 42, 117, 123, 128
leper 16–17
leprosy 27, 58, 70, 155, 170n. 33
līlā (play) 32, 124, 157, 159
Lo ma gyon ma 61 *see* Parṇaśavarī
lymph 135–6

Maḍhkeda 59
Madhya Pradesh (Madhya Pradeś) 59, 61–2, 69
Mahābhārata 3, 6, 37n. 35, 48, 146n. 7
Mahābrahmāmantra 6, 7, 35n. 11
Mahādevī 46, 161, 187
Mahākālasaṃhitā 7
Mahākālayogaśāstra 7
Maheśvara 23, 186 *see* Śiva
Mahiṣāsuramardiṇī 60, 145n. 2, 162–3, 167
mālākār 133 *see mālin*
malaria 132, 152, 158–9
mālin (class of gardeners, garland makers and flower sellers) 52, 133–4
Mālinīvijayottaratantra xxii
mallāh (class of boatmen and fishermen) 114–17, 145n. 4, 166–7
māṁjhī (boatman, fisherman) 114, 166
  see mallāh
Manasā 3, 23, 26, 39n. 67, 43, 55, 58, 81n. 2, 89
Manasāmaṅgalkāvya 169n. 10
mānasik (promise to a deity) 93
mandir (temple) 3, 42–3, 115, 162, 163–5
maṅgal gān (auspicious song) 27
Maṅgalā (appellative of Śītalā) 3, 5, 88
Mangala (character of CC) 156–9
maṅgalkāvya 34, 121, 172, 147n. 24
Mānikrām Gāṅgulī 24, 38n. 61, 128
Mañjuśrīmūlakalpa 6–7, 35n. 11
mantra (ritual formula) xxi, xxiiin. 2, 6, 7, 9, 11, 16–17, 20–3, 34, 38nn. 55, 57, 50, 98, 134, 143, 153, 180, 185–7, 188nn. 9, 22
  bījamantra (seed mantra) 22, 78
  dhyānamantra (meditation formula) 7, 19, 20, 26, 39n. 64, 67, 68, 79, 82n. 23, 92, 177, 186, 188n. 28
mārgīya (doctrinal) 20, 130
Marglin, Frédérique A. 94, 136, 140, 148n. 45, 149n. 50, 171
mārjana (broom) 50
masān (whooping cough) 46
Masān 46
Masani village 46, 48, 82n. 15
Masānī 3, 42–9, 81n. 7, 82n. 20
masānī (kind of spirit) 46
mass media 71, 88, 101–2, 104, 109n. 35, 117, 145, 151–2, 154–5, 160, 167–8, 169nn. 13, 15
masūrikā (smallpox) xxii, xxiiin. 5, 4–5, 10
Mātaṅgī 42, 68–9, 82nn. 14, 20, 110n. 39
māthā (head) 51–2, 54
Mathura (Mathurā) 69
mauli (cotton thread) 12, 42, 50, 83n. 25
measles 43, 94, 100, 124, 143, 152, 162
medicine xxi, xxiiin. 6, 10, 16, 72, 84, 106, 113, 121, 128, 133, 135–6, 138, 141–3, 148nn. 40, 46, 156 biomedicine xxii, 155 folk medicine 72, medicine men xxi, xxiiin. 2, 121 tantric medicine xxii Vedic medicine xxi. 118
Meister, Michael 52–3, 60
Mejo Mā 55–6
Merutantra 21–3, 38nn. 56, 58

middle class 3, 87–8, 95, 98–9, 103, 105, 140, 148n. 39, 160
migration 93, 99
milk 6, 12, 21–2,42, 49, 72, 78, 85n. 59, 134, 136, 170n. 32, 172, 175
misfortune xix, 4, 32, 84n. 52, 85n. 53, 148n. 45
Moḍherā 61
mokṣa (liberation) 9, 13, 80, 87, 168n. 6
monsters 126
mudrā (gesture) 19, 60–1, 63, 186
Mūlasarvāstivādavinaya 69
mule 69–70
mumps 43
muṇḍan (head shaving) 44
mūrti (image; icon) 3, 26, 35n. 15, 39n. 67, 40n. 83, 41–3, 45, 48–9, 52, 54–5, 59, 74–5, 78, 82nn. 21, 22, 83n. 32, 89, 91, 107n. 5, 134, 157, 163–6, 170n. 35, 172, 180, 188n. 11
  aniconic *mūrti* 41–3, 45, 51, 165
  anthropomorphic *mūrti* 3, 25, 41, 42, 55, 78, 82n. 21, 100, 172
  cephalomorphic mūrti 41, 51–2, 55, 83n. 32, 172
  equestrian *mūrti* 1, 41, 59–67, 172
  phytomorphic *mūrti* 41, 57–9, 172
  zoomorphic *mūrti* 41, 57–9, 172
Mūtēvī 84n. 52
myth-making 155, 167
mythologisation 151, 155

nāī (class of barbers) 133 *see nāpīt*
naivedya (food offering) 12, 175, 179, 188n. 29
najar (lit. sight; evil eye) 6, 51, 52, 109n. 25
Najīb Khān 47, 82n. 16
namaskāra (salutation) 61, 92
nāmḍāk (invocation; calling the name loudly) 89, 91
nāpit (class of barbers) 133, 148
Nāradapurāṇa 9, 12, 36nn. 18, 24, 37n. 35
Navadurgā 161
navarātrī (nine nights; festival celebrating Durgā) 31–2, 78–9, 80, 114
Nepal xix, 46, 85n. 56, 168n. 1
New Loknath Opera 121–2
Nicholas, Ralph 5, 8, 24, 35n. 3, 36n. 26, 38n. 63, 85n. 62, 110n. 38, 119, 128, 146n. 10, 147n. 31, 148n. 45, 157, 159
Nīlkāṇṭa Bandhyopādhyāy 24
nīm (*Azadirachta indica*) 13, 14, 49, 58–9, 74, 83n. 25, 115, 134, 162, 165
Nirṇayasindhu 37n. 33
Nirṛti 67–8, 71
Niṣāda (tribal kingdom; boatmen) 114–15, 145nn. 1, . 4
Nityānanda Cakravartī 24, 131, 146n. 7, 147n. 30

ojhā (exorcist; healer) 31
Olā Bibi 3, 26, 39n. 68, 40n. 80, 43, 81n. 2
Olāi Caṇḍī 26, 43 *see* Olā Bibi
olāuṭhā (cholera) 39n. 72
Orientalism xx, xxiii, 113, 142, 144, 160, 172
Osiañ 60

pacrā (devotional song to a goddess) 27, 31–3, 40n. 81, 161
paddhati (guidebook for ritual) 38n. 51, 39n. 74, 127
Pakistan xix, 46, 105, 168nn. 1, 3
Pāla (dynasty) 61, 83n. 39
pālā (story of a drama; section) 24–5, 37n. 46, 39n. 71, 72, 98, 113, 118, 120–3, 125–6, 128, 131–2, 144, 146n. 14, 147n. 31, 151, 155–6, 158–9, 172
palanquin 51, 54–6, 91n. 3, 175, 177
pālki (palanquin) 54
pañcakrośīyātrā (a circumambulatory pilgrimage) 74, 80
pāñcāmṛta (five nectars) 49
Pañcānan 27, 43, 55, 81n. 2, 89
Pañcānanda 39n. 67
Pañcatantra 71–2
pañcopacāra (offering of five items) 67, 187, 188n. 29
pandemic 152–3
paṇḍit (scholar) 48, 102, 111n. 51, 137, 167
pāpa (demerit) xxi, 87, 106n. 1, 179–80
parikrama (circumambulation) 9
Parṇaśavarī 61, 63–5, 84n. 43
Parpola, Asko 71–3
Parvatī 3, 33, 117, 183
paśubali (animal sacrifice) 87, 91n. 6, 104–6, 106n. 3 *see balidān*

pathologization xx, 106, 151
Patiala (Paṭiyālā) 88, 100, 109n. 35
pativratā ([woman] devoted to the husband) 13, 34, 182–3
Patna (Paṭnā) 6, 52, 54, 107n. 5, 111n. 46
paṭuyā (class of singers and scroll painters) 154–5, 169nn. 11, 13
peasantry 2–3, 87, 99, 105, 129, 140, 144, 151, 172
Picchilātantra 6, 10, 20, 26, 38n. 51, 67, 82n. 23, 87, 92, 105, 107n. 7, 185–7
pilgrimage xxii, 9, 38n. 62, 83n. 26, 98, 109n. 27, 153 *see parikrama*; *yātrā*
pipāl (*Ficus religiosa*) 53
pīr (Sufi teacher; Muslim saint) 94, 109n. 25
piśāca (class of flesh-eating demon) 69, 70, 177
piśācinī (female of *piśāca*) 46
pitcher 1, 16, 35n. 1, 41–2, 49–51, 53, 61, 78, 81n. 4, 114–15, 117, 122, 162, 166, 172, 179–80, 185–6
plague 25, 24, 70, 123, 155, 169n. 8, 172
pop culture 161, 173
possession 51, 88, 93–5, 98–9, 101, 103–4, 105–6, 107n. 10, 109nn. 24, 25, 112n. 52, 147n. 25, 160, 172
  devotional 3, 87, 94, 98–9, 101, 104
  and gender 96, 104
  invited 24, 101
  malignant 11, 112n. 52
  negative 6, 69, 109n. 25, 159
  and social class 98–9
  therapeutic 94
Prabhāsakhaṇḍa 8
prāṇapratiṣṭhā (rite of infusing life) 51, 186
prasād (offering [of food]) 12–13, 19, 32, 58, 92, 96, 117, 183
Pratāpasiṃha Sāha 21
pratimā (image; icon) 3, 26, 42, 48, 52, 55, 60–1, 74–5, 77, 82n. 23, 87n. 71, 107n. 5, 114–15, 163, 175 *patthar pratimā* (stone icon) 42
Pringle, Robert 3, 135
prophylaxis 44, 113, 127, 136, 141
Propp, Vladimir 156
protective-cum-malign 119, 140
pūjā (worship)
pūjak (ritual specialist) 89, 91, 187
pūjārī (ritual specialist) 3, 14, 37n. 37, 48–52, 80, 81n. 4, 76n. 75, 88–92, 99, 103, 105, 107nn. 6, 15, 115–16, 147n. 25, 166–7
pulses 2, 14, 27, 41, 51, 72, 83n. 33, 118, 123–4, 172
Punjab (Pañjāb) xxiiin. 1, 42, 50, 82n. 21, 88, 100–1, 106n. 2, 152
puṇya (merit) 177, 181, 185
purāṇa xix, 9, 17, 34, 37n. 35, 84n. 44, 117, 137, 171, 188n. 14
Puraścaryārṇava 21–3, 38n. 58, 65
pustule 4, 27, 73, 132–4, 142
Pūtanā 6, 35n. 8

quarantine 59, 132, 147n. 34

rajakī (washer-lady) 23
Rajasthan (Rājasthān) 12, 40n. 75, 47–8, 53, 60–1, 73, 81n. 1, 83n. 38, 106n. 1, 111n. 46, 140, 152
rakṣasa (a class of demons) 69–70
rakṣasī (fem. of *rakṣasa*) 6
Raktāpriyā 26, 187 *see* Raktāvatī
Raktāvatī 26, 39nn. 70, 71, 69, 118, 125, 187
Raktāvatīkā 26 *see* Raktāvatī
Rāma 18, 21, 69, 78, 115, 128, 145n. 5
Rāmāyaṇa 3, 69–71, 160, 170n. 18
Rāmnārāyaṇ Bhaṭṭācārya 24
Rāmsundar Prabhudās 16, 37n. 40
Rāvaṇa 69, 128
ṛddhi (prosperity) 17, 185
Reṇukā 100, 110n. 39
Ṛgveda xx, xxi, xxiiin. 2, 58, 67, 72
rice 12–14, 21–2, 27, 36n. 29, 51, 78, 111n. 50, 124–5, 133–4, 175–6, 178, 179–80
Rog Rāy 3
roga (disease) xxi, xxii, 4–5, 9–10,
Roger Rāja/Rāy 122
Rogeśvarī 3, 123, 131
Rudra 21, 25, 33, 39n. 64, 78
Rudrayāmala 38n. 55 *see* *Rudrayāmalatantra*
Rudrayāmalatantra 22–3, 38nn. 55, 56
rurdasarovar (Rudra's pond) 78

Śabdakalpadruma 3, 68, 137
Saccikamātā (alt. Sacciyamātā) 60

sacrifice 123, 129, 186
animal sacrifice xxiiin. 2, 3, 24, 26, 42, 57, 87–93, 103–4, 105–6, 106nn. 2, 3, 107nn. 7, 9, 108n. 17, 111nn. 48, 51, 112n. 52, 120, 147n. 25, 160, 172, 185, 187 see *balidān* and *paśubali*
ass sacrifice 68, 71
fire sacrifice 19
grain sacrifice 21–2
human sacrifice 147n. 25, 176–7
pumpkin sacrifice 91, 108n. 17
Sacrifices Prohibition Act 111n. 46
self-sacrifice 107n. 13, 169n. 10
sādhana (accomplishment; [ritual] performance) 19, 23, 78
sādhu (ascetic) 20, 44, 78, 93, 102, 166
Sāhibakaula 20
Saiban Bibi 143, 149n. 53
śākta (devoted to the Goddess) 8, 18, 23, 68, 74, 87, 104, 111n. 51, 160
Śakti (an aspect of the goddess) 3, 18, 23, 47, 68, 80, 82n. 21, 118, 131, 162
śakti (power) 15, 19, 100, 107n. 5
śaktipīṭha (seat of the goddess) 44, 46, 167, 186
Śāktism 104, 154 *see śākta*
Salkia (Sālkiyā) 54–7, 70, 83n. 28, 88–90, 92–9, 106, 107n. 6, 126
Saṃvara 69 *see* Heruka
sāmya (peaceful) 124, 131, 157
Śani 26, 55, 69–70, 83n. 32, 89, 94, 152
saṅkalpa (oath) 179, 185, 188n. 19
Śaṅkar 24
Śaṅkarabhaṭṭa 13, 37n. 33
saptā matṛkā (seven mothers) 52
Sarasvatī 3, 15, 52, 100, 160, 186
Saraswati, Dayananda 40n. 80
sarcoid 73
Sarkar, Benoy K. 20
Śarma, Jīvanāth 22
SARS 152, 155
Ṣaṣṭhī 3, 23, 43, 58, 81n. 2, 152
sāt bhagiṇī (seven sisters) 42
sāt bibi (seven ladies) 42–3
sāt caṇḍī (seven Caṇḍīs) 42
sāt kanyā (seven virgins) 42, 162
sāt mā (seven mothers) 42, 46 *see saptā matṛkā*
saubhāgya (good fortune; the state of a married woman) 179, 182
Śavara 61, 84n. 40
Sejo Mā 55, 57
Śeraṅvālī ('Rider of the Lion') 161–2
sevā ([devotional] service) 28, 87, 92, 94, 101
sevāit (temple priest and beneficiary) 39n. 70, 55, 83n. 32, 88–9, 92–3, 99
seven mothers 33, 42, 46, 52, 54
seven sisters 31, 41–3, 48, 52, 81nn. 4, 5, 6, 7, 162
Shaw, Miranda 64–5
Shitala Chalisa (smartphone app) 163
Shoolbred, John 134–5, 138
Shuvaprasanna 65–6, 84n. 45
siddhi (accomplishment; success) xxii, 8, 17, 10, 86n. 77, 102
śilā (slab stone) 42, 52, 81n. 1
sindūr 12, 37n. 32, 51, 74, 83n. 25, 108n. 21, 146n. 15
śīt (cold) 1, 5–6
Sītā 78, 115, 128, 145n. 5
śītala (cold, calm; coldness, calmness) 1, 5, 7, 15–16, 18, 20, 35nn. 8, 11, 48, 67, 171, 179
Śītalā Dhām 53, 114–15, 117, 162, 167
Śītalā Ghāṭ 14, 31, 33, 43, 74, 168n. 2
Śītalā Mātā (movie) 163–6, 170n. 30
Śītalācālīsā 15–7, 43
Śītalāgaurī 8
Śītalāmāhātmya 9
Śītalāmaṅgalkāvya xx, 2, 23–7, 119, 147n. 30, 151, 155, 171–2
Harideva's ŚMK 26, 123, 145n. 3
Kavi Jagannātha's ŚMK 72, 122–3, 128, 158
Kṛṣṇarām Dāsa's ŚMK 72, 128, 170n. 33
Mānikrām Gāṅgulī's ŚMK 38n. 63, 72, 83n. 33, 123, 128–9
Nityānanda Cakravartī's ŚMK 24, 26, 118, 122, 125, 131, 146n. 7, 147n. 31, 156
Śītalāsaptamī (Śītalā's seventh) 11–13, 36n. 25, 37n. 46, 175, 178, 179–80, 181, 187n. 1
Śītalāsaptamīvrata(kathā) 11-3, 36n. 25, 175-8, 179-180, 181-3

Śītalāṣaṣṭhī (Śītalā's sixth) 11–13, 22, 37n. 36 *Śītalāṣaṣṭhīvrata(kathā)* 11-3, 37n. 36
Śītalāṣṭakastotra 5–6, 10–11, 13, 20, 23, 67, 85n. 66, 87, 105, 122, 127, 135, 143, 189n. 31
Śītalāṣṭamī (Śītalā's eighth) 12, 36nn. 20, 27, 41, 54, 100 *Śītalāṣṭamīvrata* 12, 41
Śītalāsthāna 10
śītalikā (or *śītalā*) (a type of fever) 5, 10, 21, 23, 35nn. 6, 7, 61
Śītapūtāna 6
Śiva 10, 16–18, 21, 23, 25, 26–7, 32, 34, 39n. 64, 55, 58, 78, 81n. 2, 82n. 21, 86nn. 77, 80, 94, 186
Skandapurāṇa 6, 8–9, 11, 13, 20, 35nn. 12, 13, 36n. 20, 38n. 51, 87, 105, 109n. 25, 110n. 39, 115, 137, 142, 179–80, 188, 189n. 31
skin disease 27, 58, 73–4, 85n. 66, 118, 155, 172
Smallpox Eradication Program (SEP) 58, 113, 140–1, 143, 145, 149nn. 50, 51, 151, 154, 172
smallpox xix–xx, xxii, 2–4, 6, 8, 10, 16, 18, 22–3, 26, 34, 35n. 6, 42–3, 58, 61, 63, 70, 72–4, 81nn. 5, 8, 84n. 42, 108n. 23, 113, 119–20, 123, 128, 132–3, 135, 137–9, 140–5, 147n. 37, 148n. 48, 149n. 53, 152–3, 155–6, 158–9, 165, 172, 188n. 16
  black pox 26
  Certification of Smallpox Eradication 119
  deification of xix, 4, 145, 149n. 51
  epidemics of 3, 26, 52, 100, 108n. 23, 130, 137–8, 143–5, 157, 159
  eradication of 36n. 25, 140, 143, 152, 163, 168n. 3
  germs 41, 50, 70, 117–18
  goddess xix, 4, 6, 113, 118, 120, 143–4, 172
  goddess of xix, 2, 5–6, 100, 108n. 23, 113, 116, 118–19, 125, 130–1, 135–6, 138, 140–5, 146n. 9, 151, 172
  haemorrhagic 26, 39n. 69
  myth xx, 35n. 4, 113, 117, 119, 130–1, 143, 145, 155, 159, 168, 171
  outbreaks 2, 130, 139, 149n. 53
  and possession 94, 159
  Smallpox Commission 137–9
  ulcers/pustules 4, 27, 63, 73, 84n. 42, 132–4, 142
  victims of xix, 2, 24, 38n. 63, 58, 133, 135, 165, 169n. 13
  warriors 113, 140
Snān Yātrā (bathing pageant) 54, 88–9
sohar (devotional song) 27–9, 31
śraddhā (faith) xxii, xxiiin. 7, 1, 11
śrāddha (funeral rites) 8, 50
Śrī Ādi Śītalā Stotram 13, 18, 43, 187n. 1
Śrī Devī 70 *see* dPal-ldan Lha-mo
Śrī 18, 84n. 52
Śrītattvanidhi 21
Śrīvidyā 74
śrīyantra 78, 80
stava (eulogy) 20, 187
Stewart, Duncan 134–9
stotra (hymn) xxii, 5, 10–11, 13, 105, 188n. 23, 189n. 31
śūdra (impure classes) 72
Surāj Māl 47, 82n. 16
Sūraj 17, 58 *see* Sūrya
Suriname 33, 81n. 7
śūrpa (winnower) 10, 20, 51, 60–1, 65, 75, 82n. 22, 176, 186
Sūrya 13, 17, 33, 58, 152, 185–6
Suśrutasaṃhitā xxi–xxiii, 5, 6, 10, 73, 86n. 67, 148n. 40
svapnadarśana (dream vision) 98, 114
svapnādeś (command in a dream) 98, 114
sweepers 3, 23, 156 *see bhaṅgī*
Swine Flu 152, 155

Tamil Nadu 83n. 38, 84n. 42, 100–1, 111n. 46, 117, 168n. 3
tantra 19, 34, 38n. 55, 88, 171
tapasyā (austerity) 78, 101–2
ṭhākur (lord) 42–3
Ṭhākurāni (title of the great goddess) 3, 43, 132
thān (open-air shrine) 3, 31, 42, 53, 58
theatre 20, 132
  open theatre 108n. 21, 113, 121, 131
  folk theatre 121
ṭikā (B.)/*ṭīkā* (H.; Bhp.) ([auspicious] mark) 52, 74, 84n. 49, 166

ṭikā (variolation/inoculation) 113, 132, 134
ṭikadār (inoculator; variolator) 132, 134, 137, 139, 144–5, 151
ṭikāit (inoculator; variolator) 132
tīmiti (fire-walking) 101
tīrtha (ford) 8–9, 20, 35n. 13, 78
triśūla (trident) 25, 52, 61, 160, 162–3, 165

ugra (fierce; excessive) 6, 19, 41, 80, 88, 107, 124, 131, 157
upper class 3, 89, 140
utsav (celebration, festival) 102–3
Uttar Pradesh (Uttar Pradeś) 27, 51, 85n. 59, 106n. 2, 114, 152, 161

vaccination xix, 113, 133, 135–41, 143–4, 148nn. 38, 44, 172 Jennerian vaccination 113, 133, 144
vaccinifer 135, 140
vāhana (vehicle; mount) 11, 18, 26, 36n. 28, 61, 67, 69, 72–3, 75, 84n. 50, 172
vaidya (āyurvedic physician) 22, 10, 132
Vaiṣṇavakhaṇḍa 8
Vaiṣṇo Devī 3, 100, 152, 160–2, 168
Vallabha (Kavi) 24
vāṇ phõṛā (devotional austerity) 24
Varanasi (Vārāṇasī) xxii, 31, 36n. 25, 37n. 38, 41, 86n. 77, 167, 168n. 2, 170n. 37 *see* Banaras, Kāśī
variolation 113, 132–3, 135, 137–8, 147nn. 35, 37 *see* inoculation; *ṭikā*
variolator 132–3, 135–7, 140, 172 *see* inoculator; *mālin*; *mālākār*; *nāī*; *nāpīt*
varṇa (lit. color; class) 72
vasanta (Spring season) 4, 73
Vasanta Rāy 3, 26, 131
vasanta roga (spring fever; smallpox) 3–5, 73, 121, 148n. 48
Veda xx, 15, 17, 71, 182
vēl (arrow) 101
vessel 1, 21–2, 50, 96, 128, 185
vidhi (rule; injunction) 13, 87
vijaya (victorious hymn) 11, 15, 18, 132
Vindhyāvāsinī 15, 32, 40n. 83
viratam (vow) 102
Virāṭapālā 118, 125
visitation xix, 5, 47, 94–5, 109n. 25, 114, 123, 139–40, 163
visphoṭa(ka) (smallpox) xxii, 3–5, 9–11, 17, 19–20, 36n. 23, 65, 72–3, 185–7
Visphoṭak (name of smallpox demon) 16
Viśvanātha 10, 12–13, 37n. 33
viśvāsa (belief) xxii, 94
vitiligo 27, 96, 58
vomit 6, 26, 39n. 72, 43, 125
vrata (ritual vow; fast) 9–15, 36nn. 19, 25, 26, 40n. 74, 80, 96, 102, 105, 127, 131, 148n. 41, 151, 159, 178, 180, 182–3, 188n. 19
vratakathā (story of a *vrata*) xix, 12–13, 19, 28, 34, 36n. 19, 127, 171, 175, 187n. 1
Vratarāja 10, 12–13, 36n. 25, 179–83
Vratārka 13, 37n. 33
vyādhi (disease) xxi

Wadley, Susan W. xx, 2, 4, 36n. 26, 37nn. 36, 46, 119, 188nn. 12, 16
water xix, xxi, 1, 3, 6, 9–10, 12–13, 16, 21, 23, 41–2, 48–9, 58–9, 72, 78, 92, 96, 152, 175–8, 179–80, 185–7
  cold 1, 12, 14, 34, 42, 49, 72, 98, 100, 118, 134–5, 142, 165–6
  Ganges 49, 109n. 28, 117, 166
  healing 34, 50, 109n. 28
  rain 12, 100
  goddess 3, 114, 162, 166, 145
  gods 175–8
  oblation 18, 21–3, 185–7
West Bengal 26, 36n. 26, 39n. 71, 41, 43, 51, 54, 69n. 5, 81nn. 2, 6, 104, 106n. 2, 108n. 16, 111nn. 44, 47, 49, 152–3, 161, 168nn. 1, 3, 169n. 11
WHO (World Health Organization) 58, 113, 136, 140, 145, 151, 172
whooping cough 43, 46
Wikipedia 118
winnower 1, 7, 10, 21–2, 34, 41, 50–1, 58, 65, 69, 84n. 42, 114, 172, 186, 188n. 27 *see śūrpa*
winnowing fan 7, 50, 80, 118 *see śūrpa*
winnowing tray 51, 61, 122–3 *see śūrpa*
witchcraft 67, 71
working class 3, 44, 87–8, 98–9, 105, 128, 140
worm 73–4, 86n. 70 *see kṛmi*

Yama 39, 58, 69, 71, 177, 185
Yāmalatantra 21 *see Rudrayāmalatantra*
yantra (ritual diagram) 20–3, 34, 38n. 54
yātrā (Bengali open theatre) 108n. 21, 113, 121, 146n. 14
yātrā (pageant; pilgrimage) 93, 109n. 28, 131, 144, 146n. 12, 151
yogin (yoga practitioner) 20, 86nn. 73, 76
yoginī (female yoga practitioner; witch; magician) 7, 16, 19, 30, 65, 68, 84n. 42, 123

www.ingramcontent.com/pod-product-compliance
Lightning Source LLC
Chambersburg PA
CBHW052032300426
44117CB00012B/1787
* 9 7 8 1 4 4 1 1 6 3 8 0 6 *